RENAL DISEASE
Classification and Atlas of
INFECTIOUS AND TROPICAL DISEASES

RENAL DISEASE

Prepared by the World Health Organization Collaborating Centre
for the Histological Classification of Renal Diseases

Classification and Atlas of
INFECTIOUS AND TROPICAL DISEASES

RAJA SINNIAH   JACOB CHURG
                    LESLIE H. SOBIN

and pathologists, nephrologists, and microbiologists in nine countries

ASCP PRESS • AMERICAN SOCIETY OF CLINICAL PATHOLOGISTS • CHICAGO

Cover: Figure 12–3. Hematogenous candidal nephritis.

Library of Congress Cataloging-in-Publication Data

Renal disease : classification and atlas of infectious and tropical
  diseases / prepared by the World Health Organization Collaborating
  Centre for the Histological Classification of Renal Diseases ; Raja
  Sinniah, Jacob Churg, Leslie H. Sobin and pathologists,
  nephrologists, and microbiologists in nine countries.
     "WHO series on the classification of renal diseases"—Pref.
     Bibliography: p. 247
     Includes index.
     1. Kidneys—Infections—Classification.   2. Kidneys—Infections
  Atlases.   3. Tropical medicine—Classification.   4. Tropical
  medicine—Atlases.   I. Sinniah, Raja.   II. Churg, Jacob.
  III. Sobin, L. H.   IV. World Health Organization. Collaborating
  Centre for the Histological Classification of Renal Diseases.
     [DNLM: 1. Communicable Diseases—classification—atlases.
  2. Kidney Diseases—classification—atlases.   3. Tropical Medicine—
  classification—atlases.   WJ 17 R3929]
  RC918.I53R46   1988
  616.6'1—dc19
  DNLM/DLC
  for Library of Congress   88-3460
                                                          CIP
     ISBN: 0-89189-258-3

Printed in the United States of America.

92 91 90 89 88   5 4 3 2 1

CONTRIBUTORS

World Health Organization Collaborating Centre for the Histological Classification of Renal Diseases, Department of Pathology, Mount Sinai School of Medicine, New York, New York, USA

EDITOR-IN-CHIEF

Dr. Jacob Churg, Head of the Collaborating Centre; Mount Sinai Medical Center, New York, New York; Barnert Memorial Hospital Center, Paterson, New Jersey, USA

PARTICIPANTS AND EDITORIAL COMMITTEE

Dr. Zilton A. Andrade, Centro de Pesquisas Goncalo Muniz, Salvador-Bahia, Brazil, South America

Dr. Jay Bernstein, Department of Anatomic Pathology, William Beaumont Hospital, Royal Oak, Michigan, USA

Dr. Vijitr Boonpucknavig, Department of Pathology, Ramathibodi Hospital, Bangkok, Thailand

Dr. J. Stewart Cameron, Renal Medicine, Guy's Hospital, London, England

Dr. K.S. Chugh, Department of Nephrology, Postgraduate Medical Institute, Chandigarh, India

Dr. Vaclav Houba, World Health Organization (WHO), Geneva, Switzerland; formerly WHO Immunology Research and Training Center, University of Nairobi, Kenya, East Africa

Dr. John W. Kibukamusoke, formerly Universities of Makerere (Kampala) and Zambia, East Africa

Dr. Kendrick A. Porter, Department of Pathology, St. Mary's Hospital Medical School, London, England

Dr. Hiroshi Sakaguchi, Department of Pathology, School of Medicine, Keio University, Tokyo, Japan

Dr. Raja Sinniah, Department of Pathology, National University of Singapore, Singapore, (Chairman)

Dr. Visith Sitprija, Division of Nephrology, Chulalongkorn Hospital Medical Center, Bangkok, Thailand

Dr. Liliane (M. M.) Striker, Clinical Nephrology Services, National Institutes of Health, Bethesda, Maryland, USA

Dr. Viqar Zaman, Department of Microbiology, National University of Singapore, Singapore

INVITED CONTRIBUTORS

Dr. Edward J. Bottone, Mount Sinai School of Medicine, New York, New York, USA

Dr. Francis W. Chandler, Center for Infectious Diseases, Centers for Disease Control, Atlanta, Georgia, USA

Dr. Arthur H. Cohen, Department of Pathology, Harbor-UCLA Medical Center, Torrance, California, USA

Dr. David P. Earle, Department of Medicine, Northwestern University Medical School, Chicago, Illinois, USA

Dr. Kent J. Johnson, Department of Pathology, University of Michigan Medical School, Ann Arbor, Michigan, USA

Dr. Gary G. Knackmuhs, Barnert Memorial Hospital, Paterson, New Jersey, USA

Dr. Hyun Soon Lee, Department of Pathology, College of Medicine, Seoul National University, Seoul, Korea

Dr. Domingos de Paola, Federal University of Rio de Janeiro, Brazil, South America

Dr. Elizabeth V. Potter, Department of Medicine, Northwestern University Medical School, Chicago, Illinois, USA

Dr. John C. Watts, Department of Anatomic Pathology, William Beaumont Hospital, Royal Oak, Michigan, USA

AT LARGE

Dr. Leslie H. Sobin, Armed Forces Institute of Pathology, Washington, DC, USA; formerly Pathologist, World Health Organization, Geneva, Switzerland

EX OFFICIO

Dr. V. I. Grabauskas, World Health Organization, Geneva, Switzerland

CONTENTS

FIGURES

PREFACE

The World Health Organization convened several committees of recognized experts to classify renal diseases with international agreement. Criteria for diagnosis, a standardized nomenclature, and a uniform system for classification were needed for comparative geographic studies of kidney diseases. The first three volumes of this study dealt with the classifications of glomerular, tubulointerstitial, and congenital and vascular diseases of the kidneys.

The classifications for most of the diseases were based on morphologic features, as the etiology was unknown in the majority of disease states. Ideally, the classification of renal diseases should be based on etiology. In glomerular diseases, due to limited current knowledge of the etiology and pathogenesis, such a classification was not possible.

However, the association between parasitic infections and kidney disease has been well recognized. Though not as great a scourge as in the earlier part of the century, many parasitic kidney infections are still major problems in parts of Africa, South America, and Asia. In some of these countries, the commonest cause of nephrotic syndrome is malaria, with immune complexes deposited in the glomeruli in response to infection by *Plasmodium malariae*. Changes in the kidneys in parasitic diseases have been due to different mechanisms—for example, deposition of antibodies and antigen-antibody complexes causing glomerulonephritis or hemodynamic changes, hyperviscosity of blood, and hemolysis secondary to systemic infection. The changes have also been found to affect the tubulointerstitial tissues and blood vessels, and some infectious agents damage the kidneys by direct invasion.

Schistosoma haematobium causing bilharzia with lower urinary tract disease leading to infection and the development of bladder cancer is a major problem in some countries of the tropics. Special tropical neoplasms such as Burkitt's lymphoma are known to affect the kidneys. It therefore appears that, unlike the problems of kidney diseases encountered in the northern hemisphere, the classification of tropical and infectious kidney diseases could be based on etiological agents when known. It is proposed that such a classification be adopted in this book.

The anatomy and histology of the normal glomerulus and tubules are described and illustrated in Volumes I and II, the blood vessels and interstitium in Volume III, and the lower urinary tract in Volume V (to be published) in this WHO Series on the Classification of Renal Diseases.

Acknowledgments

Most of the illustrations in this volume were supplied by the members of the World Health Organization Collaborating Centre and by the Invited Contributors. Some illustrations came from friends and colleagues, whose contributions are gratefully acknowledged: Doctors M. Akisada, T. Antonovych, P. Banks, W.D. Bradford, A.S. Cologlu, D.H. Connor, I. Damjanov, A. Date, J.L. Duffy, J. Farsh, S.S.E. Fernando, T. Fujikura, M. Gerber, D.W. Gibson, P. Gikas, R.D. Hackman, S.B. Halstead, H. Ito, R.B. Jennings, Y.S. Kanwar, E. Larson, A.D. Loveday, R.B. Nagle, M. Needle, S.K. Nordeen, W. Ober, A.V. Oliveira, J.M. Pletcher, B.F. Rosenberg, V. Sakhuja, D.J. Silverstein, H.J. Sobel, S. Thung, R. Whitaker. If any contributor's name has been inadvertently omitted, our gratitude is no less sincere.

The following illustrations were contributed by, or reprinted with permission from, the institutions and publishers listed below.

World Health Organization. Figures 2.1, 7.11, 7.12 from "Vaccination Certificate Requirements and Health Advice for International Travel, 1986" (maps 3,1,2 (adapted); Figure 2.17 (adapted); Figure 7.20 from *Bulletin of the World Health Organization* 58(1):1–21, 1980; Figure 11.1 (adapted).

Armed Forces Institute of Pathology (AFIP). *Department of Infectious and Tropical Pathology* (corresponding AFIP negative numbers in parentheses): Figure 3.10 (83–9520), 3.11 (83–9518), 3.12 (83–7936), 3.13 (84–8502–3), 3.14 (73–4627), 3.15 (75–3276), 4.9 (86–1122), 7.2 (51–6069), 7.9 (65–4431), 7.10 (65–430), 7.13 (83–9637), 7.14 (79–674), 8.4 (84–7551), 8.5 (85–11269), 18.7 (76–4497), 18.8 (66–3065–52), 18.9 (54–10234). *Department of Veterinary Pathology*: Figures 4.7 (86–10286), 4.8 (86–10291), 4.10 (86–10290).

Figures 18.8 and 18.9 from Figs. C–10–1–C4 and C5, Binford and Connor (see p 247).

Igaku-Shoin Medical Publishers. *Renal Disease: Classification and Atlas of Glomerular Diseases* (original illustration numbers in parentheses): Figures 4.12 (10–11), 4.13 (10–12), 4.14 (10–17), 7.26 (16–5), 15.4 (16–9), 15.5 (16–11), 15.6 (16–12), 15.9 (16–23), 19.3 (12–7, 19.4 (12–21). *Renal Disease: Classification and Atlas of Tubulo-Interstitial Diseases*: Figures 10.26 (4–36), 10.35 (4–32), 15.1 (8–5), 15.2 (8–6).

Pathological Society of Great Britain and Ireland. Figures 13.4 and 13.5 from Date and Shastry (Figures 8 and 10). (See complete reference citation on p. 259 of this volume.)

Illustrations of life cycles have been adapted from multiple sources.

Appreciation is also expressed to all the technical personnel, especially Tan Tee Chok (for the photographs), Matsuni bin Hamzah (for the illustrations of world maps and life cycles of parasites), and Claire Lim of the Department of Pathology, National University of Singapore.

WHO Classification of Infectious and Tropical Diseases of the Kidney

I. Renal Diseases Caused by Protozoa
1. Malaria
2. Visceral leishmaniasis
3. American trypanosomiasis (Chagas' disease)
4. Toxoplasmosis
5. Amebiasis

II. Renal Diseases Caused by Filarial Nematodes
1. Bancroftian filariasis and Brugian filariasis
2. Loiasis
3. Onchocerciasis

III. Renal Diseases Caused by Other Nematodes
1. Trichinosis
2. Dioctophymiasis
3. Others
   a. Strongyloidiasis
   b. Enterobiasis
   c. Ascariasis
   d. Ancylostomiasis
   e. Trichuriasis

IV. Renal Diseases Caused by Trematodes
1. Schistosomiasis

V. Renal Diseases Caused by Cestodes
1. Echinococcosis
2. Cysticercosis

VI. Renal Diseases Caused by Viruses
1. Bunyaviridae (Hantavirus)
   Hemorrhagic fevers with renal syndrome (epidemic nephropathy; nephropathia epidemica; muroid virus nephropathy; Korean hemorrhagic fever; hemorrhagic nephrosonephritis; Songo fever; epidemic hemorrhagic fever; Tula fever)
2. Arenaviridae (Junin and Machupo viruses) South American hemorrhagic fever (Argentine hemorrhagic fever; Bolivian hemorrhagic fever)
3. Togaviridae (Alphavirus and Flavivirus)
   a. Yellow fever
   b. Chikungunya fever
   c. Dengue hemorrhagic fever
4. Viral hepatitis
   a. HBV glomerulonephritis
   b. Mixed cryoglobulinemia
   c. Polyarteritis nodosa (necrotising vasculitis)
5. AIDS virus (HIV: human immunodeficiency virus)
6. Other Viral infections of the kidney
   a. Landry-Guillain-Barré-Strohl syndrome
   b. Infectious mononucleosis (Epstein-Barr virus disease)
   c. Varicella
   d. Cytomegalovirus

RENAL DISEASE
Classification and Atlas of
INFECTIOUS AND TROPICAL DISEASES

General Immunologic and Inflammatory Mechanisms

Immunologic Mechanisms

The possibility that immunologic mechanisms might be involved in the pathogenesis of renal injury associated with infectious diseases was suspected at the beginning of this century, when nephritis was listed as one of the scarlatinal *Nachkrankheiten*, and the time between infection and onset was declared as a period necessary for the production of active sensitization or immunization.

This hypothesis was later related to the tissue injury described in serum sickness because of similarities characterized by (1) a latent period between exposure to the antigen and development of disease; (2) interactions between antigens and antibodies leading to formation of immune complexes in the circulation; (3) similar patterns of immunoglobulin and complement depositions in kidneys; (4) depression of complement levels in serum; and (5) glomerular hypercellularity, reflecting proliferation of mesangial and endothelial cells with infiltration of polymorphonuclear leukocytes and monocytes. Although both humoral and cellular aspects were studied in the pathogenesis of renal lesions, the demonstration of soluble immune complexes in the circulation and the time sequence related to their detection in kidney tissue directed research toward the humoral aspects; the cellular involvement was for a long time considered only in terms of different mediators or phagocytic function of cells. However, more recent studies in experimental models suggest that cell-mediated immunologic mechanisms can lead to glomerular and/or tubulointerstitial renal injury, with or without concomitant antibody-mediated reactions. Accumulation of monocytes/macrophages and, to a lesser extent, lymphocytes, necrosis, and proliferation of intrinsic glomerular cells are characteristic of glomerular lesions; tubulointerstitial lesions may show numerous lymphocytes, often with macrophages, sometimes with invasion of tubules and tubular cell damage. Although different subsets of T lymphocytes have been identified using monoclonal antibodies in several renal diseases and their role in the initiation of renal lesions has been suggested by transfer of cells, there is as yet no direct evidence that T cells participate in the pathogenesis of human glomerulonephritis. Further evidence is obviously required to establish the role of cellular immunity in human renal diseases. For this reason only humoral mechanisms, whose pathogenetic role has been quite well documented in human disease, will be described in this review.

If we accept as likely that most human glomerulonephritis is immunologic in origin, we have to admit our ignorance of the nature of the responsible antigen(s) in most cases. The evidence relies on the demonstration and detailed analysis of immune complexes in glomerular deposits studied in kidney biopsy specimens, in which the identification of the antigens is often difficult.

Much better evidence comes from animal experimental models where defined antigens were applied and IC-induced renal lesions well documented.

Initiation of Lesions

In general, there are at least three mechanisms by which the interaction of Ab with Ag can induce renal lesions: (1) Ab from the circulation can react with the components of the intercellular structures (bound immune complexes), (2) immune complexes preformed in the circulation can localize in tissues (deposition of circulating immune complexes), and (3) Ags (Abs?) can be deposited in the tissues first and react with Abs (Ags?) subsequently in situ (local formation of immune complexes).

Bound Immune Complexes. The nephritogenic potential of heterologous Abs to the glomerular basement membranes (GBM), causing an acute glomerular injury of varying severity and duration, has been clearly defined and confirmed in many experimental studies. Once these antibodies have bound to the glomerular capillary walls, they serve as "planted" Ags for the further development of the lesions in which the recipient's immune response plays an important role.

The nature of the nephritogenic GBM Ags has been ascribed to a macromolecular glycoprotein from which two major antigenic fractions have been isolated; however, peptide mapping suggests a high degree of their homology and does not exclude the possibility that one may be a subcomponent of the other.

The mechansim of the injury involves the activation of either humoral (eg, complement and other systems) or cellular (eg, neutrophils, macrophages) mediators.

The interactions of Abs with the components of basement membranes (BM) in general, and with GBM in particular, can cause a variety of diseases. In man, the glomerulonephritis in Goodpasture's syndrome, defined as an antibasement membrane Ab-induced lesion, is perhaps the best example of this group. Specific Abs to the components of tubular BM have also been detected, and these can be associated with severe tubulointerstitial nephritis. Many other components of kidney tissue have been identified as Ags reacting with autoantibodies produced, such as tubular brush border antigens and fibronectin, some of which might be potentially pathogenic for renal lesions in man. All of the autoantibodies discussed above should be distinguished from Abs reacting with components of glomerular immune deposits (eg, anti-immunoglobulins, immunoconglutinins, anti-idiotypic antibodies), that contribute to the progression of renal lesions and will be discussed in relation to the perpetuation of renal lesions.

Deposition of Circulating Immune Complexes. This mechanism presumes the interaction of Abs with relevant Ags in the circulation (ie, preformed ICs) and their subsequent localization in the renal tissue with respect to the anatomic and physiologic conditions. This hypothesis has long been regarded as the main pathogenic mechanism in the initiation of IC-induced renal lesions, and it is still valid.

The fate of circulating immune complexes (CICs) depends on their composition, size, the ratio of Ag to Ab, and other factors. Under normal circumstances more than 99 percent of CICs are eliminated by phagocytes (Kupffer cells, mononuclear and polymorphonuclear cells). The overload of these cells or the blockade of their Fc and C receptors may inhibit the elimination of CICs from the circulation and significantly contribute to their localization. This may be particularly important in the tropics, where the CIC levels are rather high and various other conditions may impair the activity of phagocytes.

The size of CICs has been recognized by all investigators as the important factor for their localization. They are classified arbitrarily into three classes according to their size and solubility: Class I—small, soluble complexes; Class II—intermediate-size, poorly soluble complexes; Class III—large, insoluble complexes. The hydrodynamic forces are sufficient to explain the penetration of CICs through the GBM, and there are two main pathways for their localization. The small and soluble CICs of Class I, composed usually from IgG antibody in excess of antigen, penetrate easily through the GBM. During this transit they aggregate progressively and are finally deposited in the epithelial slits and subepithelial spaces, where they can be detected by immunofluorescence and electron microscopy. This pathway corresponds to that of transmembranous (diffuse) glomerulonephritis in man. The second pathway presumes the presence of larger and less soluble CICs of Class II, which penetrate the GBM with difficulty and aggregate within the subendothelial-mesangial system, giving rise to deposits detectable either within the subendothelial parts of the GBM or in the mesangium. This mechanism corresponds to that of endocapillary (mesangiocapillary, lobular, focal) glomerulonephritis. Even though attractive, the theory of the passive penetration of CICs through the GBM seems too mechanistic and naive in the light of more recent observations.

Dixon and his group stress also the importance of the size of CICs based on the ratio of Ag to Ab for their pathologic effects in the tissues. According to their hypothesis, CICs formed in a substantial excess of Ag are not pathogenic because they are too small and do not activate C. Complexes formed in large excess of Ab are too big, are insoluble, and are rapidly removed by phagocytosis. Only complexes formed at the appropriate balance of Ag and Ab (medium size in slight excess of antigen) that are soluble and react with complement are potentially pathogenic. In their view, the activation of C was the main cause of damage to the GBM by production of chemotactic factors attracting polymorphonuclear leukocytes to the GBM. The proteolytic enzymes and basic proteins released from these cells do the actual damage.

A strong correlation was observed between the release of vasoactive constitutents from platelets that required polymorphonuclear leukocytes (but not complement) and the deposition of CICs in blood vessels with subsequent injury to the glomeruli. According to these experimental results in rabbits, the Ag excess in CICs reacts with sensitized blood leukocytes, which release the vasoactive amines (histamine, serotonin) from the platelets in absence of complement. This hypothesis, presuming an increased vascular permeability, was further supported by findings that the deposition of CICs can be prevented by the administration of antagonists of histamine and serotonin or by the depletion of the circulating platelets.

Although principally all immunoglobulins can react with different Ags to form CICs, the main representatives detected in the glomerular lesions in man are IgG, IgM, and sometimes IgA, whigh is more closely related to specific diseases (eg, IgA nephropathies, Berger's disease). Similarly, IgE in the glomerular deposits has been occasionally reported in cases of nephrotic syndrome, and these patients show minimal changes in histology and respond well to steroid therapy. IgE in the glomerular deposits is of special interest in some parasitic diseases, in which blood levels of IgE are known to be high; specific IgE antibodies in CICs (as in schistosomiasis) are of interest as well.

There are controversial reports about the distribution of IgG subclasses in the glomerular deposits. In several studies, all subclasses were present, with a predominance of IgG_1 and IgG_3 in mesangiocapillary glomerulonephritis, positive also for C3, whereas a predominance of IgG_4 was found in membranous nephropathies. However, other studies did not confirm these findings. In children with severe nephrotic syndrome associated with quartan malaria, IgG_2 deposits distributed in a fine, granular pattern along the glomerular vessels (negative for C) may have prognostic value.

The affinity of antibodies seems to have an important role for the localization of CICs. CICs formed in mice producing low-affinity Abs localized preferentially in the GBM, whereas ICs with high-affinity Abs localized in the mesangium. Some of the mice with low-affinity Abs produced at the beginning of antigenic stimulation showed affinity maturation, whereas others failed to do so; it was the latter group of mice in which daily injections of Ags produced more rapid and severe glomerulonephritis. However, the localization of CICs was also influenced by the density of antigenic epitopes on the Ag molecules and by the levels of Abs available for reaction, as demonstrated by passive administration of ICs.

Other physical or physicochemical reactions that might explain the localization of IC in the glomeruli were also studied. The glomerulus, as a barrier for circulating macromolecules, has highly negatively charged surfaces and, therefore, can attract and bind positively charged antigens or ICs. This has been demonstrated by application of polycationic antigens (polysaccharides, proteins), Abs, and/or relevant ICs that localized mainly in the GBM, whereas similar compounds with a negative net charge were deposited more in the mesangium. However, the size of the preformed ICs remained an important factor for the localization. It has been speculated that cationic proteins (eg, those released from the activated leukocytes or platelets) may neutralize glomerular permeability and facilitate the deposition of ICs.

Local Formation of Immune Complexes. The possibility of Ags localized first in the tissues and their subsequent reaction with Abs coming from the circulation (local formation of ICs) has been considered for some time as a possible mechanism for IC-induced injury. A classic experimental model for this type of injury is the Arthus reaction, in which the Ag is injected into the skin of the host previously immunized with the same Ag; antigen-antibody interactions can be demonstrated in and around the blood vessels that carry the antibody to the injection site.

How relevant is this mechanism to the initiation of renal injury? For a long time, immunoglobulins, alone or together with complement in glomerular deposits, were the usual findings in most patients with poststreptococcal glomerulonephritis; and the Ags were detected only in some studies. Subsequent studies demonstrated different localization of immunoglobulins and Ags in the glomeruli, suggesting that free antigens may be present during the early stage of acute poststreptococcal glomerulonephritis. Microbial antigens without any immunoglobulins were further demonstrated in the glomeruli of patients with glomerulonephritis due to other infections, such as *Streptococcus pneumoniae* and *Staphylococcus aureus*. In addition, parasitic antigens have been detected in urine in at least two infections, namely schistosomiasis (man, baboon) and onchocerciasis (man, dog). Schistosomal antigens were also detected in the kidney tissue of baboons infected with *Schistosoma mansoni* without any presence of immunoglobulins or complement.

All these examples indicate that the circulating Ags may be trapped in the GBM during the filtration and that they may subsequently react with the circulating Abs to form ICs and to initiate the lesions. However, this hypothesis may be limited to some situations only. An intensive search in malaria confirmed the early deposits of malarial antigens in the glomeruli of mice and monkeys 7 to 10 days after infection with appropriate parasites, but the antigens were always accompanied by immunoglobulins and in many cases also by complement. The same observations were reported in human cases, but here the biopsies could be taken too late for demonstration of antigens deposited alone.

Although definite evidence for the local formation of ICs in the glomeruli and for their significance in the initiation of renal lesions in man is still lacking, convincing evidence for this mechanism has been described in animal models with characterized antigens: injection of mice with small amounts of heat-aggregated bovine serum albumin resulted in deposition of this antigen within glomeruli. The injection of rabbit Ab to the same Ag when all circulating bovine serum albumin had been cleared resulted in the formation of ICs in the glomeruli.

Perpetuation of Lesions

The renal lesions initiated by autoantibodies reacting with fixed components of the tissue (eg, GBM) will progress until the final stages of kidney dysfunction (uremia) if the autoantibodies are continuously produced. Their cross-reactivity with the BM in other organs (eg, alveoli in the lung) may cause serious complications (pulmonary hemorrhage) leading to death.

The progress of lesions initiated by depositions of ICs (either preformed in circulation or formed locally) depends on supply of antigens, immunologic reactivity of the organism, and several other factors.

The "one-shot" serum-sickness type of lesions presumes supply of a large amount of Ag into nonimmune subjects during a relatively short period. The renal lesions appear during the immune elimination of Ag, usually between 7 and 10 days, as documented in experimental models of this condition. The injury is self-limited, and, if no more Ag is supplied, the disease resolves. Serum sickness in man was observed and described after injection of large amounts of heterologous sera (usually of horse origin) for the treatment of toxic infections (eg, diphtheria); it is rather rare now. An example of a similar condition in man is acute *Plasmodium falciparum* malaria infection. Acute glomerulonephritis, compatible with IC-induced lesions, may develop, especially after effective antimalarial treatment, which releases large amounts of Ag from dying parasites. Once the malaria is completely cured, there is no further supply of malarial Ags, and the renal involvement spontaneously regresses.

In conditions with a constant supply of Ags (eg, systemic lupus erythematosus, nontreated schistosomiasis), the ICs are continuously formed, and their fate depends on the immunologic capacity of the organism (eg, affinity of Ab produced), on the removal of CICs from the circulation (eg, conditions of the phagocytic system), and on the extent of the renal injury.

The CICs may continue to localize within the damaged capillary walls or in the mesangium (according to their properties discussed above) by nonspecific trapping and to increase the size of deposits. However, experimental observations on mice and rabbits indicate that the perpetuation of lesions by the additional localization of ICs is not a passive, nonspecific process due to the injury but an active, specific interaction between relevant components. The circulating Ags and/or CICs in Ag excess react with the free Ab binding sites of the deposited ICs and vice versa; the Abs and/or the CICs in Ab excess from circulation react with antigenic epitopes in IC deposits, leading to the increased size of deposited ICs. The reversibility of antigen-antibody reactions and the faster turnover of Ab molecules (as compared with Ags) may allow the replacement of low-affinity by higher-affinity Abs in the deposited ICs. The best evidence for the continued interactions of Ags with previously deposited ICs comes from experiments in which large amounts of Ags were applied to dissolve ICs and to remove them from the kidneys.

The mechanisms described above have presumed the continuous supply of the original Ag involved in the initiation of the lesions. However, in some instances, the original Ags are no longer detectable after a certain period of time (eg, cured infections), but the renal lesions progress into a chronic stage. Typical examples of this category are nephropathies associated with quartan malaria in children; malarial antigens together with immunoglobulins (and complement in many cases) could be detected in the glomerular deposits during the first period of renal involvement. An intensive antimalarial treatment followed by antimalarial prophylaxis clears the parasites from blood and from tissues. In spite of this and other treatment (corticosteroids, etc), the renal lesions progress into a chronic stage during which the depositions of immunoglobulins (and complement in some cases) are present in the glomeruli but without detectable Ags. Several mechanisms have been considered as possible candidates for the perpetuation of these lesions in terms of IC injury.

Deposition of ICs at the beginning may damage tissue components released and recognized by the immune system as "nonself." As a result, autoantibodies can be produced and can react with the tissue components involved. Investigations focused on the components of GBM and/or mesangium did not confirm this possibility because the eluates from the deposits of chronic lesions did not react with glomeruli from normal kidney in immunofluorescence. In addition, results of sensitive assay to demonstrate the autoantibodies to GBM in sera of these patients were also negative. Antibodies reacting with proximal tubular cells were occasionally demonstrated, as were antibodies to other tissue components (eg, collagen, fibronectin).

Autoantibodies to the components of ICs have been demonstrated in sera of patients with nephropathies, and these could participate in the perpetuation of the lesions. These are antiglobulins (rheumatoid factor type and perhaps others?) and immunoconglutinins. Their reaction with ICs in the circulation may alter the localization of deposits into mesangium, as shown in mice. Their reaction with deposited ICs may increase the size of deposits. However, direct evidence for their contribution to the perpetuation of the lesions is still lacking. The formation of idiotype–anti-idiotype complexes should also be considered in this group. These may be a possible source of a variety of ICs that would not depend directly on the release or the persistence in the circulation of the antigens involved in the original immune responses.

A similarity of epitopes between antigens in ICs initiating the lesions and some autologous substances might cause cross-reactivity, which would lead to the progression of lesions. A typical example is the deoxyribonucleic acid (DNA) in many microorganisms as well as in the host. It has been shown that DNA has a particular affinity to the collagenous substances in the GBM, and the possibility of local formation of DNA–anti-DNA complexes in systemic lupus erythematosus has been proposed. Therefore, the DNA or DNA–anti-DNA complexes of microbial origin could initiate the lesions, and the cross-reactivity of Abs with host DNA might contribute to the progression. The involvement of DNA in renal pathology was confirmed in schistosomiasis and should be further studied in other infectious diseases.

Other autoantibodies (eg, antinuclear, anti–smooth muscle, antimitochondrial) in the sera of patients with different infectious diseases reflect the polyclonal activation of B cells without any evidence of their association with renal pathology.

Summary

Glomerular damage induced by IC (either preformed in the circulation or formed in situ) constitutes the vast majority of kidney lesions observed during or after infectious diseases, as documented by several hundred publications. Tropical parasitic infections have made a significant contribution to these immunopathologic studies.

The reactivity of antibodies (autoantibodies?) with the components of the BM in general and of the GBM in particular has been well documented.

Cell-mediated immunologic mechanisms received little attention when compared with humoral mechanisms, but several experimental studies suggest their possible pathogenic role in glomerular and especially in tubulointerstitial injury. Their significance in human diseases has not been established, and more direct evidence will be required to clarify their role in initiation and/or perpetuation of renal lesions.

A possibility that both humoral and cellular mechanisms are involved in the development and progression of renal disease cannot be excluded.

INFLAMMATORY MEDIATORS IN GLOMERULONEPHRITIS

With the hypothesis that most types of human as well as experimental glomerulonephritis appear to be mediated by immune mechanisms with evidence of immune complex deposition in the glomeruli, the search has been under way to determine how these deposited immune complexes cause glomerular injury. Early on, it became apparent that immune complex deposition per se did not directly cause the glomerular injury; rather the host's immune inflammatory response had to be activated. The development of several animal models of glomerulonephritis has revealed much about the pathogenesis of glomerular injury, particularly immune complex formation and deposition in the glomerulus. However, there is still relatively little information on the inflammatory mediators involved in the pathogenesis of glomerular injury. With this in mind in the following discussion, we will concentrate on what is known about the sequence of the inflammatory response in the renal glomerulus, with particular emphasis on the role of leukocytes.

Complement System in Glomerular Injury

The complement system has long been thought to be critically involved in the evolution of glomerulonephritis, and experimentally was the first relevant mediator system found to be required for the development of some models of acute glomerular injury.

Many types of human glomerulonephritis appear to require the participation of the complement system, but it must be stressed that the evidence for this is inferential rather than direct. First, many types of glomerulonephritis are associated with low levels of total serum hemolytic complement (CH_{50}), with evidence of both classical as well as alternative pathway activation. Second, complement deposition along with immune complex deposition is also observed in the glomeruli. Thus, some types of human glomerulonephritis, most notably systemic lupus erythematosus, are associated with glomerular deposition of the early complement components such as C1q, C4, and C2, suggesting activation of the classical pathway of complement. By comparison, other types of glomerulonephritis, such as IgA nephropathy and mesangiocapillary (membranoproliferative)

glomerulonephritis, have complement deposits of C3 and properdin, suggesting that these types of glomerulonephritis activate complement through the alternative pathway. C3 deposition alone in the absence of immune complex deposition has also been observed in some types of glomerulonephritis, mostly notably mesangiocapillary glomerulonephritis. Therefore, in many types of human glomerulonephritis, complement involvement appears critical to the development of the glomerular injury.

Experimentally, an intact complement system is also required for some models of glomerulonephritis. Complement is required for the development of the early or heterologous phase of the anti-GBM nephritis model. However, the later or autologous phase of this model was found to be complement-independent, as was the model of acute serum sickness. The exact role that complement plays in the anti-GBM nephritis model is not entirely clear, but it appears to relate to the generation of chemotactic peptides, presumably C5a, with the subsequent attraction of neutrophils into the glomeruli. This hypothesis is supported by histologic studies showing the accumulation of neutrophils in the glomeruli as well as more convincing studies using techniques of neutrophil depletion. Other possible ways in which complement can attract neutrophils into glomeruli include immune adherence mechanisms with C3b receptors on glomerular epithelial cells.

Recently, it has become apparent that complement may also initiate glomerular injury directly. Using the Heymann nephritis model studies, Couser and others found that the complement system is involved in this model via the generation of the C5b–9 terminal complement components, otherwise known as the membrane attack complex (MAC), which presumably has a direct "membranolytic" effect on the glomerular basement membrane. This direct attack on the basement membrane by the MAC is analogous to complement-mediated red cell lysis, where "holes" are produced in the red cell membrane by the MAC.

As illustrated in Figure 1.1, the complement system appears to be critically involved in the mediation of some types of glomerular injury by at least two different mechanisms. In the classic model of anti-GBM nephritis, local complement activation presumably leads to C5a generation and the subsequent attraction of neutrophils into the glomeruli, which are in turn responsible for glomerular injury. C3b may also be involved in attracting neutrophils into the glomeruli. With the de-

FIGURE 1.1 The role of complement in glomerulonephritis.

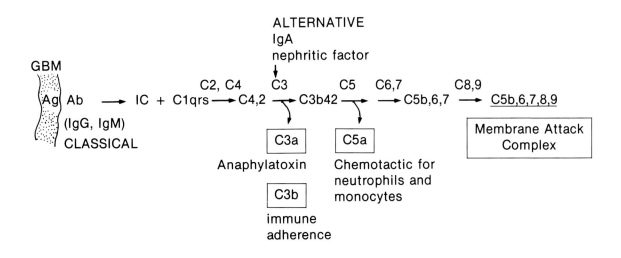

velopment of complement-dependent but neutrophil-independent models, evidence is accumulating that complement may also directly damage the glomerular basement membrane via the formation of the terminal MAC. Thus, MAC formation may play a critical role in the development of noninflammatory proteinuria associated with subepithelial immune complex formation.

Role of Leukocytes

It has long been recognized that the migration of leukocytes, specifically phagocytes, to a site of injury is critical to the development of inflammation. These phagocytic cells, which engulf and destroy foreign invaders such as bacteria, constitute the primary defense mechanism of the host. However, leukocytes can damage as well as protect the host, and intensive research has been done to determine how leukocytes damage tissue.

Role of Neutrophils

Neutrophils are the critical effector cells in acute inflammation and are the first line of defense against the invasion of foreign pathogens such as bacteria. Yet the host's dependence on the neutrophil is a two-edged sword, in that neutrophils can also induce tissue injury. When immune reactants collect in tissues (such as those

of the renal glomerulus), neutrophils are attracted to the site and attach themselves to the immune deposits; during phagocytosis or attempted phagocytosis they damage surrounding structures, including cells as well as connective tissue matrix.

Some experimental models of glomerulonephritis clearly illustrate that the neutrophil can induce glomerular injury and proteinuria. In the acute or heterologous phase of anti-GBM nephritis, depleting circulating neutrophils largely prevent glomerular injury and subsequent proteinuria. At least two other models of neutrophil-dependent glomerular injury also illustrate the phlogistic potential of the neutrophil in the renal glomerulus.

The way in which neutrophils cause tissue injury, specifically glomerular injury, has been the focus of extensive investigation. As Table 1.1 indicates, neutrophils can produce a whole array of biologically active inflammatory mediators, perhaps the most important of which are reactive oxygen products, lysosomal enzymes, and arachidonate products. Traditionally, most of the interest has centered on the lysosomal enzymes. When neutrophils are activated, these lysosomal enzymes, or proteases, are released into the extracellular milieu, where they hydrolize various extracellular matrix proteins, including collagen, elastin, and hyaluronic acid.

TABLE 1.1 INFLAMMATORY MEDIATORS PRODUCED
BY THE NEUTROPHIL

Proteases

Neutral proteases
  Elastase
  Cathepsin G
  Proteinase 3
  Collagenases

Acid hydrolases
  Cathepsin B
  Cathepsin D

Other proteases
  Thrombin-activating protease
  Kinogenase
  Surface proteases

Reactive oxygen products

Superoxide anion (O_2^-)

Hydrogen peroxide (H_2O_2)

Singlet oxygen ($1O_2$)

Hydroxyl radical ($\cdot OH$)

Hypochlorous acid (HOCl)

Arachidonic acid metabolites

Cyclo-oxygenase products (endoperoxides, prostaglandin, thromboxane)

Lipoxygenase products (hydroperoxy derivatives, [5 and 15 Hete], leukotrienes)

Cationic proteins

Arginine-rich band protein (vasopermeability)

Protein bands 1, 3, and 4 (vasopermeability)

Chemotactic factor for monocytes

Leukocyte inhibitory factor

Proteases will also hydrolize glomerular basement membranes in vivo. In in vivo models of immune complex injury with glomerulonephritis, degranulation of neutrophils is observed at the site of tissue injury, and GBM fragments are excreted in the urine. Thus there seems to be little doubt that proteases are involved in inflammation, particularly chronic inflammation, in terms of their documented ability to alter connective tissue matrix proteins such as elastin.

There is, however, increasing evidence that proteases do not appear to be the inflammatory mediators primarily responsible for acute tissue injury. There is little evidence that proteases are directly cytotoxic. In vivo inflammatory models have also consistently failed to show a primary role for proteases in acute injury. A variety of protease inhibitors have failed to protect animals from tissue injury in various acute inflammatory models, including immune complex–induced injury. Therefore, while proteases may be important in the evolution of chronic diseases such as emphysema, where connective tissue breakdown is involved, they do not appear to be the primary cause of acute tissue injury.

In view of the above studies, attention was then directed at neutrophil products other than proteases that could be responsible for acute tissue injury.

Specifically, attention was directed to reactive oxygen products. Reactive oxygen products have long been thought to be involved in certain types of injury in biological systems, and most interest has centered on the phlogistic potential of oxygen species possessing an unpaired electron, the so-called oxygen radicals. As shown in Table 1.2, there are numerous potential sources of oxygen radicals in biological systems. The first biological system in which oxygen radicals were implicated in tissue injury was radiation injury, where radiolysis of water has long been thought to be responsible for cellular injury. Subsequently, many in vitro studies have demonstrated the toxicity of oxygen radicals against both cell targets and connective tissue matrix.

TABLE 1.2 SOURCES OF OXYGEN RADICALS
IN BIOLOGICAL SYSTEMS

From autoxidation reactions (ADP-Fe^{2+}, hemoglobin, electron transport, cytochrome C)

Photoxidation reactions (neucleosides, K Flavanol, melanin)

Enzymatic oxidations

  Xanthine oxidase, dehydrogenases

  Membrane-associated NADPH Oxidase (phagocytic cells only)

Radiolysis of H_2O

Babior, in 1974, found that the phagocytic cells (neutrophils and macrophages), in addition to having the capacity like all cells to make oxygen radicals in the mitochondria and cytosol, are unique in that they possess a plasma membrane associated NADP/NADPH oxidase system, which generates large amounts of reactive oxygen products. The phagocytic cells use these reactive oxygen products to kill bacteria and other pathogens, but during cell activation large quantities of reactive oxygen products diffuse into the extracellular milieu. Of the products formed, perhaps the important are the superoxide anion (O_2-), hydrogen peroxide (H_2O_2), the hydroxyl radical ($\cdot OH$), and myeloperoxidase products such as hypochlorous acid ($HOCl-$) (Figure 1.2). While the formation of these reactive oxygen products is necessary for the destruction of microorganisms, there is also clear evidence that in many instances they are toxic to the host. A wealth of in vitro studies illustrate the cytotoxic potential of these products to a variety of nucleated and nonnucleated eukaryotic cells. In addition, they can alter collagen structure, oxidize lipids, aggregate gamma globulins, and inactivate various enzymes. Clearly, these reactive oxygen products produced by the phagocyte are potentially very destructive.

Within the last few years many in vivo experimental studies have also illustrated the toxicity of phagocyte-derived oxygen radicals. Either superoxide dismutase (SOD) or catalase, naturally occurring enzymatic inhibitors of O_2- and H_2O_2, respectively, has markedly inhibited the tissue injury in many acute models of inflammation. In additional studies, therapeutic inventions designed either to suppress $\cdot OH$ formation, which is a metabolic conversion product of H_2O_2, or to use specific scavengers of this radical have provided evidence that $\cdot OH$ radical formation is also apparently involved in the pathogenesis of acute immune complex–induced tissue injury.

Within the last 2 to 3 years, evidence that neutrophil-derived oxygen radicals injure the renal glomerulus is emerging. In two models of neutrophil-dependent acute glomerular injury (including the heterologous anti-GBM nephritis model), the administration of catalase but not SOD to the animals resulted in marked amelioration of the glomerular injury as assessed by reduced proteinuria levels and morphologic evidence of glomerular injury. Therefore, in the glomerulus, as well as elsewhere in the body, neutrophil-derived oxygen radicals appear to cause much of the tissue damage. Figure 1.3 illustrates

FIGURE 1.2   Reduction sequence of oxygen by the plasma membrane–associated NADPH oxidase system of the phagocytic cell.

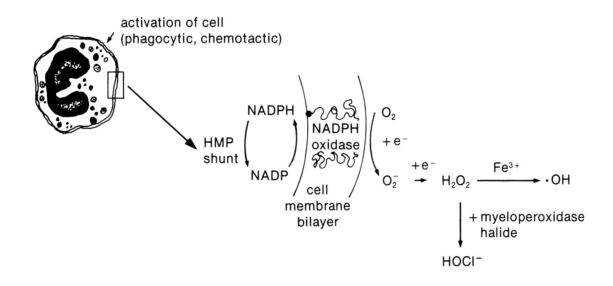

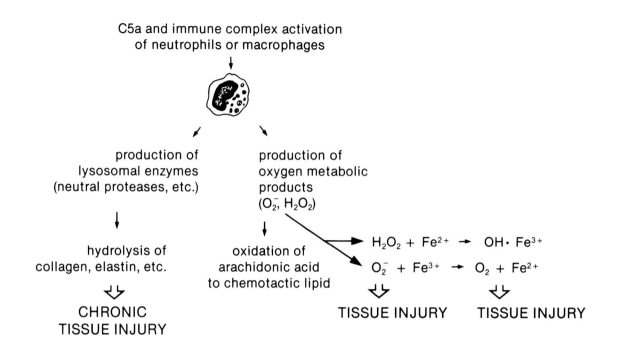

the postulated sequence of events occurring in neutrophil-dependent, immune complex–induced tissue injury.

Role of Monocytes/Macrophages

Evidence has been increasing that these cells are perhaps the most important mediator of glomerular injury in proliferative types of glomerulonephritis. Depending on the species examined, normal glomeruli contain resident macrophages within the mesangium, and these may be the cells responsible for the phagocytic capability of the mesangial region. During inflammation, macrophages accumulate in the glomeruli, and sometimes in the space around them; in most types of experimental and human glomerulonephritis, macrophages recruited from the circulation constitute the increased cellularity seen in acute glomerulonephritis.

There is experimental evidence that the macrophage can induce glomerular injury with proteinuria. Macrophages are required for the development of proteinuria in the late phase of the accelerated anti-GBM nephritis model, and in another study mononuclear cell populations containing T cells sensitized to glomerular antigens induced focal glomerular hypercellularity and necrosis. In the serum sickness models of glomerulonephritis, the macrophage appears critical to the development of the hypercellularity and proteinuria. In both the anti-GBM nephritis as well as the serum sickness model, depletion of circulating monocytes prevented proteinuria. This monocyte/macrophage infiltration into the glomeruli is independent of the complement system and suggests that macrophage accumulation, unlike neutrophil accumulation in glomeruli, does not depend on the generation of the C5a chemotactic peptide. Thus in both humans and animals the monocyte/macrophage cell appears responsible for much of the early proliferative changes, and experimentally they have been shown to be largely responsible for injury to the glomerulus.

The exact way in which macrophages induce glomerular injury is not clear. As shown in Table 1.3, mac-

TABLE 1.3 INFLAMMATORY MEDIATORS PRODUCED BY THE MACROPHAGE

Lysozyme

Neutral proteases

   Elastase

   Collagenase

   Plasminogen activator

Arachidonic acid metabolites

   PGEs

   $F_{2\alpha}$

   PGI_2

   TXB_2

   leukotrienes

Reactive oxygen products

   Superoxide anion

   Hydrogen peroxide (H_2O_2)

   Singlet oxygen ($1O_2$)

   Hydroxyl radical ($\cdot OH$)

   Hypochlorous acid (HOCl)

Others

   Tumor cell necrosis factor

   Interleukin 1

   Interferon

   Complement components

   Growth factors (for fibroblasts, blood vessels, and myeloid progenitor cells)

   Coagulation factors (Factor V, thromboplastin)

---

rophages, like neutrophils, can produce a whole array of biologically active mediators. Macrophages, being phagocytic cells, possess a membrane-associated NADP/NADPH oxidase system that allows production and release of large quantities of reactive oxygen products into the extracellular milieu. There is increasing evidence in vivo in experimental models of acute and chronic lung injury that macrophages can cause tissue injury by oxygen-dependent mechanisms.

Currently there are insufficient data to assess whether macrophage-derived oxygen radicals are involved in the pathogenesis of glomerular injury. However, it is reasonable to expect that in the kidney, as in other organs, the production of oxygen radicals by leukocytes (macrophages and neutrophils) appears critical to the development of the tissue injury.

Role of Platelets

Over the last two decades, there has been considerable interest in the potential role of the platelet in glomerulonephritis. Besides being critical to coagulation, platelets also contribute to inflammation by their release of such biologically active substances as vasoactive amines, various lipid mediators (including arachidonate products), and platelet-derived growth factor (PDGF), which induces chemotaxis, cell division, and collagen deposition by smooth muscle cells and fibroblasts. This knowledge could be directly relevant to the study of cell replication and collagen formation within the glomerulus.

It has been postulated that the platelet aids immune complex deposition in the glomerulus by generating vasoactive amines. Platelet factor 4 can neutralize the glomerular charge barrier, and intrarenal platelet activation produces a glomerular lesion resembling focal sclerosis. Antiplatelet drugs have been shown to diminish protein excretion in both serum sickness and nephrotoxic nephritis models.

In man, there is evidence of platelet activation in many types of glomerulonephritis, particularly the hemolytic uremic-thrombotic thrombocytopenic purpura syndromes. There is also some evidence that antiplatelet drugs may be useful therapeutically, but it remains to be determined whether they alter the eventual disease progression.

Role of Lymphocytes

Traditionally, glomerulonephritis has been considered a prime example of humoral immunity, with damage resulting from immune complex deposition. However, this is not to say that lymphocytes, particularly T lymphocytes, are not involved in this process. T cells may be indirectly involved by their stimulation or suppression of B cell activity, with subsequent antibody formation. In the spontaneous model of murine lupus there appears to be a specific decrease in T suppressor cells associated with an increase in B cells and B cell activity. Some studies have suggested that macrophage accumulation and activation in the glomerulus is a T cell–dependent process, with macrophage accumulation following earlier T cell infiltration. Prior T cell depletion prevented much of the macrophage accumulation. It also seems likely that glomerular injury may sometimes occur directly from cytotoxic T cells rather than from just macrophage recruitment and activation. In humans with various types of proliferative glomerulonephritis, T cells in the circulation are sensitized against modified basement membrane components. One study associated a loss of the negative charge of glomeruli in anti-GBM nephritis with the direct effect of nonsensitized lymphocytes, perhaps natural killer cells. Thus, it seems likely that under certain conditions lymphocytes are involved in the pathogenesis of glomerular injury both from the standpoint of the regulation of antibody formation and macrophage recruitment and activation as well as, perhaps, direct cytotoxic effects.

Role of Arachidonate Metabolites

The normal glomerulus can metabolize arachidonic acid through both cyclo-oxygenase (mainly PGI_2) and lipoxygenase (mainly 12-Hete) pathways. Experimentally, there are suggestions that thromboxane A_2 is involved in the regulation of glomerular blood flow and filtration. Neutrophils, macrophages, and platelets produce significant levels of arachidonate metabolites; the macrophage in particular is an important source of these products during chronic inflammation. There is a wealth of data illustrating the importance of these products in the inflammatory response. It appears that PGI_2 and PGE_2 inhibit inflammatory cell activity presumably by raising levels of cyclic AMP in the cells, whereas thromboxane A_2, $PGF_{2\alpha}$ and the leukotrienes are proinflammatory. In two models of acute glomerular injury, treatment with PGE_1 inhibited the injury. The exact mechanism responsible for this inhibition is not clear, but in one model delays in antibody formation suggested a suppression of B cell activity. Another possible mechanism relates to the fact that prostaglandins (specifically PGI_2 and PGE) under certain conditions inhibit the generation of oxygen radicals and release of lysosomal enzymes by phagocytic cells. Thus, prostaglandins appear to inhibit the inflammatory response by more than one mechanism. Although there is no evidence at present to indicate that inhibition of arachidonate products is beneficial in treating glomerular disease in man, such inhibition may potentially be beneficial.

CONCLUSION

There has been a great deal of research over the past few years on the pathogenesis of tissue injury in glomerulonephritis. Starting with the preliminary evidence of the mediators involved in the anti-GBM nephritis model, further research has considerably extended our understanding of the role of these mediators. For example, we now know that the complement system appears to be involved in the pathogenesis of glomerular disease by a variety of mechanisms. In terms of neutrophil-dependent acute tissue injury, we now have a much more complete understanding of the role of the various inflammatory mediators produced by these cells; the generation and release of reactive oxygen products by these cells appear to be critical to the development of the injury.

Finally, recent animal as well as human studies have emphasized the critical role that monocytes/macrophages play in the evolution of glomerulonephritis. They appear to be the main inflammatory cell present in most types of glomerulonephritis and experimentally appear responsible for much of the glomerular injury in complement-independent proliferative models of glomerulonephritis. The exact macrophage product(s) responsible have not been identified but initial studies suggest an important pathogenic role for oxygen radicals and arachidonate products. The challenge in further studies will be to more precisely map out in a sequential fashion the mediators involved in the initiation and prolongation of glomerular injury.

PROTOZOAL INFECTIONS

MALARIAL NEPHROPATHY

Malaria is an infection caused by the protozoan parasite belonging to the genus *Plasmodium*. There are four species that affect man: *P. falciparum, P. malariae, P. vivax*, and *P. ovale*. However, renal manifestations have been studied in two species only, *P. falciparum* and *P. malariae*.

P. falciparum is widely prevalent in many tropical areas of the world and is of greatest clinical importance because of the possibility of serious complications. Chloroquine-resistant strains, now widely encountered, require greater use of quinine. This in turn has resulted in the re-emergence of blackwater fever after it had almost disappeared. *P. malariae* is common in tropical Africa, parts of the Indian subcontinent, Burma, Sri Lanka, Malaysia, and Indonesia.

P. falciparum can invade erythrocytes of any age, and very high infection rates of 50% or more can result. The young trophozoites form delicate rings, sometimes with two nuclei. Multiple infection of red cells is common. The infected red cells may show coarse stippling known as Maurer's clefts. Schizogony results in the formation of an average of 16 merozoites, and this stage usually develops in the blood vessels of the internal organs of the body. The gametocytes are typically crescent-shaped and can be easily distinguished from other species.

P. malariae tends to invade older erythrocytes and infection rates are generally low, rarely exceeding 1 percent. The trophozoites are often solid and ribbon-like in shape and are therefore known as "band forms." The infected red cells may show fine irregular stippling known as Ziemann's dots.

Schizogony results in the formation of 6 to 12 merozoites that are generally symmetrically arranged in rosette form. The gametocytes are circular and fill the red cell. They have a large nucleus and coarse granules of pigment.

Malaria is transmitted naturally by the bite of mosquitoes belonging to the genus *Anopheles*. Infection is initiated by the mosquito's injection of sporozoites, which develop into the pre-erythrocytic stages in the liver. Merozoites liberated from the liver then initiate the erythrocytic cycle. Some of these merozoites become gametocytes and, when taken up by the mosquito, start the sexual cycle. On completion of the sexual cycle, sporozoites are produced.

Clinical Manifestations

The incubation period of falciparum malaria varies between 9 and 12 days and of malariae malaria from 13 to 30 days. Classic stages of fever consist of the cold stage, hot stage, and sweating stage. Following the sweating stage there is an apyrexial interval, which lasts from 12 to 36 hours in falciparum malaria and about 60 hours in malariae malaria. These patterns may vary with simultaneous infections by more than one species and in hyperendemic areas where immunity levels are high. Falciparum malaria causes two types of renal manifestations, transient nephritis and acute renal failure.

Mild and transient proteinuria with few cellular elements occurs in as many as 50 percent of cases. Proteinuria is usually less than 1 gram per 24 hours, disappearing shortly after the disease is brought under control. Renal function invariably remains normal, with occasional mild elevations of urinary N-acetyl-beta-D-glucosaminidase. Hyponatremia occurs commonly; hypocalcemia and hypophosphatemia, occasionally. The disease is an immune complex–induced nephritis and responds well to antimalarial therapy.

Acute renal failure occurs in fewer than 1 percent of cases but accounts for about 60% of the complications of falciparum malaria. It typically develops in patients with heavy parasitemia or intravascular hemolysis. Associated with either blackwater fever or G6PD deficiency, it also occurs in patients with light parasitemia as a reaction to quinine, chloroquine, and pyrimethamine. Renal failure is often accompanied by jaundice with rapid development of azotemia. Alarming progressions of hyperkalemia may be associated with intravascular hemolysis. Nonoliguric renal failure is not uncommon.

The acute renal failure is due to renal ischemia resulting from hypovolemia, blood hyperviscosity, and sludging of erythrocytes, catecholamine effects, intravascular hemolysis, and intravascular coagulation. Free oxygen radical release further contributes to cellular injury.

Quartan malaria (*P. malariae* infection) causes severe nephritis that can progress to chronic glomerulonephritis; most patients do not respond to antimalarial therapy. Although rapid progression of infection may quickly lead to chronic renal failure in adolescents and young adults, slow progression is well recognized and resolution may occur after successful treatment. Transient nephritis also occurs in quartan malaria and resolves in the same way as in falciparum infections.

Children often suddenly develop nephrotic syndrome, with poorly selective heavy proteinuria, hematuria, hypoproteinemia, edema, and severe ascites. Creatinine clearance remains normal, and there is no azotemia. Blood pressure also usually remains normal.

Progression of renal failure and nephrotic syndrome in adolescents and adults is the rule rather than the exception. They have nonselective proteinuria, hematuria, azotemia, and hypertension. The glomerular lesion is associated with the urinary loss of large quantities of malarial antibody in both children and adults.

Pathologic Manifestations: Transient Glomerulonephritis

Light Microscopic Findings. The glomerular mesangium is mildly hypercellular, with increased matrix. Capillary lumens contain lymphocytes, plasmacytes, and malarial pigment-laden monocytes. Glomerular capillary walls are occasionally thickened. Parasitized erythrocytes are rarely present in the glomerular capillaries but are numerous in peritubular capillaries and interlobular veins. Although fibrin-platelet thrombi are present in interlobular veins and arteries, they are hardly detected in glomerular capillaries. Giant nuclear masses may occasionally appear in capillaries, especially in patients with disseminated intravascular coagulation.

Electron Microscopic Findings. Mesangial and subendothelial deposits are associated with widening of foot processes. The capillary lumens contain deformed erythrocytes and phagocytes, and deformed erythrocytes are trapped together with amorphous and fibrillary material within the spaces formed by endothelial cytofolds and paramesangial areas.

Immunomicroscopic Findings. Granular deposits of IgM and C3 are present in mesangial areas and along some capillary loop walls, and IgG and IgA are occasionally present. The eluates from glomeruli of renal autopsy tissue react with *P. falciparum* antigens, confirming the presence of specific antibodies.

Pathologic Manifestations: Acute Renal Failure

Light Microscopic Findings. Tubular degeneration, necrosis, and regeneration affect the distal and collecting tubules more than the proximal tubules. Eosinophilic, granular, hyaline, and hemoglobin casts are present mostly in medullary ducts and to a lesser degree in convoluted tubules. The casts cause tubular obstruction, leading to dilatation of Bowman's spaces and the proximal parts of tubules.

Peritubular capillaries and interlobular veins may be congested with parasitized erythrocytes, pigmented macrophages, lymphocytes, and plasma cells. Cells are also focally present in the interstitium. Platelet-fibrin thrombi are commonly present in cases complicated by disseminated intravascular coagulation.

Pathologic Manifestations: Quartan Malarial Nephritis

Light Microscopic Findings. The basic lesion consists of thickening of the glomerular capillary walls, which in the earliest cases affects only a few glomeruli in a segmental manner. Most glomeruli in such cases appear normal on light microscopy. PASM stain reveals double contour or a plexiform arrangement of argyrophilic fibers. Crescents are occasionally present. As the disease progresses, it involves an increasing number of capillaries and causes further narrowing and eventually total obliteration of the capillary lumens.

The glomerular abnormalities are less severe in children than in adults. Mesangial hypercellularity in children tends to be segmental, against a background of normal or mildly hypercellular glomeruli. Segmental mesangial sclerosis in the adult is more likely to progress to global sclerosis and contracted kidneys. The glomerular abnormality may be static for many years, with neither progression nor healing.

Electron Microscopic Findings. The essential abnormalities are thickening of the glomerular basement membrane and the presence of electron-dense deposits. Patients with mild symptoms and short duration of the disease have usually had irregular thickening of the glomerular basement membrane with only a few dense deposits beneath the epithelium, whereas patients with progressive disease have had enormous thickening of the glomerular basement membrane and massive intramembranous deposits. The epithelial foot processes can be distinct at the beginning of the disease, but they are usually widened and, in progressive disease, coalesced or obliterated. Subendothelial aggregates of electron-dense material may impinge upon the lumen.

Immunomicroscopic findings. Deposits of immunoglobulins IgG and IgM, either alone or in combination, were detected in 96 percent of African patients, both children and adults. IgA was found only exceptionally and always in combination with IgG or IgM. The deposits were present along the glomerular capillary loops and sometimes in the mesangium, with a distribution varying from segmental and focal to global and diffuse. The deposits were granular, sometimes coarse to medium and sometimes exceedingly fine. These two patterns may be important because of their relation to the effects of therapy. The coarse granular pattern, even if mixed with fine granules, was always positive for subclass IgG_3, either alone or in combination with other subclasses of IgG and with IgM and complement. The fine granular pattern was associated with a predominance of subclass IgG_2, often in the absence of complement.

About 60% of biopsy specimens positive for immunoglobulin were also positive for the third component of complement (C3). Granular C3 was less widely distributed than immunoglobulin, even in the same glomerulus. It was associated with IgM and with the coarsely granular pattern of IgG.

P. malariae antigens were detected in about 25 percent of biopsy specimens, always in combination with immunoglobulin. *P. falciparum* antigens, on the other hand, have not been demonstrated in the glomeruli of any nephrotic children, even with double infection, although they have been found in one adult infected with both *P. falciparum* and *P. malariae*.

The few patients who responded very well to corticosteroids, cyclophosphamide, or azathioprine showed negative findings on immunofluorescence in biopsies repeated 12 months or more after the first biopsy. Patients with poor or no response to treatment showed either no significant changes in glomerular fluorescence or a progression of staining from segmental to global, focal to diffuse involvement. Antigens of *P. malariae* were never found in repeated biopsies.

The coarsely granular pattern of deposits by immunofluorescence correlated with circumscribed intramembranous or epimembranous deposits by electron microscopy; all patients who responded to treatment had this pattern. The finely granular deposits were subendothelial; these patients did not respond to therapy and had a poor outcome.

VISCERAL LEISHMANIASIS

Visceral leishmaniasis is a systemic infection caused by a protozan parasite, *Leishmania donovani* and its subspecies.

The disease may appear in various parts of the world in endemic, sporadic, or epidemic forms. *L. donovani* occurs in the Indian subcontinent, parts of eastern Africa, and China. *L. donovani infantum* occurs in the Mediterranean region and *L. donovani chagasi* in South and Central America and Mexico.

Organisms in the genus *Leishmania* have only the promastigote and the amastigote stages in their life cycles. The promastigote has a single flagellum arising from the anterior end without an undulating membrane. The amastigote is a round or an ovoid body, 1.5 to 3.0 μm in diameter and containing a single nucleus and a kinetoplast. The kinetoplast is not always visible in tissue sections because of the orientation of the parasite.

The vectors are sandflies of the genus *Lutzomyia* (new world) and the genus *Phlebotomus* (old world). The infective stages of the parasite (promastigotes) are inoculated into the host by the sandfly. In the host the parasites enter the macrophages, and other phagocytic cells transform into amastigotes and multiply by binary fission. Dogs appear to be an important animal reservoir in many endemic areas. Jackals, foxes, and rodents have also been implicated. In India, no animal reservoir has been discovered so far.

Clinical and Pathologic Manifestations

The incubation period is extremely variable, ranging from 10 days to 1 year, and the onset of the disease is insidious. Children are commonly involved in the Mediterranean region, China, and Latin America. The usual symptoms are pyrexia, weight loss, malaise, and anorexia. The usual signs are splenomegaly, anemia, moderate hepatomegaly, and lymphadenopathy. Darkening of the skin of some parts of the body also occurs in the Indian form, hence the name Kala-azar which means "black disease." Renal changes in such cases are usually mild and are indicated by moderate proteinuria and hematuria. After chemotherapy and cure of leishmaniasis, kidney functions return to normal, and no sequelae of glomerular damage have been documented.

Light Microscopic Findings. The changes in the glomeruli are predominantly in the mesangium, ranging from minor mesangial widening to diffuse mesangial sclerosis and diffuse proliferative glomerulonephritis. Membranous changes associated with the diffuse mesangial sclerosis may be seen in some cases, especially in patients dying of visceral leishmaniasis. These probably result from protein entrapment within the mesangial matrix. Interstitial nephritis with mononuclear cellular infiltrations, tubular degeneration, and amyloidosis have been observed in some cases. In most cases, however, the tubular lesions are restricted to protein casts, sometimes with a multilaminated appearance, and multiple hyaline droplets within the proximal tubular cell cytoplasm.

Electron Microscopic Findings. The few cases recorded have revealed electron-dense deposits in mesangial areas and some subepithelial humps, as well as thickening and irregularities in the lamina densa of the basement membrane. These changes are clearly demonstrated in the glomeruli of hamsters with experimental *L. donovani* infection.

Immunomicroscopic Findings. All classes of immunoglobulins and complement and fibrin have been detected by immunofluorescence microscopy in patients with visceral leishmaniasis. The immunoproteins are localized predominantly in the mesangium. However, all attempts to detect leishmanial antigens in such cases have so far been unsuccessful. Recently, both immunoglobulin and leishmanial antigen have been detected in the glomeruli of hamsters experimentally infected with *L. donovani*.

AMERICAN TRYPANOSOMIASIS (CHAGAS' DISEASE)

Chagas' disease is caused by a protozoan parasite, *Trypanosoma cruzi*, the distribution of which is confined to Central and South America, where it is a typical zoonosis. The animal hosts include a variety of wild mammals.

No direct parasite-related renal changes are found in Chagas' disease. However, during the course of chronic cardiac failure due to this disease, the kidney is frequently involved by marked passive congestion and by thromboembolic phenomena.

TOXOPLASMOSIS

Toxoplasmosis is caused by an intracellular protozoan, *Toxoplasma gondii*. It is a very common parasite of man and animals, and it is estimated that more than one third of the world's population is infected by it.

In humans, two stages are seen—the proliferative intracellular stage (tachyzoite) and the slowly developing intracystic stage (bradyzoite). The tachyzoites are crescent-shaped, 4 to 8 μm long, and 2 to 3 μm wide. The cysts formed in chronic infection vary in size and have an argyrophilic wall. The bradyzoites are strongly PAS-positive and can be easily recognized in tissues when this stain is used.

Humans and other animals are the intermediate hosts of the parasite. The domestic cat and members of the family Felidae are the definitive hosts. The sexual stages develop in the intestinal tissues of the cat, resulting in the formation of oocysts. Humans become infected by ingesting oocysts from the cat or by eating improperly cooked meat containing the cysts. Human-to-human transmission can occur through the placenta, giving rise to congenital toxoplasmosis.

Clinical and Pathologic Manifestations

Toxoplasmosis is less severe in its acquired form unless the individual is immunocompromised. Patients with clinical toxoplasmosis may show involvement of the eye and the lymphatic system. Rarely, myocarditis or myositis may be seen. The disease is more severe in its congenital form and may lead to abortion, stillbirth, and deformities of various organs of the body.

Renal involvement is uncommon but is part of the disseminated disease. *Toxoplasma gondii* organisms are seen in the renal parenchyma and in foci of tubulointerstitial inflammation. There may be impaired renal function and onset of nonoliguric renal failure. It is one of the causes of congenital nephrotic syndrome in the newborn.

AMEBIASIS

Amebiasis is caused by a protozoan parasite, *Entamoeba histolytica*. It is cosmopolitan in distribution but is seen more often in tropical countries with poor sanitary conditions.

There are four stages in the life cycle: the trophozoite, precyst, cyst, and metacyst. The trophozoite varies in size from 12 to 30 μm, although occasionally larger forms may be seen. It has a single spherical nucleus with a darkly staining karyosome. If the parasite is invading tissues, red cells are generally present in the cytoplasm. Before encysting, the parasite rounds up and becomes a precyst that ceases to ingest food and begins to secrete a cyst wall. The cyst, when it matures, has four nuclei. It may also contain other inclusions, including glycogen and chromatoid bodies.

Infection results from ingesting a mature cyst by the fecal-oral route, usually through contaminated food or water. The trophozoites invade the intestinal tissues, giving rise to varying degrees of pathology. Some strains appear to be more invasive than others and can be differentiated by their isoenzyme patterns. The trophozoites from the intestinal tissues may be carried to other organs, most commonly the liver, via the portal circulation. From the liver, the parasites can spread directly or hematogenously to other organs of the body. In hu-

mans, encystation occurs in the large bowel, and cysts are passed in the feces. Cysts do not form in sites other than the intestine.

Clinical and Pathologic Manifestations

The severity of infection varies from asymptomatic to acute fulminating cases. Acute dysentery presents as diarrhea with blood, mucus, and tenesmus. Most cases subside after 1 or 2 weeks, but many develop chronic forms of colitis. Liver involvement may result in abscess formation, usually the principal cause of death in endemic areas. The kidney may be involved by direct extension through the capsule of the liver or by the hematogenous route.

Cystitis, hematuria, and nephritis, with albuminuria and urine casts attributable to infection with *E. histolytica*, have been reported. Urine at 37°C is lethal to *E. histolytica*, and the organism is therefore unable to survive and proliferate in the urinary tract. The organisms, when found in the urine, may be from an amebic vaginal or penile lesion, a colovesical fistula, or liver abscess draining into the renal pelvis.

Metastasis to the urinary tract via the bloodstream is a rare occurrence.

Macroscopic Findings. Usually there is evidence of extension of the amebic lesion from the liver or the bowel to involve the perinephric tissues and form an abscess. There are single or multiple foci of destruction of the renal parenchyma, involving the cortex and capsule, with medullary involvement in the late stages. The abscess contains yellow or gray opaque liquid and has a shaggy, fibrinous wall. Hemorrhages into the abscess cause the typical "anchovy sauce" appearance. If there is secondary bacterial infection, frank suppuration occurs.

The bladder is involved via a colovesical fistula, with typical necrotic lesions of amebic infiltration in the mucosa and wall.

Light Microscopic Findings. When the renal lesion is due to direct extension through the capsule from the adjacent liver abscess, the pathology is predominantly in the cortex. There is destruction of both glomerular and tubular elements, with formation of an abscess with a fibrinous lining. The inflammatory cells in the surrounding vascularized granulation tissue are predominantly lymphocytes and monocytes. In secondary infection, polymorphonuclear neutrophils may predominate. Erosion of blood vessels with hemorrhage into the abscess is frequently seen. The trophozoites are seen in clusters in the abscess wall, especially with PAS stain. Trophozoites of E. *histolytica* can be identified within the lumen of glomerular capillaries and peritubular blood vessels bordering the abscess wall. There is mild mesangial proliferation in the early stage. Later, the tro-phozoites attack the glomerular capillary loops and eventually destroy the entire glomerulus, including Bowman's capsule, and extend into the surrounding tubulointerstitium. Trophozoites within the distended vessels cause vascular necrosis and interstitial inflammation with lymphoplasmacytic cells; in advanced stages the lesions progress toward complete tissue destruction and abscess formation.

MALARIA

FIGURE 2.1 Epidemiological Assessment of Status of Malaria, 1984. (Courtesy of World Health Organization.)

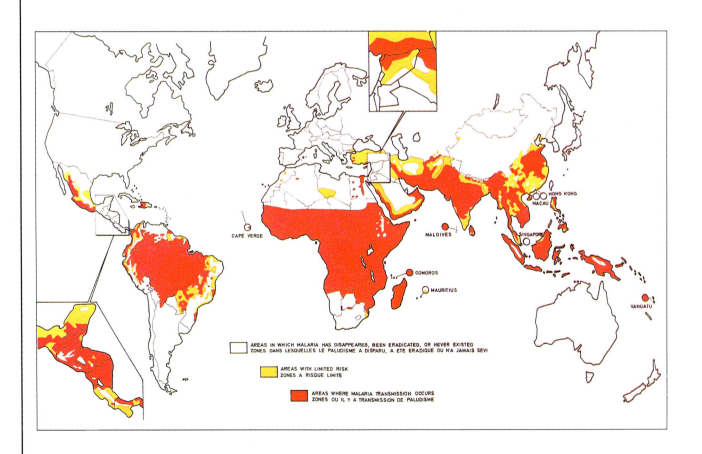

AREAS IN WHICH MALARIA HAS DISAPPEARED, BEEN ERADICATED, OR NEVER EXISTED
ZONES DANS LESQUELLES LE PALUDISME A DISPARU, A ETE ERADIQUE OU N'A JAMAIS SEVI

AREAS WITH LIMITED RISK
ZONES A RISQUE LIMITE

AREAS WHERE MALARIA TRANSMISSION OCCURS
ZONES OU IL Y A TRANSMISSION DE PALUDISME

MALARIA

FIGURE 2.2   Life cycle of *Plasmodium falciparum*.   (*1*) Sporozoites enter host tissues with the saliva of the mosquito.   (*2*) Sporozoite enters liver cells to initiate the development of the pre-erythrocytic stage. (*3, 4*) Pre-erythrocytic stage undergoing development.   (*5*) Merozoites form as a result of schigozony in the liver cell.   (*6*) Merozoites are liberated into the bloodstream and invade red cells.   (*7*) Merozoites from red cells reinvade other red cells.   (*8*) Microgametocyte (male).   (*9*) Macrogametocyte (female). (*10*) Exflagellation giving rise to microgametes.   (*11*) Macrogamete.   (*12*) Fertilization of the macrogamete. (*13*) Ookinete.   (*14*) Oocysts on the stomach wall of the mosquito.   (*15*) Sporozoites liberated from the oocyst.   (*16*) Sporozoites entering the salivary gland of the mosquito.

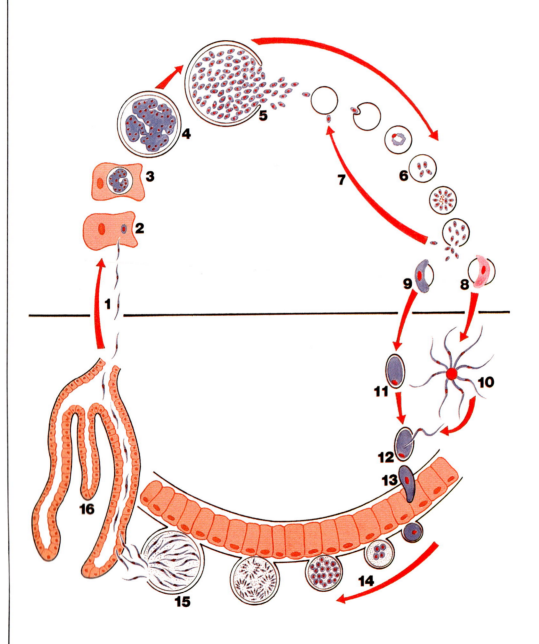

MALARIA

FIGURE 2.3   *Plasmodium falciparum.* Trophozoites in red blood cells. (Acridine orange × 950)

FIGURE 2.4   Falciparum malarial nephropathy. The cut surface of the kidney shows severe medullary congestion and petechial hemorrhages in the cortex.

FIGURE 2.5   Glomerular capillaries are congested and contain malarial pigment-laden macrophages, lymphocytes, and plasma cells. (H & E × 235)

FIGURE 2.6   Glomerulus shows mesangial cell proliferation and increased amount of matrix. There is a giant nuclear mass in the capillary lumen (right lower area). (H & E × 380)

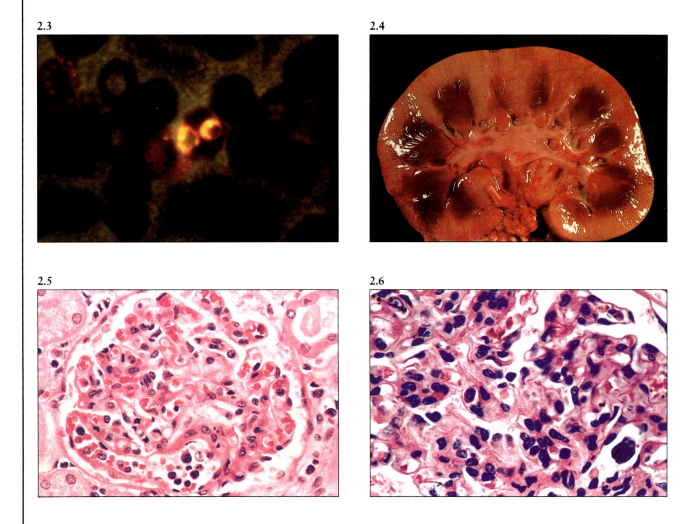

2.3

2.4

2.5

2.6

MALARIA

FIGURE 2.7 Immunofluorescence microscopy. Same case as in Figure 2.4, showing granular deposits of IgM in mesangial areas and along some capillary walls. (× 260)

FIGURE 2.8 Peritubular capillaries contain parasitized erythrocytes. (H & E × 760)

FIGURE 2.9 Renal tubules contain hemoglobin, hyaline, and granular casts. There is focal necrosis of epithelial lining cells. (H & E × 190)

2.7

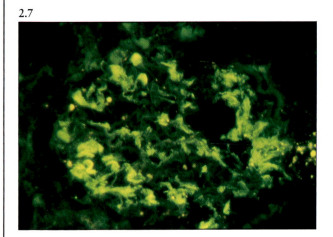

2.8

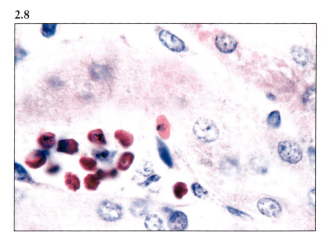

2.9

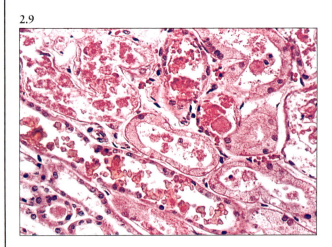

MALARIA

FIGURE 2.10 Peritubular capillaries are congested and contain malarial pigment-laden macrophages, lymphocytes, and plasma cells. These cells also infiltrate the interstitial tissue. (H & E × 190)

FIGURE 2.11 Small fibrin-platelet thrombi are present in dilated peritubular capillaries. (H & E × 190)

FIGURE 2.12 Quartan malarial nephropathy. Glomerulus showing slight mesangial widening with some increase in cells and thickening of the capillary walls. (PAS × 380)

2.10

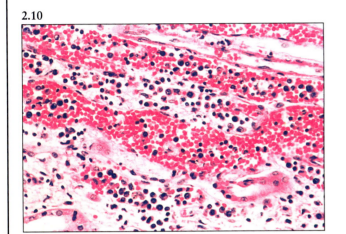

2.11

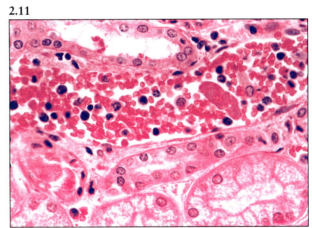

2.12

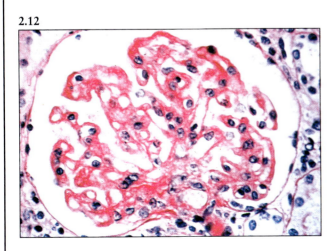

MALARIA

FIGURE 2.13 Same case as Figure 2.12 showing double outlines of glomerular capillary walls and narrowing of the lumens. (PASM × 950)

FIGURE 2.14 Immunofluorescence microscopy. There are massive coarse granular deposits of IgG, mainly along the glomerular capillary walls. (× 260)

FIGURE 2.15 Electron micrograph. There are electron-dense deposits within the glomerular basement membrane and also in the subepithelium. The epithelial foot processes are widened. *Bm* = basement membrane; *Ep* = epithelium; *En* = endothelium; *L* = capillary lumen. (× 21,000)

2.13

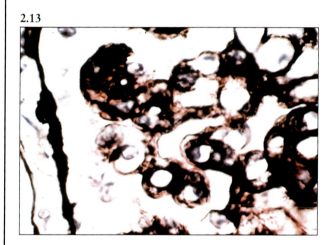

2.14

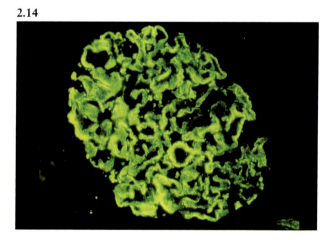

2.15

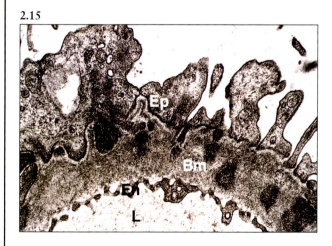

MALARIA

FIGURE 2.16 Electron micrograph. Deformed and fragmented erythrocytes and monocytes in the glomerular capillary lumen. (× 3,375)

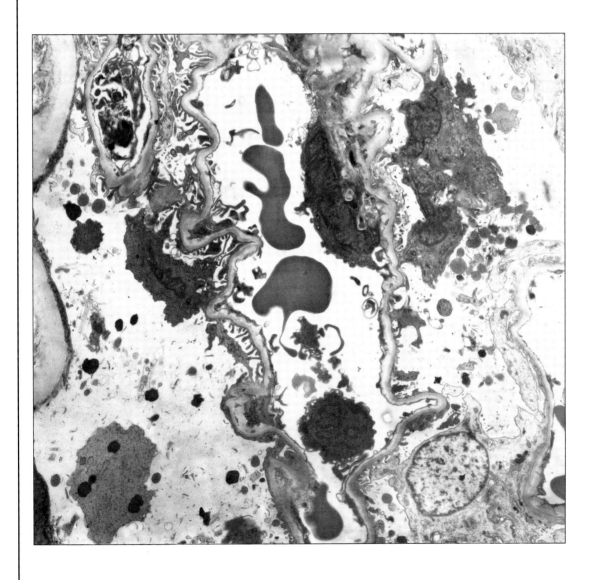

CUTANEOUS LEISHMANIASIS

FIGURE 2.17 Distribution of cutaneous and mucocutaneous leishmaniasis in the world, 1984. *Colored areas* = endemic areas; *dots* = sporadic cases. (Courtesy of World Health Organization.)

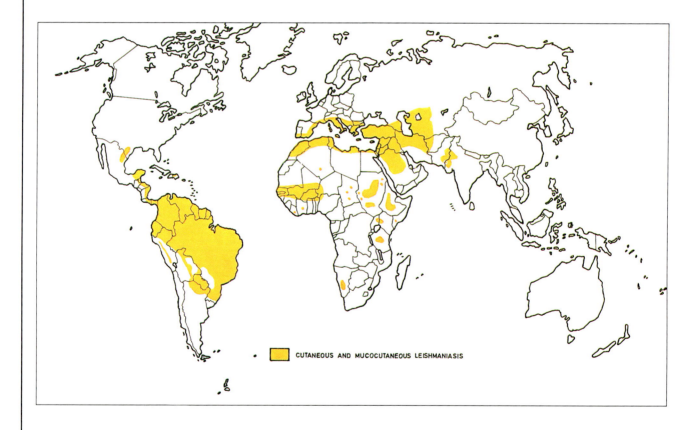

CUTANEOUS AND MUCOCUTANEOUS LEISHMANIASIS

VISCERAL LEISHMANIASIS

FIGURE 2.18 Distribution of visceral leishmaniasis in the world, 1984. *Colored* areas = endemic areas; *dots* = sporadic cases. (Courtesy of World Health Organization.)

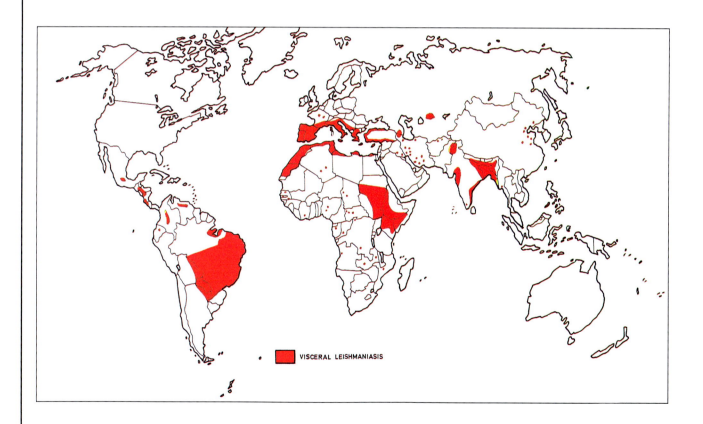

VISCERAL LEISHMANIASIS

VISCERAL LEISHMANIASIS

FIGURE 2.19   Life-cycle of leishmania.   (*1*) Development in the sandfly (vector). Amastigotes develop a flagellum and become promastigotes.   (*2*) Promastigote entering a host macrophage. Entry occurs by the flagellar end.   (*3*) Promastigote loses the flagellum and becomes an amastigote.   (*4*) Amastigotes underto asexual division and fill the cell.   (*5*) Infected macrophage ruptures and liberates amastigotes in the surrounding tissues.   (*6*) Liberated amastigotes ingested by other macrophages.   (*7*) Asexual development occurs in the newly infected macrophages, and this cycle is repeated many times. Some infected cells are ingested by sandflies, initiating development in the sandfly.

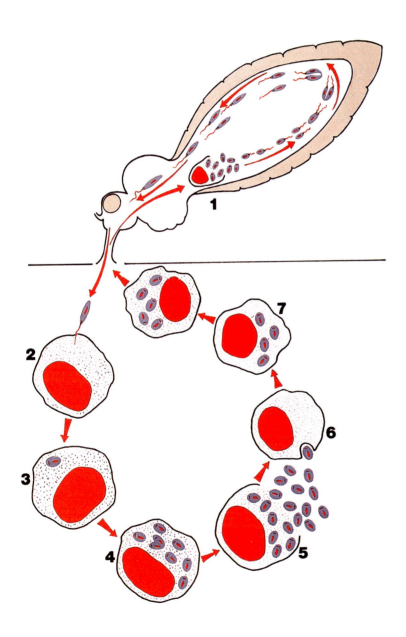

VISCERAL LEISHMANIASIS

FIGURE 2.20   Leishmania. Smears from the bone marrow show parasites (*L. donovani chagasi*) in macrophages within the cytoplasm, and some free. (Giemsa × 760)

FIGURE 2.21   Visceral leishmaniasis. There is diffuse mesangial thickening with moderate mesangial cell proliferation in the glomerulus of a patient dying of visceral leishmaniasis. (H & E × 235)

FIGURE 2.22   Same case as in Figure 2.21. The trichrome stain shows moderate thickening of the centrilobular stalks of the glomerular mesangium. (Masson trichrome × 235)

2.20

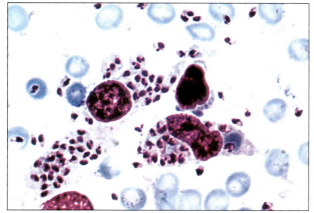

2.21

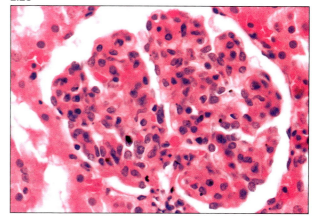

2.22

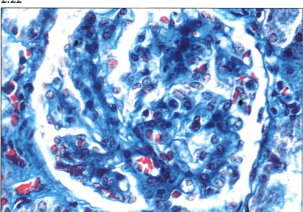

Visceral Leishmaniasis

FIGURE 2.23   Visceral leishmaniasis. There is an acute interstitial nephritis with mononuclear cellular infiltration, predominantly lymphocytes. (H & E × 140)

FIGURE 2.24   Visceral leishmaniasis. Foci of tubular epithelial cell degeneration, interstitial lymphocytic, and mononuclear cellular infiltration and protein casts in the tubular lumen. (H & E × 235)

FIGURE 2.25   Immunofluorescence microscopy. Immunoglobulin deposits localized mainly within the mesangial areas in the glomerulus of a hamster experimentally infected with *L. donovani*. (× 235)

2.23

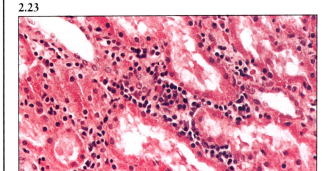

2.24

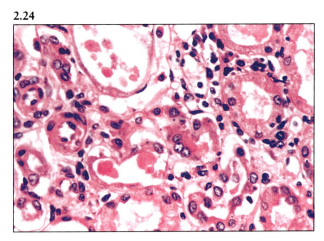

2.25

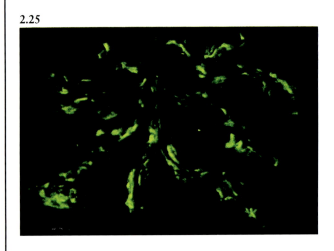

VISCERAL LEISHMANIASIS

FIGURE 2.26 Immunofluorescence microscopy. Deposits with specific fluorescence for leishmanial antigen in the glomerulus of a hamster with 21-day-old *L. donovani* infection. The biopsy also showed proliferative glomerulonephritis. (× 235)

FIGURE 2.27 Immunofluorescence microscopy. Human case of kala-azar showing deposition of IgA in the glomerular mesangium. (× 235)

FIGURE 2.28 Immunofluorescence microscopy. Same case as in Figure 2.30, showing predominantly mesangial localization of IgG. (× 235)

2.26

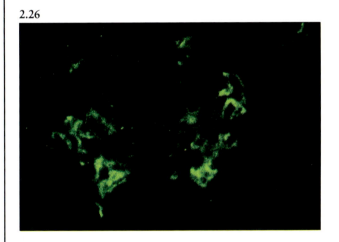

2.27

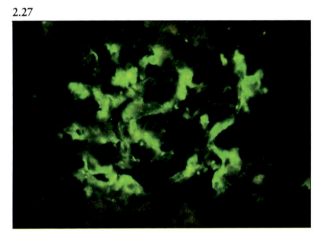

2.28

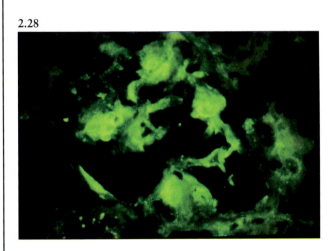

VISCERAL LEISHMANIASIS

FIGURE 2.29   Electron micrograph. Electron-dense deposits in the glomerular mesangium (arrowhead). (× 15,900)

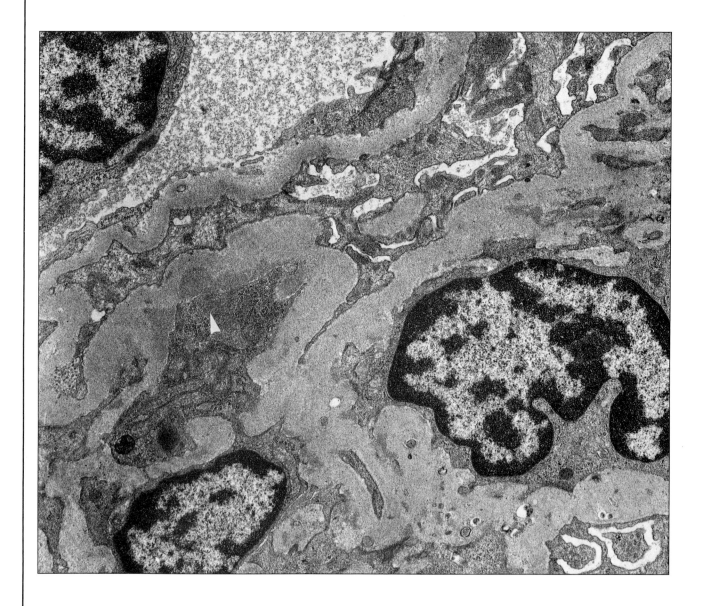

Visceral Leishmaniasis

FIGURE 2.30   Electron micrograph. Small intramembranous and mesangial deposits in the glomerulus (arrows). The mesangium and some cells also contain small vacuoles that suggest severe hyperlipidemia (arrowheads). (× 11,900)

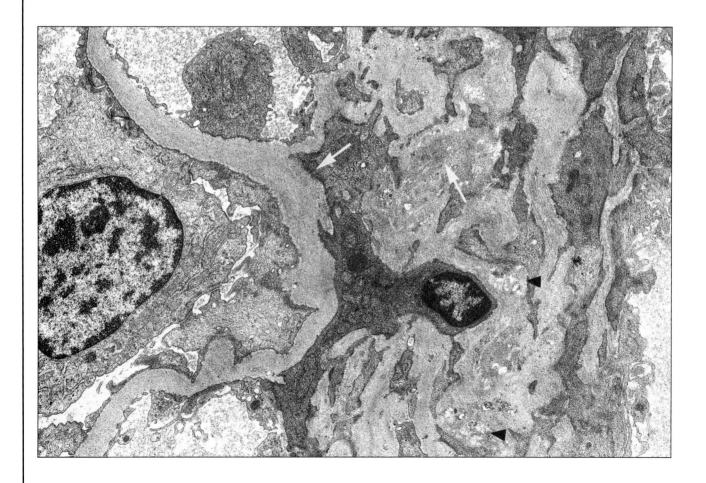

AMERICAN TRYPANOSOMIASIS (CHAGAS' DISEASE)

FIGURE 2.31   Blood smear with trypomastigote of *Trypanosoma cruzi*. (Giemsa × 760)

FIGURE 2.32   The characteristic aneurysmal dilatation of the left ventricular apex of the heart and mural thrombosis in a case of chronic Chagas' myocarditis.

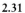

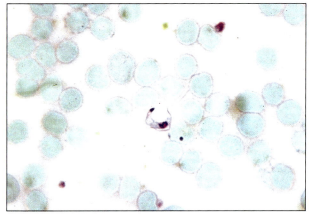

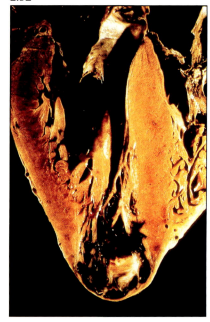

AMERICAN TRYPANOSOMIASIS (CHAGAS' DISEASE)

FIGURE 2.33   Passive congestion and embolic infarction are the main lesions affecting the kidneys in cases of chronic Chagas' disease, as illustrated in this picture.

FIGURE 2.34   Necrosis and hemorrhage involving the renal tissue. These changes resulted from a recent embolic infarction during the course of chronic Chagas' disease. (H & E × 940)

2.33

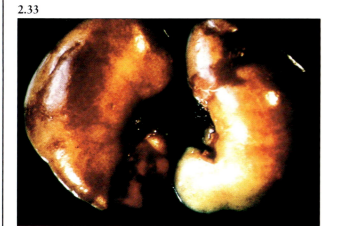

2.34

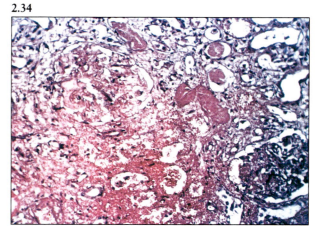

Toxoplasmosis

FIGURE 2.35 Life cycle of *Toxoplasma gondii* in the cat. (*1*) Immature oocyst in cat feces, showing a single sporoblast. (*2*) Oocyst with two sporoblasts. (*3*) Oocyst with two sporoblasts. (*4*) Mature oocyst with four sporozoites in each sporocyst. (*5*) Mouse and other rodents are infected by ingesting oocysts. (*6*) Zoites are liberated from rodent tissue when it is eaten by a cat and enter the cells of the small intestine. (*7*) Parasites undergo schizogony, which results in the formation of merozoites. (*8*) Some merozoites enter the extraintestinal tissues by the hematogenous route. (*9, 10*) Other merozoites re-enter the cells of the small intestine and initiate the sexual cycle. (*11*) Microgametes fertilize the macrogametes, giving rise to the oocyst.

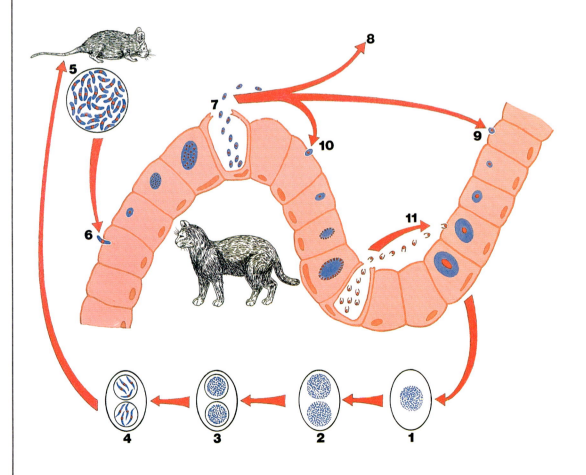

Toxoplasmosis

FIGURE 2.36 Mode of infection in humans: (*1*) Cat feces. (*2*) Oocysts from feces. (*3*) Host animals. (*4*) Tissue cyst. (*5*) Human. (*6*) Congenital transmission.

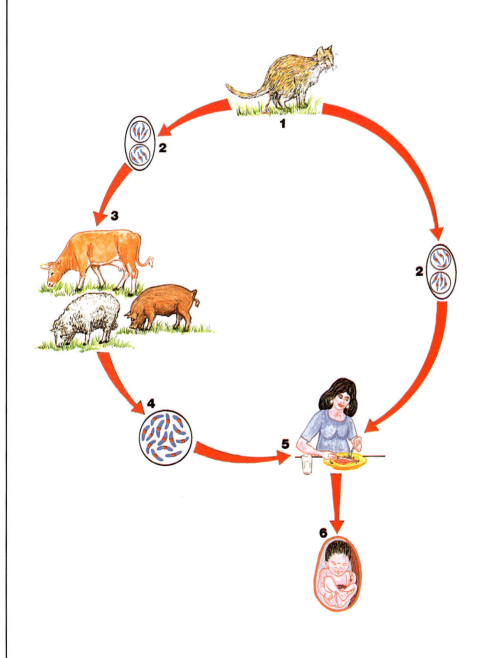

TOXOPLASMOSIS

FIGURE 2.37   Toxoplasma. Endozoites (tachyzoites) in macrophage. (Giemsa × 760)

FIGURE 2.38   Toxoplasma endozoites (tachyzoites) lying free after breaking out of macrophage. (Acridine orange × 760)

FIGURE 2.39   Toxoplasma cyst in brain. Impression smear. (Acridine orange × 285)

2.37

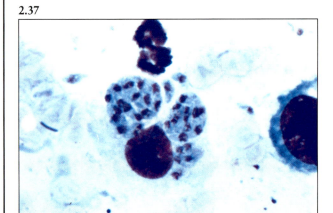

2.38

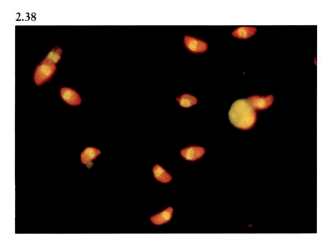

2.39

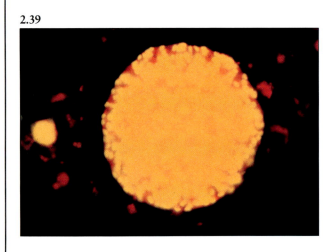

TOXOPLASMOSIS

FIGURE 2.40   Toxoplasmosis. Cluster of toxoplasma organisms in the kidney, together with tubulointerstitial inflammation consisting of mononuclear cells, lymphocytes, plasma cells, and eosinophils. (H & E × 235)

FIGURE 2.41   Same case as in Figure 2.40. Higher magnification of the same field showing toxoplasma organisms. (H & E × 950)

AMEBIASIS

FIGURE 2.42   Amebiasis. Section through the margin of an amebic abscess of the kidney. Extensive necrosis, fibrinous exudate, and several trophozoites are seen. (H & E × 60)

2.40

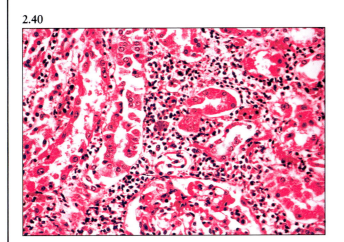

2.41

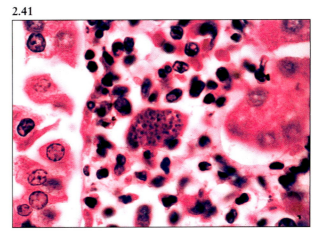

2.42

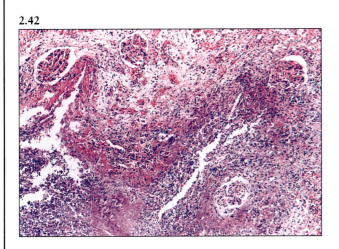

AMEBIASIS

FIGURE 2.43   Same case as in Figure 2.42. There is a trophozoite of *Entamoeba histolytica* within the lumen of a glomerular capillary (lower left) and mononuclear cells infiltrating the glomerulus. Several trophozoites are present within an adjacent peritubular capillary (right). (H & E × 235)

FIGURE 2.44   Same case as in Figure 2.42. Clusters of amebic trophozoites are seen within the glomerulus and in a peritubular capillary. Extensive tissue necrosis involves the glomerulus, tubules, and interstitium. (PAS × 235)

FIGURE 2.45   Same case as in Figure 2.42. The peritubular blood vessels are dilated and contain clusters of trophozoites. There is tubular necrosis and tubulointerstitial inflammation, with lymphocytes, plasma cells, eosinophils, and monocytes. (H & E × 235)

2.43

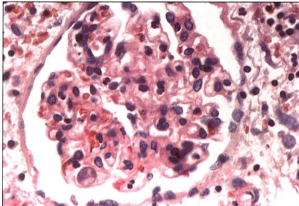

2.44

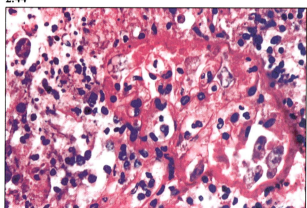

2.45

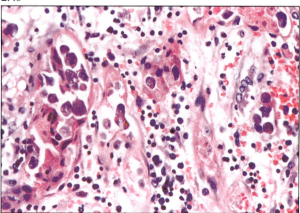

CHAPTER **3**

FILARIAL NEMATODE INFECTIONS

The principal filarial species parasitic in man are *Wuchereria bancrofti, Brugia malayi, Brugia timori, Onchocerca volvulus, Loa loa, Mansonella perstans, Mansonella streptocerca,* and *Mansonella ozzardi.* Occasionally, Dirofilaria spp from animals infect man. In terms of distribution and pathogenecity, the most important species are *W. bancrofti, B. malayi, O. volvulus,* and *L. loa.*

BANCROFTIAN AND BRUGIAN FILARIASIS

These infections are caused by the nematode parasites *Wuchereria bancrofti* and *Brugia malayi. W. bancrofti* is the most widely distributed filarial infection. It occurs in the Far East, Southeast Asia, eastern Asia, parts of the Middle East, major portions of Africa, and South and Central America. *B. malayi* is restricted to the eastern regions of the Indian subcontinent and to Southeast Asia.

The adults are elongated, thread-like worms that live in the lymphatics of various parts of the body. The female is viviparous and liberates sheathed microfilariae. The microfilariae are 200 to 300 μm long and show "nuclei" in their bodies after staining. The shape and arrangement of these nuclei are used for differentiating species.

The life cycles for *W. bancrofti* and *B. malayi* are similar, and transmission occurs through mosquitoes.

After the microfilariae are ingested by the mosquito, they moult twice to become the third stage or the infective larvae. The infective larvae emerge from the labium of the mosquito during feeding and enter the wound produced by the biting mouth parts. After entering the host tissues, the larvae migrate to the lymphatics, where they become adults. The microfilariae liberated in the lymph find their way into the thoracic duct and then to the bloodstream.

Clinical and Pathologic Manifestations

A large number of patients in endemic areas remain asymptomatic and without patent microfilaremia.

The acute stage of the disease manifests when the worms develop in the lymphatics, and the patient may have lymphangitis of the limbs; transient skin swellings; and recurrent inguinal, axillary, or epitrochlear lymphadenitis. Sometimes lymphangitis is severe and is accompanied by high fever, headache, and chills requiring hospitalization. In addition to lymphatic involvement, some patients may present with epididymitis and orchitis. Microfilariae appear in the blood during this stage.

The chronic stage may take a number of years to appear. Meanwhile, repeated attacks of acute lymphangitis may continue. The classic symptoms of this stage are elephantiasis, hydrocele, and chyluria. Microfilaremia begins to decline during this stage, and in long-standing cases of elephantiasis there is often no microfilaremia.

Adult worms within dilated lymphatics cause thickening of the endothelial lining and vessel walls with a chronic inflammatory infiltrate of lymphocytes, histiocytes, plasma cells, and eosinophils. Granulomatous inflammation may occur.

In biopsy and autopsy specimens, microfilariae may be found within blood vessels or within lymphatics of any organ. Degenerating microfilariae may be present in microabscesses or granulomatous reaction sites. There may be focal vasculitis and thrombosis.

Light Microscopic Findings. Microfilariae of *W. bancrofti* may be seen within the glomerular capillaries. Viable microfilariae do not usually cause lesions, but degenerating organisms evoke inflammation with lymphocytes, plasma cells, and eosinophils. Some reports suggest that chronic antigenemia results in glomerular lesions with mesangiocapillary (membranoproliferative) glomerulonephritis type I and acute eosinophilic glomerulonephritis. Patients present with acute nephritic syndrome, marked eosinophilia of 20 percent in the peripheral blood, and circulating microfilariae. The glomerular lesions are essentially those of acute diffuse proliferative glomerulonephritis. Among the cells infiltrating the glomerular capillary lumens are large numbers of eosinophils. Large numbers of microfilariae are present within the glomeruli.

Some cases may show acute interstitial nephritis with lymphocytes, plasma cells, monocytes, and eosinophils. Granulomatous inflammation may occur in the presence of degenerating organisms.

Immunomicroscopic Findings. Immunofluorescence shows the pattern characteristic of acute postinfectious glomerulonephritis, with granular discontinuous and diffuse deposits of IgG and C3 along the glomerular capillary walls.

In one case the glomerular deposits stained with an antibody directed against filarial antigens derived from *B. malayi*. Although the acute glomerulonephritis may have been caused by acute infestation by microfilariae, the relationship may have been coincidental.

LOIASIS

Loiasis is an infection caused by the filarial nematode *Loa loa*, also called the African eyeworm. It is widely distributed in the rain forests of western Africa, south of the Sahara. Although a strain of *L. loa* is found in various monkeys and baboons in the African rain forests, it is now regarded as distinct from the human strain.

The female worms measure 50 to 70 × 0.45 to 0.60 mm, and the male worms measure 30 to 40 × 0.35 to 0.40 mm. The cuticle is covered with minute bosses. The microfilariae are sheathed, and the body nuclei are coarse and tend to overlap each other.

The vector is the mango fly of the genus *Chrysops*. The ingested microfilariae develop in the fat body of the insect and become infective larvae in about 10 days. They enter the tissues of the definitive host during feeding by the female *Chrysops*. The prepatent period is about 6 months, and the adults may live up to 17 years. The microfilariae circulate in the blood and show diurnal periodicity. During the night they inhabit the pulmonary blood vessels.

Clinical and Pathologic Manifestations

Infection may persist for years without signs or symptoms. Migration of the worm beneath the conjuctiva or skin causes swelling of the lids, congestion, itching, and pain. Hypersensitivity reactions in the skin are called calabar swellings. The onset is sudden, but the swellings regress gradually and tend to recur at the same sites. There is marked eosinophilia.

Renal involvement is unusual. A few cases of nephrotic syndrome have been reported. Several varieties of glomerular disease have been reported in association with filarial infection.

Light Microscopic Findings. The kidneys, when involved, show mononuclear cell infiltrates and foci of microinfarction around obstructed blood vessels. The glomeruli invariably show membranous lesions with diffusely thickened peripheral capillary walls and a mild increase in the number of endocapillary cells. By light microscopy, these cases do not differ from idiopathic membranous glomerulonephritis. Other glomerular lesions seen in patients with overt filariasis range from mild to advanced renal damage, with minor change, mesangial proliferation, mesangiocapillary proliferation (membranoproliferation), and extensive sclerosing glomerulonephritis. Microfilariae may be seen in the lumens of some glomerular capillaries. The older lesions show varying degrees of glomerular sclerosis. In the glomeruli with partial sclerosis and thickened capillary walls, microfilariae of *L. loa* can be seen within the lumens of the capillaries.

Interstitial microinfarction and inflammation occur

around obstructed renal blood vessels. Degenerating microfilariae of *L. loa* are seen in the fibrin.

Electron Microscopic Findings. Electron microscopy reveals changes of membranous glomerulonephritis. Capillary basement membranes are irregularly thickened by widely spaced subepithelial and intramembranous deposits of varying density, along with basement membrane spiking. Sheath and lateral cuticular ridges characteristic of *L. loa* may also be visible.

Immunomicroscopic Findings. By immunofluorescence, cases studied show IgG, IgM, and complement C3 distributed in a granular pattern along the glomerular capillary walls and in the mesangium. Filarial antigens have been found in the glomeruli and in renal tubules.

ONCHOCERCIASIS

Onchocerciasis is an infection caused by the filarial nematode, *Onchocerca volvulus*. It is endemic throughout tropical Africa, the southern tip of the Arabian peninsula (Yemen), and certain parts of Central and South America.

Female worms measure 23 to 50 cm $\times$ 0.30 to 0.50 mm, and males measure 16 to 42 $\times$ 0.125 to 0.20 mm. The cuticle is thick and has distinctive annulations, which in cross-section appear as small protuberances. The microfilariae do not have a sheath, and the body nuclei are mostly separated.

The parasite is transmitted by black flies of the genus *Simulium*. Infective larvae enter human tissues during feeding and develop into adult worms in the deep fascial planes and dermis. Microfilariae are discharged by gravid females in the subcutaneous tissues and find their way to the dermis, where they are picked up by the *Simulium*. After ingestion, the microfilariae penetrate the gut and enter the thoracic muscles, where they moult and become infective larvae. These larvae then find their way to the head and enter the proboscis.

Clinical and Pathologic Manifestations

Unlike *Wuchereria bancrofti* and *Brugia malayi*, the adult worms are relatively nonpathogenic, and microfilariae are the main cause of disease. In heavily infected individuals, microfilariae are found in the skin, eyes, lymph nodes, and various internal organs. The presenting symptoms are generally itching and scratching. Persistent itching causes secondary infection of the dermis and dermatitis. This may be followed by intradermal edema and lichenification. The loss of elastic tissue may eventually lead to a condition known as "hanging groin," in which the skin in the inguinal region hangs in folds. In Yemen, one sees a very severe form of dermatitis known as "Sowda" (meaning black), in which body parts become heavily pigmented.

The eye disorders produced by microfilariae may start as conjunctivitis, photophobia, and lacrimation. Limbitis with brownish pigmentation is often present. In chronic cases punctate keratitis, glaucoma, and optic atrophy occur. The nodules produced by the adult worms are known as onchocercomas and are generally found over bony prominences such as scapulae, ribs, skull, elbows, iliac crest, knees and sacrum. The nodules are movable, firm, and non-tender.

Invasion of deep organs by *O. volvulus*, with kidney involvement, has been documented. Proteinuria has been reported in populations hyperendemic for onchocerciasis. In some studies heavy proteinuria was detected in patients during treatment with diethylcarbamazine; however, it was transient and disappeared within a month of completion of treatment.

Light Microscopic Findings. Microfilariae of *O. volvulus* are present in the glomeruli, tubules, and interstitium. Many microfilariae degenerate, especially within microabscesses. Focal collections of lymphocytes, plasma cells, and polymorphonuclear neutrophils are distributed throughout the renal glomeruli. The microfilariae provoke acute inflammation; some glomeruli show increased cellularity, and others some degree of hyalinosis.

The proximal tubules are dilated and the distal convoluted tubules may contain granular and hyaline casts.

Immunomicroscopic Findings. Studies are in progress in western Africa to detect and characterize the depositions of immune complexes in renal tissue obtained by biopsies. Preliminary results have shown a high incidence of immunoglobulins accompanied by complement in the glomerular deposits. Antigens have been detected in some of them.

LYMPHATIC FILARIASIS

Although chyluria is a well-recognized and common complication of chronic infection in filariasis, it has been assumed until recently that it was unaccompanied by specific renal lesions. Chyluria is caused by an abnormal connection between lymphatics and the urinary tract. A case of an immune complex type of focal proliferative glomerulonephritis with mesangial deposits has recently been documented.

Bancroftian Filariasis and Brugian Filariasis

FIGURE 3.1   Vectors and their filarial parasites.

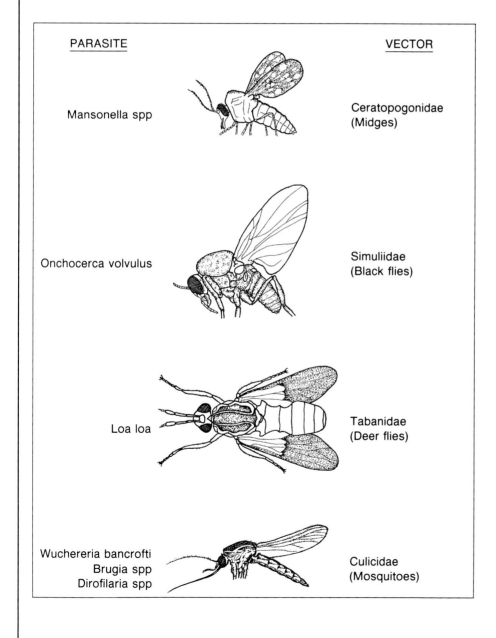

PARASITE   VECTOR

Mansonella spp   Ceratopogonidae
                                                  (Midges)

Onchocerca volvulus   Simuliidae
                                                  (Black flies)

Loa loa   Tabanidae
                                                  (Deer flies)

Wuchereria bancrofti
    Brugia spp   Culicidae
Dirofilaria spp   (Mosquitoes)

BANCROFTIAN FILARIASIS AND BRUGIAN FILARIASIS

FIGURE 3.2   Life cycle of *Wuchereria bancrofti*.   (*1*) Skin showing the entry of the infective larvae through the space left by the mosquito proboscis.   (*2*) Entry of the parasites into the lymphatics. (*3*) Development of the parasite in the region of the lymph gland.   (*4*) Blockage of the lymphatics, leading to elephantiasis.   (*5*) Microfilariae being discharged via the thoracic duct into the bloodstream. (*6*) Microfilaria in blood.   (*7*) Development of the parasite in the mosquito.

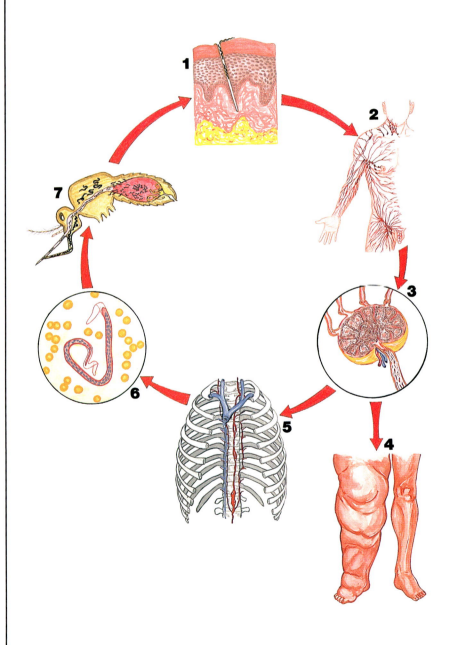

BANCROFTIAN FILARIASIS AND BRUGIAN FILARIASIS

FIGURE 3.3   Distribution of Bancroftian filariasis in man. (Adapted from several sources.)

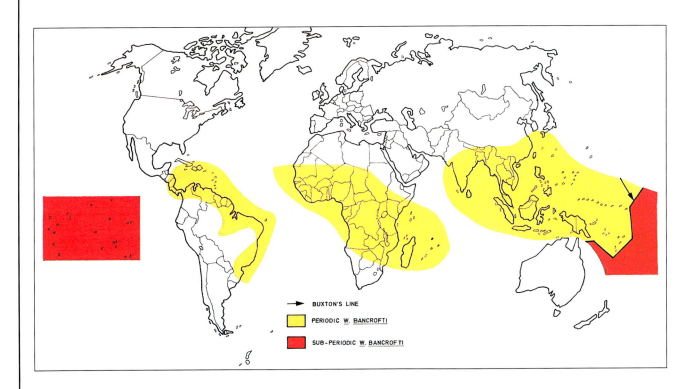

→ BUXTON'S LINE

🟨 PERIODIC W. BANCROFTI

🟥 SUB-PERIODIC W. BANCROFTI

Bancroftian Filariasis and Brugian Filariasis

FIGURE 3.4   Distribution of Malayan filariasis in man. (Adapted from several sources.)

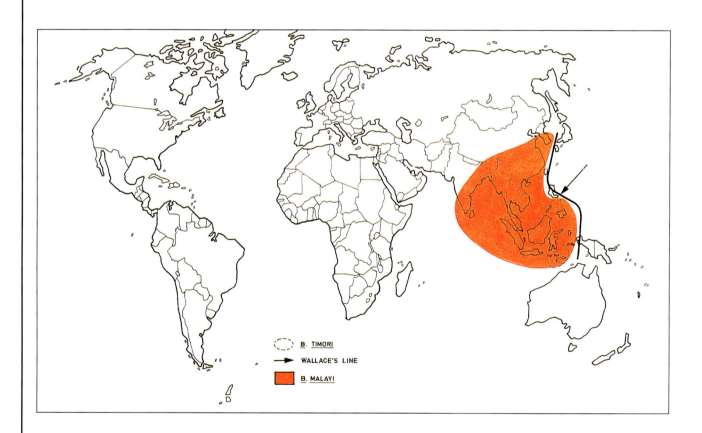

BANCROFTIAN FILARIASIS AND BRUGIAN FILARIASIS

FIGURE 3.5 Microfilariae of *Brugia malayi* in the blood vessel of the kidney of a patient at autopsy. (Giemsa × 210)

FIGURE 3.6 Microfilariae of *Brugia malayi* showing yellowish "nuclei." (Acridine orange × 780)

FIGURE 3.7 Microfilariae of *Brugia malayi* in glomerulus of a middle-aged Malay male who died in Singapore. There was macroscopic evidence of filariasis. In the glomeruli there were numerous microfilariae. (H & E × 235)

FIGURE 3.8 Filariasis. There is severe tubulointerstitial nephritis, with heavy infiltration by lymphocytes, histiocytes, plasma cells, and eosinophils. (H & E × 60)

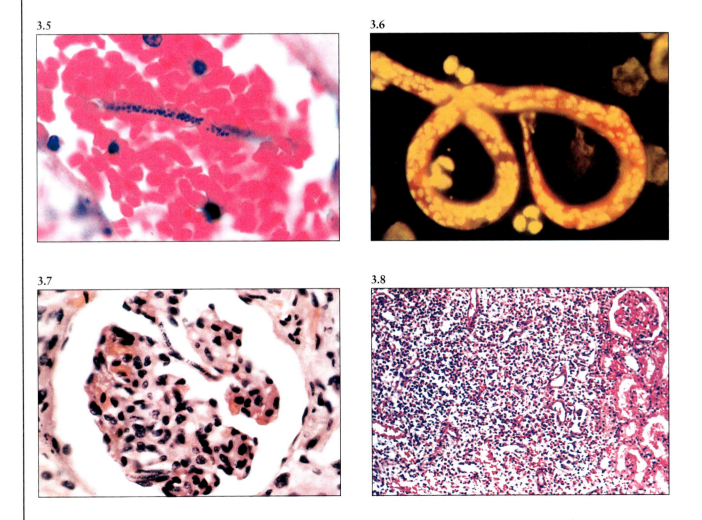

3.5

3.6

3.7

3.8

BANCROFTIAN FILARIASIS AND BRUGIAN FILARIASIS

FIGURE 3.9 Same case as in Figure 3.7. Degenerating microfilariae within an abscess evoke a granulomatous reaction. (H & E × 50)

LOIASIS

FIGURE 3.10 Loiasis. The glomerulus shows partial sclerosis of the tuft and thickened capillary walls, with microfilariae of *Loa loa* within lumen of capillary in the sclerosed area. (PAS × 165)

FIGURE 3.11 Loiasis. Interstitial microinfarction and inflammation around an obstructed renal blood vessel. Degenerating microfilariae of *Loa loa* are in the fibrin. (H & E × 165)

FIGURE 3.12 Same case as in Figures 3.10 and 3.11. Microfilariae of *Loa loa* are seen in the renal capillaries. (H & E × 165)

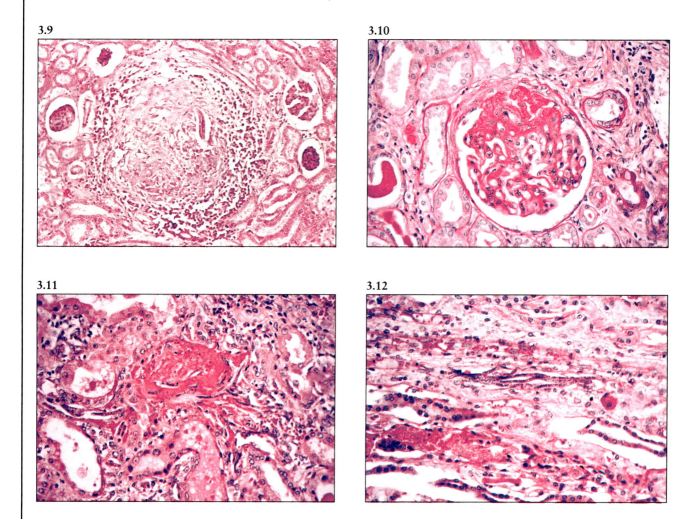

3.9

3.10

3.11

3.12

LOIASIS

FIGURE 3.13   Loiasis. Electron micrograph showing subepithelial and intramembranous deposits of varying density (arrows), and a cross-section of a *Loa loa* microfilaria in a capillary lumen. Note the sheath and the lateral cuticular ridges. (× 7,560)

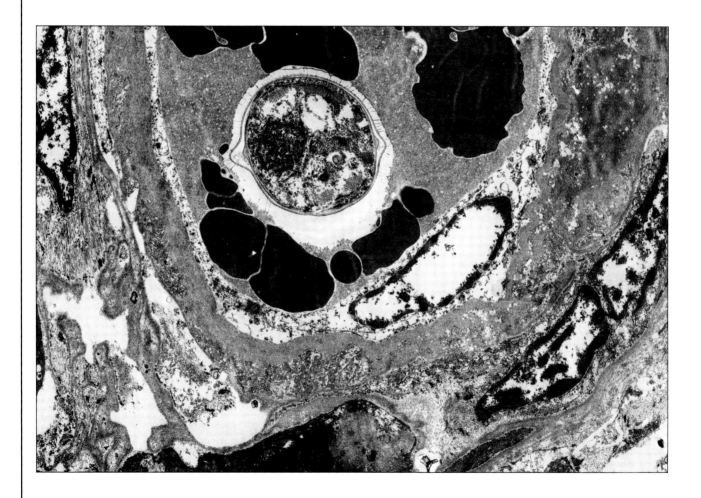

ONCHOCERCIASIS

FIGURE 3.14   Onchocerciasis. Microfilariae of *Onchocerca volvulus* in renal glomerulus, provoking acute inflammation with cellular proliferation and infiltration by lymphocytes, plasma cells, and polymorphs. The surrounding renal parenchyma is also involved. (H & E × 235)

FIGURE 3.15   Onchocerciasis. Posterior end of microfilaria of *Onchocerca volvulus* in kidney, demonstrating terminal nuclei and caudal spine. (H & E × 640)

3.14

3.15

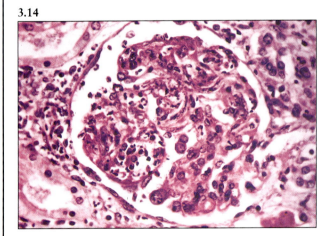
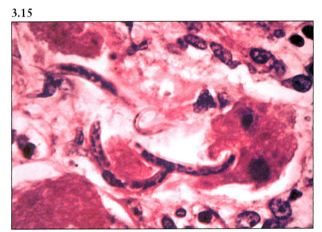

NEMATODE INFECTIONS

TRICHINOSIS

Trichinosis is caused by a nematode, *Trichinella spiralis*. This infection is endemic in many areas of the world where pork is consumed. These areas include central and eastern Europe; Central, South and North America; and parts of Africa and Asia. The infection also occurs in the Arctic and results from eating infected bear meat.

The adult male nematode is 1.4 to 1.6 mm long. The female is viviparous and about twice as long as the male. The anterior part of the body contains a row of glandular cells called stichocytes. The male worm lacks a spicule but has two conical papillae on the sides of the cloacal opening.

Humans become infected mainly by eating improperly cooked pork or pork products, such as sausages. In some parts of the world, wild boar, bear, bush pig, and walrus are heavily infected and can infect humans. After ingestion, the larvae are liberated in the small intestine and mature into adults. The female deposits larvae in the intestinal tissues, from where they find their way into the bloodstream and then into the striated muscles of the body. The most heavily infested muscles are those in the diaphragm, tongue, larynx, and abdomen. After penetration, a larva undergoes three moults and coils into a spiral-shaped body that eventually becomes enclosed in a thick-walled cyst. In this form, the larva may remain viable for many years.

Pigs become infected by eating infected scraps and garbage from slaughterhouses or farms. Occasionally they become infected by eating carcasses of infected rats. Recently, in some parts of the world horses have been found to be infected, probably from food containing remnants of infected meat.

Clinical and Pathologic Manifestations

Most individuals who are lightly infected remain asymptomatic. In cases of heavy infection, the disease is generally manifested in three clinical stages.

Invasion Stage. This is seen during the first week of infection and is due to larvae and adults burrowing into the intestinal tissues. The patient suffers from abdominal pain, nausea, vomiting, and diarrhea of varying intensity. There may be fever, profuse perspiration, and tachycardia.

Migration Stage. This usually begins after the first week of infection. During this period, the larvae are liberated into the circulatory system by the gravid female and find their way to the muscles. Symptoms occur due to toxic effects and hypersensitivity due to the liberation of parasite antigens. There is edema of the face and periorbital tissues, muscular tenderness, fever, and hypereosinophilia. Complications involving the myocardium, central nervous system, and lungs may occur due to the migrating larvae. However, the larvae do not encyst in the myocardium.

Encystment Stage. This usually begins after the third week of infection and is marked by a gradual recovery from symptoms. In a few heavily infected cases the symptoms worsen, and death results from myocardial failure and respiratory and central nervous system involvement.

Mild proteinuria with benign urinary sediment changes may occur in the course of the disease. Renal function is normal in most cases. Para-aminohippuric acid clearance may be reduced due to hypovolemia. However, glomerular filtration rate is usually normal. In severe cases, renal insufficiency may occur. This is, however, not common.

In occasional cases hyperuricemia may be observed. Myoglobinuria may be detectable in the urine. Proteinuria and urinary sediment changes usually disappear when the disease is under control.

Light Microscopic Findings. There is mild mesangial cell proliferation with increased matrix. Occasional thickening of the peripheral capillary wall is noted. Some capillaries may contain mononuclear cells. Hyaline deposition in the glomerular afferent arterioles may be noted. Dilated tubules lined by degenerated epithelial cells accompanied by edematous interstitium are seen in focal areas in some cases.

Electron Microscopic Findings. There is no specific ultrastructural change. Electron-dense deposits are present in paramesangial areas. Thickening of basement membranes is limited to the lamina rara interna.

Immunomicroscopic Findings. All glomeruli show evenly distributed granular deposits of IgM in the mesangial areas and along some glomerular capillary walls. In all cases IgG, IgA, and C3 are also present in weaker intensity than IgM. Dense deposition of C3 in arteriolar walls is rather pronounced. Occasionally, fibrin deposition is noted.

DIOCTOPHYMIASIS

Dioctophymiasis is an infection caused by a large nematode, *Dioctophyma renale*, also called the giant kidney worm, which involves and consumes the kidney, leaving only the capsule. The parasite has a cosmopolitan distribution involving a variety of mammals such as dog, cat, horse, and ox. At least 13 verified cases have been described in humans.

The worm is reddish in color. Males measure 14 to 20 cm, and females 20 to 100 cm. The eggs are ellipsoidal with blunt ends and are 60 to 80 μm in length. The surface is covered with deeply sculptured depressions.

The first-stage larva takes about a month to develop inside the egg before it hatches in the intestine of aquatic oligochaetes, where it becomes infective in about 2 months. The infective larvae are usually taken up by fish or frogs, which act as paratenic hosts. Humans become infected from eating poorly cooked fish or frogs. The infective larvae migrate through the duodenum into the mesentery and then to the pelvis of the kidney. The worms become adults in this location, and the eggs are passed in the urine.

Clinical and Pathologic Manifestations

Patients may complain of loin pain and transient attacks of hematuria and colic. Ultrasound and renal arteriography confirm a renal cystic lesion. Surgical removal of the involved kidney or segment apparently gives a cure.

Macroscopic Findings. The kidney is replaced by a large cyst wall lined by a thin layer of finely granular blood clot. At points of rupture, there are patches of fat necrosis and fibrous tissue. Renal parenchyma is destroyed by lytic action of the cytolytic enzymes in the esophageal glands of the nematode.

Light Microscopic Findings. The cyst wall is composed of fibrous tissue with scattered chronic inflammatory cells and numerous foreign-body giant cells. Eggs of *D. renale* are sometimes found in the wall. They must be distinguished from so-called Liesegang rings, which consist of precipitate of protein and calcium that form double-ringed structures with radial striations and faint birefringence under cross-polarization. Liesegang rings occur in various locations, including the kidney, and are found mainly in abscesses; in the walls of cysts, where increasing concentration of solutes precipitate in layers around a central nidus; or in fibrotic, inflamed, or necrotic tissue.

OTHER INTESTINAL NEMATODES

The most common intestinal nematodes, such as *Strongyloides stercoralis*, *Ascaris lumbricoides*, hookworms,

Ancylostoma duodenale, Necator americanus, Trichuris trichiura, Enterobius vermicularis, usually do not cause any renal injury. Patients with nephrotic syndrome and mild asymptomatic *Strongyloides* infection may develop hyperinfective and severe diarrheal disease, especially when submitted to steroid therapy. This is a major problem in all immunocompromised individuals (eg, patients with AIDS). Hydropic, granular, or vacuolar degenerative changes may thus appear in renal tubules, probably reflecting marked electrolyte imbalance (hypokalemia).

Rarely *Ascaris* may be found in the kidney after anomalous erratic migration through the intestinal wall. Such migration may also occur with *E. vermicularis*; this helminth may reach the urethra and even ascend toward the urinary bladder, ureters, and renal pelvis, causing inflammation along its migratory path.

Severe hypoproteinemia with anasarca may occur in severe ancylostomiasis as a consequence of a protein-losing enteropathy, and the disorder may be erroneously diagnosed as nephrotic syndrome caused by ancylostomiasis.

Trichinosis

FIGURE 4.1 *Trichinella* larvae encysted in muscle. (H & E × 235)

FIGURE 4.2 *Trichinella spiralis* larvae in muscle. Fresh preparation. (Interference contrast × 330)

FIGURE 4.3 Immunofluorescence microscopy of muscle of same case as Figure 4.1, showing positive staining of Trichinella larvae. (Anti–*Trichinella spiralis* antibody × 380)

FIGURE 4.4 Trichinosis. The glomerulus shows mild mesangial cell proliferation with increased matrix. (H & E × 380)

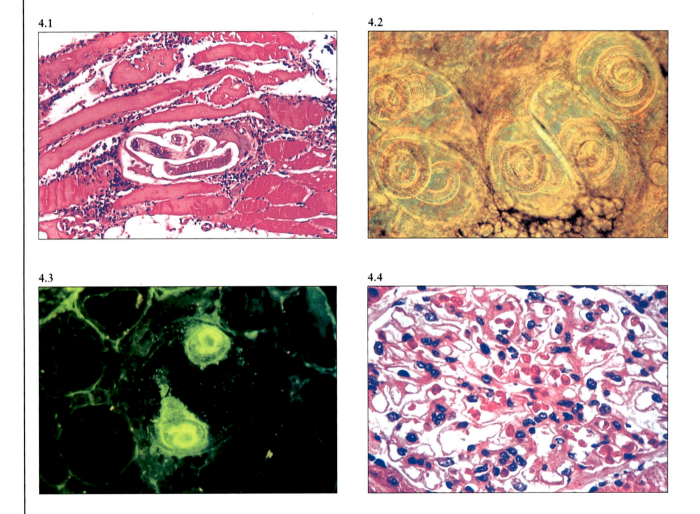

4.1

4.2

4.3

4.4

Trichinosis

FIGURE 4.5   Immunofluorescence microscopy showing diffuse fine granular deposits of IgM in mesangial areas and along some capillary walls. (× 380)

FIGURE 4.6   Group of dilated tubules with degenerated epithelial lining cells. There is interstitial edema without inflammatory cell infiltration. (H & E × 235)

Dioctophymiasis

FIGURE 4.7   *Dioctophyma renale*. Section of an adult female showing structure of the wall and numerous ova. (H & E × 40)

4.5

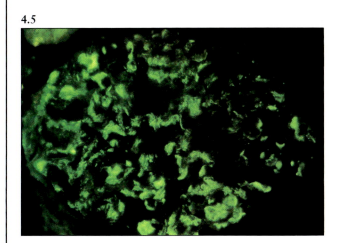

4.6

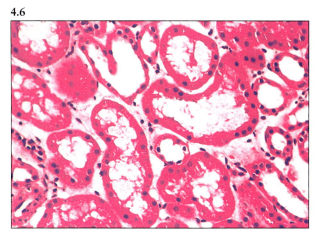

4.7

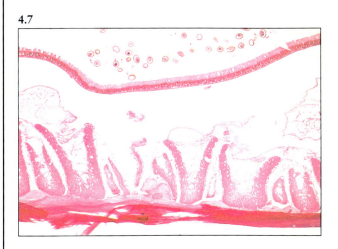

DIOCTOPHYMIASIS

FIGURE 4.8 *Dioctophyma renale.* Ova (in section) are large, measuring 60 to 80 μm long and 40 to 45 μm wide, with thick, wrinkled shells. (H & E × 425)

FIGURE 4.9 Liesegang ring in renal tissue; compare with Figure 4.8. The structure is 85 μm in diameter, and is spherical and laminated. (H & E × 275)

FIGURE 4.10 Ovum in kidney of a dog. (H & E × 425)

4.8

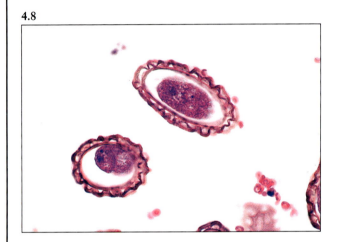

4.9

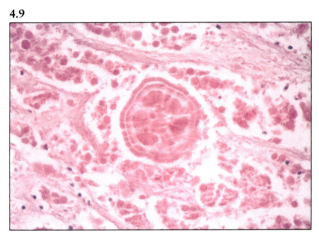

4.10

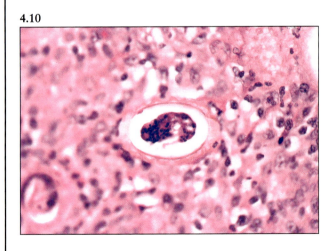

DIOCTOPHYMIASIS

FIGURE 4.11   Human kidney transformed into a cyst lined by finely granular blood clot, thought to be due to *Dioctophyma renale*.

OTHER INTESTINAL NEMATODES

FIGURE 4.12   Disseminated strongyloidosis. Glomerulus shows diffuse thickening of capillary walls. (PAS × 235)

FIGURE 4.13   Same case as Figure 4.12. Glomerulus under high magnification. Membranous change with spike formation is evident. (PAS × 950)

4.11

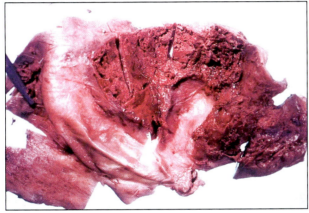

4.12

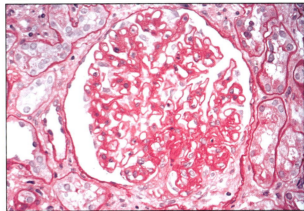

4.13

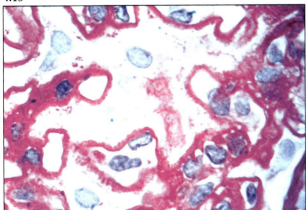

FIGURE 4.14   Electron micrograph. Same case as Figure 4.12. Part of a glomerular capillary with washed-out areas under the epithelium, suggestive of previous deposits. Projections of basement membrane (spikes) are seen between the washed-out areas. (× 19,500)

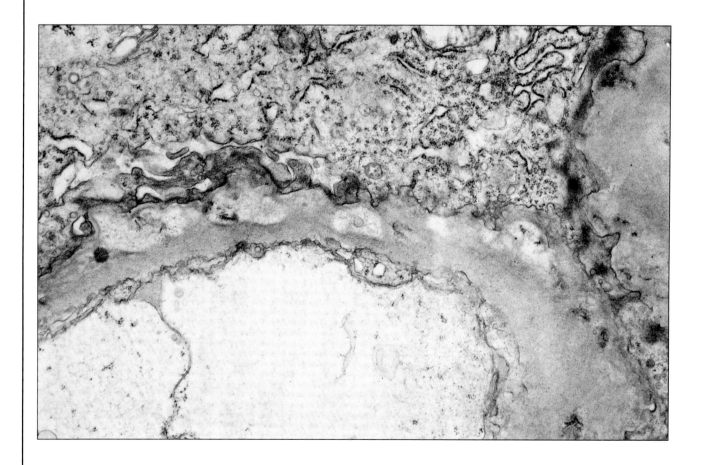

TREMATODE INFECTIONS

SCHISTOSOMIASIS

Schistosomiasis is an infection caused by trematodes of the species *Schistosoma haematobium, S. mansoni,* and *S. japonicum.* In addition, *S. intercalatum* and *S. mekongi* are also seen in some areas. *S. mansoni* causes immune complex glomerulonephritis in 12 to 15 percent of patients with hepatosplenic disease, whereas *S. japonicum* has been known to cause glomerulonephritis only in experimental animals. *Schistosoma haematobium* primarily involves the lower urinary tract.

S. haematobium is widespread in Africa and the Middle East with a small focus in India. *S. mansoni* is widespread in Africa, Brazil, Surinam, Venezuela, and some Caribbean Islands. *S. japonicum* is found in China, Taiwan, Japan, the Philippines, Sulawesi, and a few other parts of Southeast Asia. *S. intercalatum* is seen in Central Africa; and *S. mekongi* is found in islands in the Mekong River in Laos, Cambodia, and Vietnam.

Schistosomes are diecious. The adult males are 10 to 20 mm long and 0.5 to 11 mm wide. They have a deep ventral groove in which the longer and thinner females lie during copulation. Both sexes have two suckers, one situated ventrally and the other anteriorly. The eggs of *S. mansoni* are ellipsoidal with a lateral spine. *S. haematobium* eggs are also ellipsoidal but with a terminal spine. *S. japonicum* eggs are spheroidal with a much smaller spine or a knob.

Eggs that leave the body in urine or feces contain fully formed miracidia that hatch when they come in contact with water. The miracidium swims actively to penetrate an appropriate snail host, where it develops through various stages to become a cercaria. The cercariae emerge from the snail and infect animal hosts by penetrating the skin. All schistosome cercariae have a bifid tail that is shed during penetration, and the parasite is transformed into a schistosomula inside the host tissues. The schistosomula first enters the systemic circulation and then finds its way into the portal circulation. *S. mansoni* and *S. japonicum* worms mature in the mesenteric veins of the portal circulation. *S. haematobium* worms generally remain in the systemic circulation and mature in the blood vessels of the ureteric and vesical plexus. The eggs produced by *S. mansoni* and *S. japonicum* are discharged mainly in the feces, and those produced by *S. haematobium* mainly in the urine.

Clinical and Pathologic Manifestations

The adult worms do not multiply, and the eggs are the main cause of pathology. Complete immunity does not develop, and repeated infections result in the gradual building up of the worm load. The extent of damage is generally related to the number of eggs present in the tissues.

The disease passes through three distinct stages.

Invasive Stage. Cercarial dermatitis, also known as

swimmer's itch, may appear on parts of the body that have come in contact with water containing cercariae. The dermatitis often develops 24 hours after exposure and appears in the form of a pruritic, papular rash.

Acute Stage. This stage generally begins 5 to 10 weeks after infection and is also known as Katayama fever. The syndrome consists of cough, fever, and asthma-like symptoms and is seen more often in *S. japonicum* infection. Lymphadenopathy, hepatomegaly, and splenomegaly may be present.

Chronic Stage. This may take a number of years to develop. Fibrosis of the periportal areas of the liver may lead to portal hypertension in *S. mansoni* and *S. japonicum*. In *S. haematobium* infection, fibrosis of the ureters and bladder may result in urinary obstruction and bladder malfunction.

Twelve to fifteen percent of patients may develop immune complex schistosomal glomerulonephritis. Antigens from the digestive tubes of adult worms, probably the main mediators of immune nephritis, are usually phagocytosed and denatured by Kupffer cells and do not reach the general circulation. That phenomenon appears to explain why schistosomal glomerulonephritis is restricted to patients with portal hypertension. In these patients the collateral circulation allows the schistosomal antigens and/or the immune complexes generated in the portal system to bypass the liver phagocytic system and reach the systemic circulation.

Proteinuria, usually with nephrotic syndrome, is the most frequent form of clinical presentation of schistosomal nephropathy. Proteinuria of low selectivity or nonselectivity is usually noted. IgM, α_2 macroglobulin, lipoprotein, IgG, and IgA can be detected in the urine in rather large amounts. The specific antischistosome nature of at least part of these urinary globulins has been demonstrated. Characteristically, schistosomal nephropathy presents with increased plasma globulin concentration and normal cholesterol levels in one third of patients. Therapy for schistosomiasis has so far not altered the evolution of established renal disease.

Light Microscopic Findings. There are heterogeneous glomerular lesions, with the least severe cases showing mesangial expansion due to deposition of fibrillar PAS-positive material. Other cases show diffuse mesangial cell proliferation with increased matrix and cells in the centrilobular mesangial stalks. In advanced cases, usu-

ally with nephrotic syndrome, mesangiocapillary glomerulonephritis with lobular accentuation is the most frequent type of glomerulonephritis. In some cases, focal and segmental sclerosing glomerulonephritis and occasional capillary aneurysms can be observed. In the most advanced cases there is a diffuse sclerosing glomerulonephritis. Membranous glomerulonephritis with spikes in the basement membrane and proliferating mesangial cells were seen in one case. In some cases advanced proliferative and sclerosing changes can be observed. Even an end-stage kidney associated with hypertension and severe vascular changes, tubulointerstitial inflammation, and other alterations are not uncommon with hepatosplenic schistosomiasis. The glomerular lesions in hepatosplenic schistosomiasis are similar to those observed in patients with liver cirrhosis without parasitic infestation. It is therefore possible that the renal lesions result from the effects of liver cirrhosis and are not directly related to the parasitic infection.

Electron Microscopic Findings. Electron-dense deposits and laminar bodies can be found in mesangial areas. Changes in the basement membrane are less marked and consist of subepithelial, subendothelial, and intramembranous deposits. Sometimes melanin-like schistosomal pigment can be found within the mesangial matrix.

Immunomicroscopic Findings. IgG, IgE, IgM, and IgA as well as complement C3 and fibrin have been repeatedly demonstrated in glomerular lesions associated with schistosomiasis, both in man and in experimental animals. The deposits are granular and occur mainly in mesangial areas but also along capillary walls. Schistosomal antigens have been detected in both man and animals. These antigens were detected with immunofluorescence microscopy by means of antibodies raised against whole-worm antigens, worm metabolic products, or antisera specific for the anodic polysaccharide gut antigen. Antibodies eluted from human kidneys with schistosomal glomerulopathy bound specifically to the intestinal lining of the adult worm. Schistosomiasis is a possible example of a parasitic disease with in situ immune complex formation.

SCHISTOSOMA HAEMATOBIUM

In haematobium schistosomiasis, concurrent infection with *Salmonella typhi* or *Salmonella paratyphi* may be associated with the development of heavy proteinuria and the nephrotic syndrome. The renal manifestations are thought to be related to the Salmonella infection. Clinical presentation resembles that of a febrile, toxic illness. The Salmonella organisms can be recovered from the blood and urine. Resolution of the nephrotic syndrome follows successful treatment of the Salmonella infection. The hematuria in *S. haematobium* infection is usually of lower urinary tract origin and only rarely from the kidney itself.

SCHISTOSOMIASIS

FIGURE 5.1   Life cycle of Schistosoma species.   (*1*) Humans become infected from contact with water containing cercaria.   (*2*) Adult worm.   (*3*) Eggs of *S. mansoni*, *S. japonicum*, and *S. haematobium* discharged via feces and urine.   (*4*) Miracidium.   (*5*) Snail in which further development occurs. (*6*) Sporocyst.   (*7*) Cercaria.

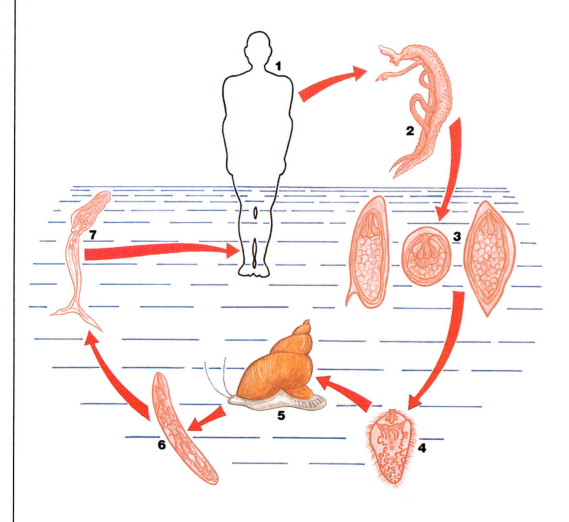

Schistosomiasis

FIGURE 5.2   World distribution of schistosomiasis infections in man. (Adapted from several sources.)

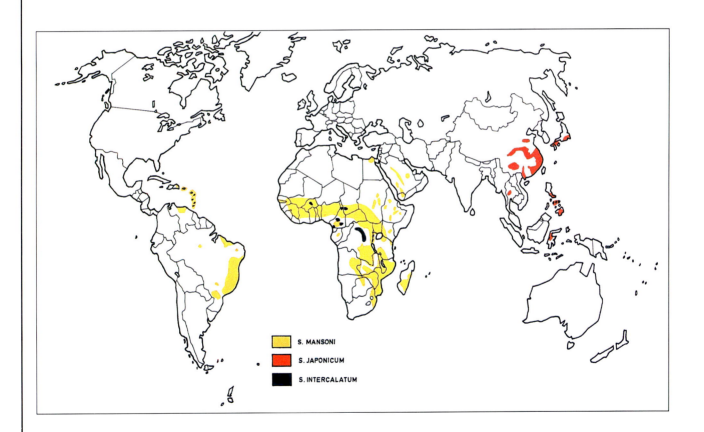

SCHISTOSOMIASIS

FIGURE 5.3   Schistosomiasis. Mild mesangial proliferation and an area of focal and segmental glomerulosclerosis with capsular adhesions. (PAS × 235)

FIGURE 5.4   Same case as in Figure 5.3. One glomerulus has a capillary aneurysm filled with red blood cells, an infrequent finding in schistosomiasis. (MSB × 235)

FIGURE 5.5   Schistosomiasis. There is a diffuse proliferative glomerulonephritis with mesangial cell hyperplasia and increased matrix. (H & E × 235)

FIGURE 5.6   In advanced cases of schistosomiasis, usually accompanied by the nephrotic syndrome, the most common lesion is mesangiocapillary (membranoproliferative) glomerulonephritis. (H & E × 235)

5.3

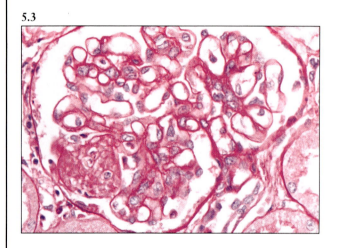

5.4

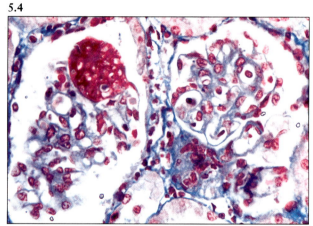

5.5

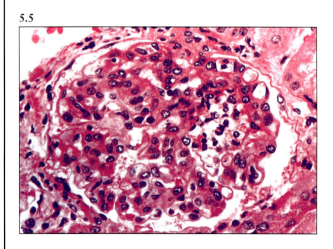

5.6

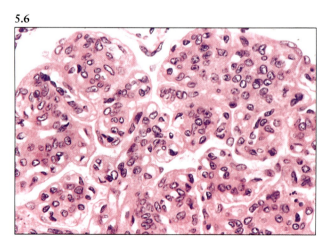

SCHISTOSOMIASIS

FIGURE 5.7 Same case as in Figure 5.6. Hepatosplenic schistosomiasis with mesangiocapillary glomerulonephritis, showing well-formed double outlines of the capillary loops and enlargement of the mesangium. (PASM × 235)

FIGURE 5.8 Schistosomiasis. Thre is tubulo-interstitial inflammation with infiltration by lymphocytes, monocytes, plasma cells, and eosinophils. Protein casts are present in some tubular lumens. (H & E × 95)

FIGURE 5.9 Immunofluorescence microscopy. Granular IgG deposits are present in glomerular mesangial areas and along some of the capillary walls. (× 235)

FIGURE 5.10 Immunofluorescence microscopy. Section of adult *Schistosoma mansoni*, showing specific fluorescence for the anodic polysaccharide antigen localized in the intestinal epithelial lining. Such antigen eliminated by the worm can be detected in the circulating blood, in Kupffer cells, in the urine, and in the glomerulus of the host. (× 50)

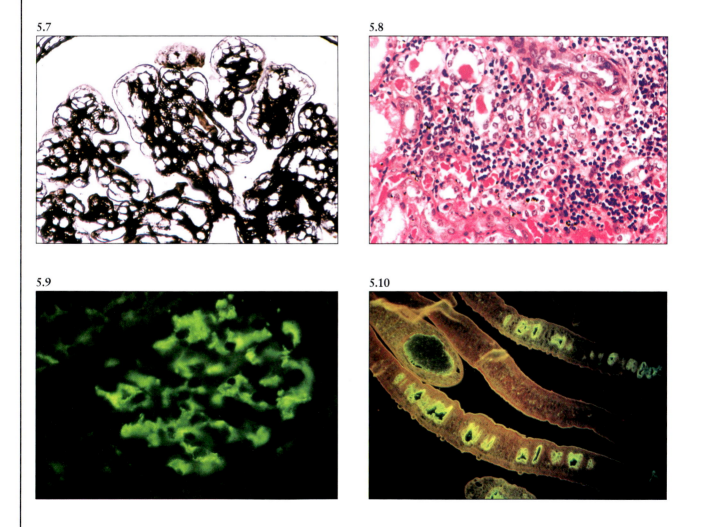

5.7

5.8

5.9

5.10

SCHISTOSOMIASIS

FIGURE 5.11   Electron micrograph. Deposits (*D*) of irregular densities in the glomerular mesangium of a mouse infected with *Schistosoma mansoni*. They probably represent immune complexes formed during the course of the schistosomal infection. *L* = capillary lumen. (× 11,800)

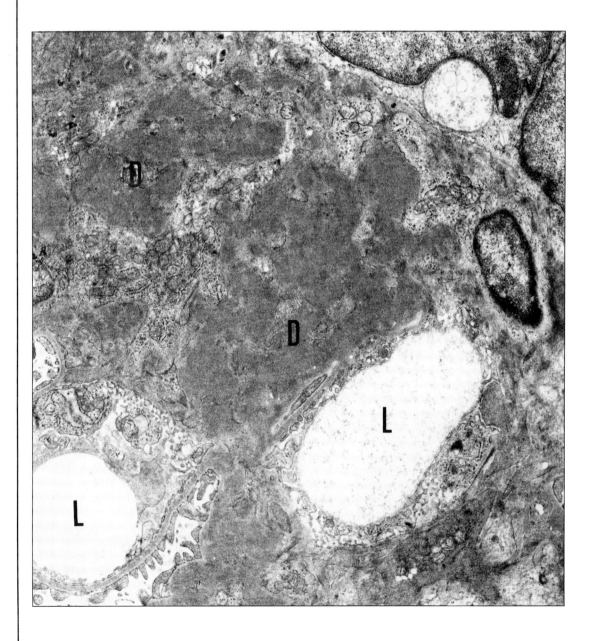

CESTODE INFECTIONS

ECHINOCOCCOSIS (HYDATID DISEASE)

Echinococcosis is an infection caused by the cestodes of the genus *Echinococcus*. At present four species are known to be capable of infecting man; of these, *E. granulosus* is the most important.

E. granulosus is found worldwide, with the main endemic areas in Argentina, Brazil, Chile, Uruguay, Peru, Sardinia, Cyprus, the Middle East, northern India, Pakistan, some eastern European countries, and Kenya.

The adults are harbored in the small intestine of the dog and other carnivores. These cestodes are 3 to 6 mm long with three to four proglottids. The spherical scolex has two rows of 28 to 40 hooks and four suckers. The worms are firmly attached to the wall of the small intestine by the scolex and suckers. The terminal segment is gravid and contains about 5,000 eggs. The eggs are identical in morphology to those of other *Taenia* spp.

The gravid proglottids disintegrate in the dog intestine, and the eggs are then discharged in the feces. If they are deposited on pasture, they are ingested by various grazing animals. The onchosphere (hexacanth embryo) hatches in the duodenum and penetrates the intestinal wall. It then reaches various organs of the body via the bloodstream. The liver is principally involved because of capillary filtering. The hooks then disappear, and the parasite begins to grow into a hydatid cyst. Hydatid fluid secreted by the parasite fills the cyst cavity. The fluid is bacteriologically sterile in living cysts and is clear or slightly yellowish in color with a specific gravity of about 1.012. The development of the cyst is slow, and protoscoleces are formed after 1 to 2 years.

In man, cysts with a non-fertile germinal epithelium are sometimes seen, and therefore no brood capsules are present. Cut sections of these cysts have a characteristic laminated layer.

Clinical and Pathologic Manifestations

These depend on the location and the number of hydatid cysts. The most common location is the right lobe of the liver, followed by the lungs. Rarely, cysts may be found in the brain, eye, kidney, muscles, and bone. The early stage of infection is generally asymptomatic. As the cyst enlarges, symptoms of a space-occupying lesion develop. Pyrexia, urticaria, multiple cutaneous eruptions, and sometimes anaphylactic shock may occur if the cyst ruptures. Rupture may also lead to the escape of scoleces into the surrounding tissues; these can then develop into further cysts.

The kidney is involved in approximately 4 percent of cases. The main renal symptoms are caused by mechanical pressure at the site of the enlarging cyst. If the cyst is very large, it may be palpable. There may be loin pain, and there is usually macroscopic hematuria and proteinuria. An instance of malignant hypertension secondary to pressure on the renal artery has been reported. Blood eosinophilia is present in about 20 percent of cases. Radiologically calcified cysts have a smooth circular outline. Radionuclide scans show a round, cold area.

Macroscopic Findings. Hydatid cysts in the kidney are usually single and vary from a few centimeters in diameter to a huge mass that fills the retroperitoneal space. *E. granulosus* cysts are unilocular, lined by a 1-mm-thick translucent white laminated membrane, and filled with clear, watery fluid. They usually also contain pale, finely granular material known as hydatid sand; sterile cysts lack this sand. In infection with *E. multilocularis* and *E. oligarthrus*, multiple daughter cysts, called alveolar cysts, invade surrounding host tissue and produce a multilocular appearance. These alveolar cysts are usually sterile and macroscopically appear solid.

Light Microscopic Findings. Renal tissue adjacent to the hydatid cyst is compressed and atrophic; immediately surrounding the cyst is a fibrous wall. The laminated cyst lining has no nuclei, and on its inner side there is a nucleated germinal layer about 20 μm thick. Within fertile cysts thre are brood capsules that have arisen from this germinal layer. Larval scolices can be seen developing from the wall of each brood capsule. Some of the brood capsules together with free scolices constitute the hydatid sand that can be seen macroscopically. Calcification is common in the walls of dead hydatid cysts.

Usually the glomeruli appear normal; but, of five patients previously treated with mebendazole, four showed diffuse mesangial proliferative glomerulonephritis and one a florid mesangiocapillary glomerulonephritis, type I. Mebendazole causes necrosis of the hydatid cyst wall, and these glomerular changes may have resulted from immune complex formation in the kidney following release of hydatid antigens. Immunofluorescence and elec-

tron microscopy were not done in this study. No specific tubular, interstitial, or vascular changes are seen in the kidney in hydatid disease.

Immunomicroscopic Findings. In untreated cases, immunoglobulins, complement components, and fibrinogen are not seen in the glomeruli.

CYSTICERCOSIS
Cysticercosis is caused by the larval stage of *Taenia solium*.

T. solium is endemic in all parts of the world where pork or pork products are eaten. Endemic areas include Latin America (particularly Mexico), South Africa, parts of the Indian subcontinent, some regions in Southeast Asia, and, more recently, West Irian (Indonesia).

The organism is typically a semitransparent fluid-filled ovoid body with an average size of 10 × 5 mm. In section, the invaginated scolex, with four suckers and a row of hooks, may be visible.

Man becomes infected by accidentally ingesting eggs of *T. solium* in contaminated food and water. It is postulated that retroinfection can occur in persons harboring the adult worm; the proglottids are regurgitated into the stomach, where they disintegrate and liberate a large number of eggs. The oncospheres (hexacanth embryos) from the eggs then find their way via lymphatics and blood vessels into various parts of the body and develop into cysticerci.

Clinical and Pathologic Manifestations
Any organ of the body may be involved, but symptoms are generally related to the involvement of the central nervous system. Occasionally cysticerci are found in the kidneys. After a period, the parasite dies and eventually calcifies.

ECHINOCOCCOSIS

FIGURE 6.1 Life cycle of *Echinococcus granulosus.* (*1*) Dog is infected by eating hydatid cyst. (*2*) Adult worms develop in the intestine. (*3*) Eggs are passed in feces and may be accidentally ingested by humans or by other animals that form the normal life cycle. (*4*) Animals involved are sheep, pigs, horses, and camels. (*5*) Intermediate stage or the hydatid cyst containing the protoscoleces, each of which can give rise to an adult worm.

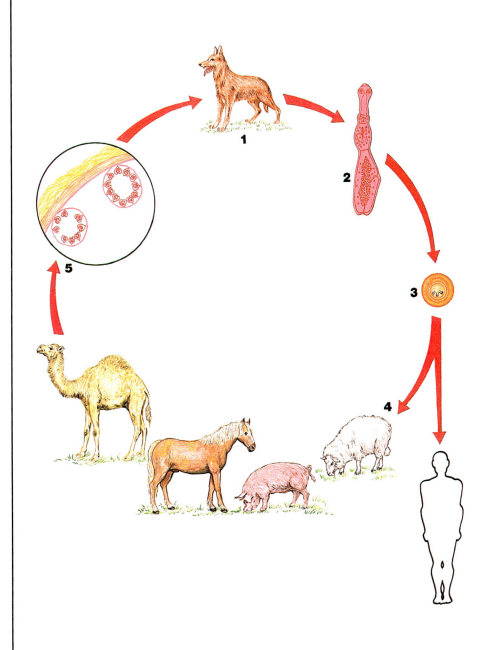

Echinococcosis

FIGURE 6.2 *Echinococcus granulosus* adult worm, showing scolex and three segments. (Acid carmine stain × 17)

FIGURE 6.3 Multilocular hydatid cyst in the kidney. Such cysts are not common.

FIGURE 6.4 Large unilocular hydatid cyst removed from kidney.

6.2

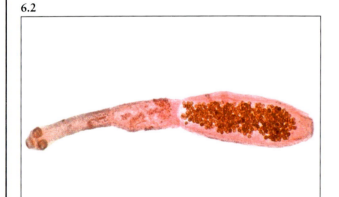

6.3

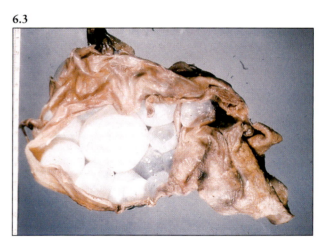

6.4

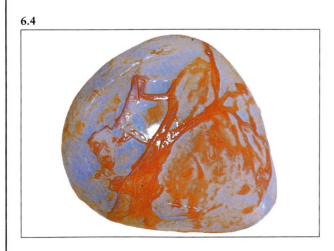

ECHINOCOCCOSIS

FIGURE 6.5   High-power view of brood capsules from hydatid sand, showing hooklets and suckers invaginated within a vesicle. (Interference contrast × 95)

FIGURE 6.6   Wall of hydatid cyst, showing inner germinal layer and laminated membrane. A brood capsule is seen in the lumen. (H & E × 190)

CYSTICERCOSIS

FIGURE 6.7   A gravid segment of *Taenia solium*. The uterus is filled with eggs. (H & E × 7)

6.5

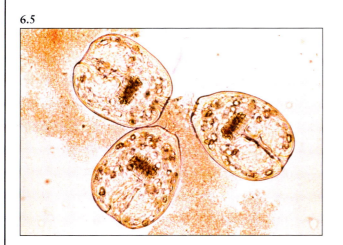

6.6

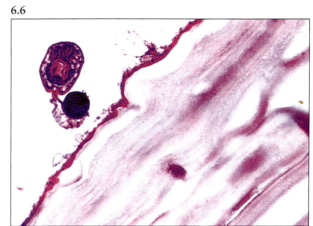

6.7

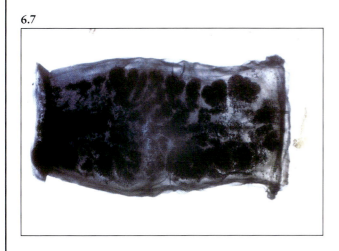

Cysticercosis

FIGURE 6.8   Scolex (head) of *Taenia solium* with suckers and symmetrically arranged row of hooklets. (Interference contrast × 70)

FIGURE 6.9   Wall of dead cysticercus in kidney. There are projections on its outer surface and surrounding the cyst is granulation and fibrous tissue. (H & E × 75)

FIGURE 6.10   Cysticercus with invaginated scolex that is surrounded by fluid and the cyst wall. (H & E × 30)

6.8

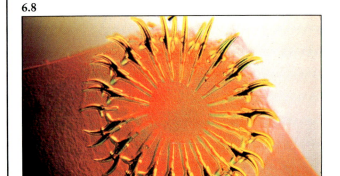

6.9

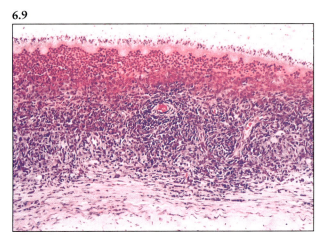

6.10

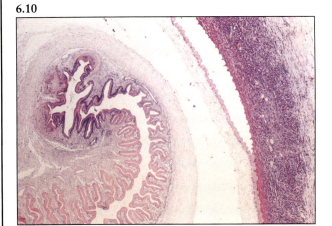

VIRAL INFECTIONS

HANTAVIRUS (BUNYAVIRIDAE)

Hemorrhagic fever with renal syndrome is a collective term for the following diseases: epidemic nephropathy, nephropathia epidemica, muroid virus nephropathy, Korean hemorrhagic fever, hemorrhagic nephrosonephritis, Songo fever, epidemic hemorrhagic fever, Tula fever. These diseases are endemic and sporadically epidemic throughout Asia (especially Korea), western Russia, the Balkans, and Scandinavia. Serologic tests indicate that these viruses exist throughout the world, and hemorrhagic fever with renal syndrome remains a major threat to human health. In China in 1982, 61,705 patients required hospitalization, and 5 percent of them died. Over the past 5 years in the far eastern part of the Soviet Union, there have been 11,000 cases. In Korea, several hundred cases occur each year with approximately 5% mortality, and in the past two years about 30 cases have been described in northeastern France.

The arboviruses responsible for this group of diseases belong to the Hantavirus (Bunyaviridae) family and consist of three single-stranded RNA segments of negative polarity contained in three nucleocapsids. The viruses are transmitted to man from healthy rodent carriers that excrete the organisms from their lungs, and in their urine, feces, and saliva. Hemorrhagic fever with renal syndrome is a predominantly rural disease transmitted by field mice and voles. The less common urban cases are due to rats. Recently there have been several reports of outbreaks in laboratory staff handling rats that were subsequently found to be infected.

Clinical and Pathologic Manifestations

There is a variable incubation period of 1 to 5 weeks from the time of contact with the virus to the appearance of symptoms. In many cases an influenza-like syndrome lasting 4 to 10 days, often with vomiting and temperature as high as 40.5°C, is followed by intense bilateral loin pain, transient oliguria, severe proteinuria, and microscopic hematuria. Dialysis is only occasionally needed, and serum creatinine levels return to normal 2 to 6 weeks after the attack. The diagnosis is confirmed by the demonstration of rising titers of antibodies to the virus, commencing after about 7 days and reaching a peak at about 3 weeks. Some patients have, in addition, conjunctival hemorrhages and petechiae in the axillae and on the face, neck, anterior chest wall, and soft palate. About 20% develop severe features such as shock, major hemorrhage and gross fluid and electrolyte imbalance; death may occur in these cases. Other patients, except those who have had central nervous system hemorrhages, usually recover and are immune to reinfection. The form of hemorrhagic fever with renal syndrome encountered west of the Ural Mountains is clinically mild and only rarely associated with gross hemorrhagic manifestations. The urban disease transmitted by rats also tends to be less severe than disease in the rural population. Cases occur in two seasonal peaks during late spring and autumn, when the rodent population is highest.

Macroscopic Findings. The kidneys are enlarged, weighing from 200 to 400 g each; and the cut surface bulges. The medulla is dark red, contrasting with the widened pale cortex. Hemorrhages are often present, particularly in the medulla, pelvis, and calices.

Light Microscopic Findings. Patients with the mild form of the disease have acute interstitial nephritis. The interstitium is diffusely edematous; and there is marked patchy, cellular infiltration of the superficial cortex, boundary zone, and medulla. The infiltrating cells are mainly lymphocytes, with some macrophages, a few plasma cells, and rare neutrophil polymorphonuclear leukocytes. There are also scattered small foci of interstitial hemorrhage. In the areas of cellular infiltration there is some tubular damage and loss. The intertubular capillaries are congested. The glomeruli, arterioles, and arteries are normal.

In the more severe disease, hemorrhage and shock occur early and as a result the changes seen in acute renal failure predominate in the kidneys. The extent and distribution of tubular damage and regeneration depend on the time of biopsy or death in relation to the onset of shock.

Electron Microscopic Findings. A study of renal biopsies from cases of the mild form of the disease that occurs in Finland (nephropathia epidemica) showed scanty focal and segmental intramembranous and subepithelial deposits on the glomerular capillary walls and in the mesangium from the fourth day onward. In contrast, the glomeruli appeared normal in biopsy samples obtained at 10 days from a sporadic case in France and at 6 days after onset of the disease in a laboratory-acquired case in Belgium.

Immunomicroscopic Findings. In the Finnish cases described under Electron Microscopic Findings, scanty focal and segmental granular deposits of immunoglobulin and C3 were detected on glomerular capillary walls, in the mesangium, and on the tubular basement membranes from the fourth to the twenty-fifth day. After the eighteenth day, the capillary wall deposits disappeared. Initially the immunoglobulin was mainly IgM, but later IgG predominated. IgA was present in 30 percent of cases. Similar changes have been reported in one study of the more severe form of the disease in China. There were no deposits of immunoglobulin, complement, or fibrinogen in the sporadic French case and the laboratory-acquired Belgian case discussed above.

ARENAVIRIDAE (JUNIN AND MACHUPO VIRUSES)

Argentine hemorrhagic fever and Bolivian hemorrhagic fever are diseases known collectively as South American hemorrhagic fever. They are endemic and sporadically epidemic in Argentina and Bolivia. Most cases show mild tubular damage associated with viral inclusions in the cytoplasm of the tubular cells. Severe illnesses are complicated by acute tubular necrosis.

Virus-associated hemorrhagic fever was first recognized in the New World in Argentina in 1953. The agent isolated from humans was designated Junin virus and belongs to the Arenaviridae family. A related virus, named Machupo, was subsequently recovered from cases of a clinically similar disease occurring in Bolivia.

Characterization of the two agents failed to show any immunologic relationship to arboviruses previously associated with Omsk and Kyasanur Forest hemorrhagic syndromes of Russia and India, respectively. Researchers did find, however, that complement-fixing antigens were shared not only between Junin and Machupo but also with a Trinidadian bat virus, *Tacaribe*, and a virus from rodents in Brazil, *Amapari*. These four viruses have therefore been designated as members of the arenavirus (Tacaribe) group. The viruses are present in small rodents such as *Calomys callosus*, *Calomys musulinis*, and others that are found in and near houses. Although remaining healthy, these animals can become chronic carriers and persistently excrete the virus in the urine. The organism is transmitted directly to humans by aerosol, urine, blood, and crushed tissues. This explains the occurrence of disease in farm workers.

Clinical and Pathologic Manifestations

The disease affects mainly young agricultural workers. Eight to ten days after infection there is malaise, high fever, severe myalgia, headache and hyperemia of the conjunctivae. Leukopenia and thrombocytopenia are found, and at about the fourth day fine petechiae appear on the neck and upper chest. More severely ill patients have epistaxis, bleeding from the gums, hematemesis, melena, metrorrhagia, and, not infrequently, secondary bacterial pneumonia. Between the seventh and ninth days some patients develop shock and a neurologic syndrome with hyporeflexia, tremors, cerebellar symptoms, and even convulsions and coma. Proteinuria is common, but renal function is rarely severely depressed unless there is shock. Ten to fifteen percent of the patients die from shock and its complications. In survivors, antibodies to the virus appear between the twelfth and seventeenth days after infection, but IgM immunofluorescent antibody may not develop for 2 to 3 weeks after clinical illness, making early serologic diagnosis difficult. Complement components C2, C3, and C5 are low during the early acute period of the disease but return to normal with clinical recovery.

Macroscopic Findings. The kidneys are enlarged, and the cut surface bulges. The medulla is dark red. Petechial hemorrhages are present in about 15 percent of cases.

Light Microscopic Findings. In patients with mild disease, the kidneys may appear normal. More severe cases manifest changes of acute renal failure. The extent and distribution of tubular damage and regeneration depends on the time of biopsy or death in relation to the onset of shock. No specific viral lesions are seen.

Electron Microscopic Findings. In the Argentine form of the disease, circular particles containing small granules and surrounded by a single membrane are present in the cytoplasm of the tubular cells. They lie in the cisternae of the endoplasmic reticulum and have been shown by immunohistochemical methods to contain Junin virus antigens.

Togaviridae and Flaviviridae

Togaviridae is a family of viruses that belong to a general category of arboviruses. These pathogens are transmitted by arthropods (mosquito, sandfly, tick, etc) to mammals or birds. Most viruses in this family that cause disease in man belong to the genus *Alphavirus* (eg, those causing Chikungunya fever). Flaviviruses (which include yellow fever and Dengue hemorrhagic fever viruses) were in the past classified as a genus of Togaviridae but now are assigned to a separate but related family of Flaviviridae.

Yellow Fever

Yellow fever is endemic and sporadically epidemic in Africa and South America and is transmitted to humans from monkeys by Anopheles mosquitoes. It is characterized by fever, bleeding, and hepatic and renal failure.

The disease is caused by an RNA-containing group B arbovirus that belongs to the *Flavivirus* genus of the Togaviridae (Flaviviridae) family. There are serologically different strains in Africa and in the New World. In both continents the virus is maintained in monkeys living in the forest canopy and is transmitted from monkey to monkey by various species of mosquitoes. Infected mosquitoes may then pass the virus to humans; and in rural areas endemic infection is widespread, although only occasional cases may be recognized. Occasionally, the endemic fever is introduced into a town by an infected traveller. If *Aedes aegypti* or other suitable mosquitoes are prevalent in the town, then man-to-man spread can produce an outbreak. Yellow fever has never been reported in Asia or Australia, even though potential vector mosquitoes abound there.

Clinical and Pathologic Manifestations

The incubation period lasts from 3 to 6 days. There is a sudden onset of continuous fever, chills, headache, and myalgia, lasting 3 to 4 days. In mild infections there may be a trace of proteinuria; but in more severe infections heavy proteinuria suddenly develops at the third day, and the urine becomes loaded with granular casts. In most patients these urinary changes last a few days and then quickly disappear, but in a few they are succeeded after another 48 hours by severe oliguria or anuria. The urine contains hemoglobin, and renal function falls. Overall mortality is 5 to 10 percent, but in individual epidemics it may be much higher. Death may be due to hemorrhage, shock, uremic coma, or myocardial failure. Massive albuminuria, severe icterus, prolonged prothrombin time, and high serum transaminase levels are poor prognostic signs. Death occurs on the third or fourth day from fulminant infections. After the tenth day, renal failure is the usual cause of death.

Macroscopic Findings. The kidneys are swollen and diffusely bile-stained. Sometimes there are small subcapsular hemorrhages. The cut surface bulges, the cortex is widened, and there is a variable amount of yellow streaking in the medullary rays and portions of the cortex. The medulla is dark red.

Light Microscopic Findings. The tubular epithelial cells, both proximal and distal, show varying degrees of acute tubular necrosis. Fatty change, hydropic change, and accumulation of bile pigment are common, particularly in the convoluted and straight parts of the proximal tubules. The distal tubules are dilated and lined by regenerating low epithelial cells with basophilic cytoplasm. The lumens of many of the tubules contain hyaline, granular, bile pigment and hemoglobin casts, some calcified. Leucine crystals are also found in the tubular lumens. The interstitium is diffusely edematous; and there are small focal collections of mononuclear cells, principally near the corticomedullary junction. Hemorrhages are infrequent. The glomeruli and blood vessels appear normal.

Electron Microscopic Findings. Glomeruli are usually normal, and there are no tubular or interstitial changes specific for yellow fever. Inclusion bodies do not occur.

Immunomicroscopic Findings. There are no deposits of immunoglobulins or complement components. Focal and segmental collections of fibrinogen are sometimes present in glomerular capillaries.

CHIKUNGUNYA FEVER

This disease is sporadically epidemic in Africa, India, and Thailand and is transmitted to humans from monkeys and other mammals by Aedes mosquitoes. Renal involvement occurs only in the Asian illness and takes the form of acute tubular necrosis and hemorrhages.

The pathogen is an RNA-containing virus of the Togaviridae family that was first isolated during an epidemic of an apparently new disease that affected many inhabitants of the Makonde plateau in Tanzania in July 1952. The virus was named "chikungunya" from the word used by the natives to describe the disease; it means "the disease that bends up joints." Chikungunya virus strains have since been isolated from patients in several parts of southern and eastern Africa. They have also been implicated in several epidemics of hemorrhagic fever in Thailand and India. The virus is transmitted to humans by the mosquito *Aedes aegypti* and in Africa also by *A. africanus*. There is also a forest cycle involving monkeys, baboons, and other mammals with transmission by *A. luteocephalus*.

Clinical and Pathologic Manifestations

The clinical syndromes produced by the African and Asian strains are different. The African disease has few sequelae, and renal involvement is rare. After an incubation period of 3 to 13 days, there is a sudden onset of high fever, malaise, crippling joint pains, and, later, a conspicuous rash. The illness generally lasts for about a week, and complete recovery with no recurrence is usual. The Asian disease form in Thailand and India affects indigenous children particularly and is often of insiduous onset. It is characterized by vomiting, abdominal pain, subcutaneous hemorrhages, and an injected pharynx. Severe shock occurs in about 7 percent of patients, half of whom subsequently die. In cases with severe shock, proteinuria, hematuria, oliguria, and anuria occur.

Macroscopic Findings. The kidneys are enlarged. On the cut surface the cortex is pale and wider than normal; the medulla is dark red and often contains hemorrhages. Hemorrhages also occur in the pelvis and calices.

Light Microscopic Findings. Severe forms of the Asian disease show the changes of acute renal failure with tubular damage and regeneration, the extent and distribution of which depend upon the time that has elapsed between the onset of shock and either biopsy or death. There are no lesions specific to the chikungunya virus. Interstitial hemorrhages are frequent, with a small amount of focal mononuclear cell infiltration.

Electron Microscopic Findings. No viral inclusions or other specific lesions are found.

Immunomicroscopic Findings. There are no deposits of immunoglobulins or complement components. Fibrinogen may be present in some glomerular capillary lumens in the severe forms of the disease.

DENGUE HEMORRHAGIC FEVER

Dengue hemorrhagic fever or dengue shock syndrome is endemic in Southeast Asia, the western Pacific region, and the Caribbean. It is a severe febrile disease affecting children predominantly and adolescents occasionally. The highest incidence is in children 3 to 5 years of age. Transient immune complex glomerulonephritis or acute renal failure may develop during the disease. The disease causes increased vascular permeability.

The disease is caused by the four dengue virus serotypes 1 to 4 of the *Flavivirus* genus of the Togaviridae (Flaviviridae) family following the bite of the *Aedes* mosquito. *Aedes aegypti* is the most important worldwide vector species.

Clinical and Pathologic Manifestations

The incubation period is usually 1 week, with a range from 4 to 15 days. The disease is characterized by a sudden onset of fever, nausea, vomiting, abdominal pain, hepatomegaly, petechiae, epistaxis, hematemesis, melena, and shock. About 80 percent of cases have effusions of yellow clear fluid in serous cavities. The clinical severity varies from mild to severe and has been classified into four clinical gradings. Severe hemorrhage and shock occur in about 40 to 50 percent of cases and are the cause of death. Microscopic hematuria and/or proteinuria are present in all clinical gradings. Acute renal failure may develop in patients with profound shock (grade IV).

Treatment is mainly supportive and is concentrated on maintenance of fluid volume. Corticosteroids may be given in certain cases.

Light Microscopic Findings. Biopsy specimens reveal transient glomerulonephritis with mononuclear cells in some glomerular capillaries. There are mild mesangial cell proliferation with increased matrix and irregular thickening of some capillary walls. Tubules may contain clusters of erythrocytes or hyaline casts. Interstitial edema with mononuclear cell infiltration may be present focally.

Electron Microscopic Findings. There are mononuclear phagocytic cells in the glomerular capillary lumen. Some of these cells degenerate and the cell membrane ruptures, releasing cytoplasmic contents, including large amounts of glycogen granules into the capillary lumens. These cell particles are trapped between endothelial cytofolds and paramesangial areas. The other prominent feature is focal splitting of the capillary basement membrane where mononuclear phagocytic cells come in contact.

Immunomicroscopic Findings. The findings depend upon the time of biopsy. There are dense deposits of IgG, IgM, and low intensity of C3 in the glomeruli during the third week of disease. The deposits are confined mainly to mesangial areas. Occasionally, they may be seen along the capillary walls. Dengue antigens are not demonstrable in the glomeruli but can be seen in inflammatory cell infiltrates in areas of skin rash.

VIRAL HEPATITIS

Glomerular and vascular abnormalities occur in patients infected with hepatitis B virus. The changes consist of glomerulonephritis (usually membranous glomerulonephritis), the glomerular lesions of mixed cryoglobulinemia, and necrotizing vasculitis.

There is a strong association between renal disease and hepatitis B virus infection. This organism is a complex DNA virus with a core (HbcAg) and an outer envelope consisting mainly of surface antigen (HbsAg). The other main components of the virus are the DNA-dependent DNA polymerase and the e antigen (HbeAg). HbeAg has recently been identified as a subunit of HbcAg. Hepatitis B infections can be complicated by simultaneous or subsequent infection with another virus, the delta agent, which can multiply only in the presence of Hbs antigen. About 5 to 15 percent of acute or inapparent hepatitis B infections develop into chronic carrier states with only minimal liver changes. The prevalence of HbsAg antigenemia varies greatly throughout the world. It is highest in Southeast Asia, China, Japan, and central and South Africa and lowest in northern and western Europe, the United States, Canada, Australia, and New Zealand. For example, the proportion of blood donors who were HbsAg-positive in one extensive study in South Vietnam was 24.5%; in Great Britain the equivalent figure was 0.1%.

HEPATITIS B GLOMERULONEPHRITIS

Most of the patients in published studies of renal disease associated with hepatitis B virus have had membranous glomerulonephritis; but mesangial proliferative glomerulonephritis, mesangiocapillary glomerulonephritis type I and type III, focal glomerulosclerosis, and diffuse endocapillary proliferative glomerulonephritis have also been reported. The relationship between membranous glomerulonephritis and persistent hepatitis B virus infection is a close one; that between mesangiocapillary glomerulonephritis and the virus is less clear because some of these cases may have been stage IV membranous glomerulonephritis, which can resemble mesangiocapillary glomerulonephritis on light microscopy. A wrong diagnosis may be made if electron microscopy is not done. However, in about one third of cases subendothelial and intramembranous deposits, disruption of the basement membrane, and stretches of mesangial interposition, in addition to the subepithelial deposits, are found (see Electron Microscopic Findings). These findings produce a mixed picture of membranous and mesangiocapillary glomerulonephritis. Mesangial hypercellularity is probably the earliest response to hepatitis B virus complexes in the glomeruli; it is usually associated with subepithelial immune deposits and progresses to predominantly membranous glomerulonephritis. The association between hepatitis B infection and focal glomerulosclerosis and diffuse endocapillary proliferative glomerulonephritis is more tenuous and may be incidental.

Clinical and Pathologic Manifestations

Glomerulonephritis caused by hepatitis B infection is most common in young children but occurs at all ages, with a marked predominance in males. About 70 percent of patients present with the nephrotic syndrome, and the remainder have asymptomatic proteinuria. In Japan, where mass screening of children by urinalysis is carried out, many cases have been detected by chance findings of proteinuria and hematuria. Approximately 50% of the Japanese patients developed nephrotic syndrome during the course of the disease. There may be associated hypertension and some renal dysfunction. Microscopic hematuria is detectable in most patients. About 30% show reduced serum C3 values. Nephrotic syndrome is unresponsive to corticosteroid therapy. All patients have HbsAg in their serum, and about 70% also have HbeAg. Antibody to core antigen (HbcAb) is almost always present, antibody to e antigen (HbeAb) is present in about 25%, but antibody to surface antigen (HbsAg) is invariably absent. In children, nephrotic syndrome usually disappears within several months of onset. Proteinuria may persist but is usually slight. Progressive renal failure and relapse are rare. Remission is usually associated with loss of HbeAg from the patient's serum and the appearance of HbeAb. A high incidence of hepatitis B virus carrier, abnormal urinalysis, and liver dysfunction among the families of the Japanese patients was reported. These findings indicate that hepatitis B virus–associated glomerulonephritis may be caused by vertical transmission infection during infancy. However, transmission may also be horizontal.

Macroscopic Findings.   The kidneys are enlarged and pale with smooth subcapsular surfaces.

Light Microscopic Findings.   The predominant lesion is usually diffuse membranous glomerulonephritis in which the glomerular capillary walls are uniformly thickened. With trichrome stain, red subepithelial deposits can sometimes be seen; and silver impregnation often reveals projections of basement membrane between the deposits. In some cases the spikes join to produce a chain. The mesangium is slightly expanded, and often the number of mesangial cells is increased to three or four per mesangial area. In early cases mesangial proliferation may be the only obvious feature. In some cases the glomeruli show the features of a mesangiocapillary type of glomerulonephritis. Small foci of tubular atrophy and interstitial lymphocytic infiltration are often present, but in general tubulointerstitial changes are slight.

Electron Microscopic Findings.   The most consistent and prominent feature is electron dense subepithelial deposits along the capillary walls. Occasionally the deposits are small and scattered (stage I) but usually they are numerous, larger, evenly distributed, and separated from each other by projections of lamina densa (stage II). In a substantial number of cases the condition is even more advanced with new basement membrane covering the deposits, some of which are rarefied (stage III). In almost a third of patients, subendothelial and/or intramembranous deposits and a degree of mesangial cell interposition into capillary loops are also present. The mesangial areas almost invariably contain electron-dense deposits. There is widespread loss of visceral epithelial cell foot processes. As the disease remits, the basement membrane is partially or completely restructured and approaches normal appearance.

Immunomicroscopic Findings.   Numerous evenly distributed granular deposits of IgG and C3 are found along the glomerular capillary walls. In about half the cases IgM is also present in a similar distribution, but IgA and early components of complement are rare. Using F(ab')$_2$ fragments of monoclonal HbeAb, e antigen (HbeAg) can often be demonstrated in the capillary walls and mesangium. Patients who do not show deposits of HbeAg usually have HbeAb in their serum. In some studies, deposits of HbcAg were found in the majority of patients. HbsAg in the glomeruli was often reported in early studies of this disease, but much of the staining was probably nonspecific since it is abolished when labeled HbsAb F(ab')₂ fragments are used in place of the whole antibody.

MIXED CRYOGLOBULINEMIA

Mixed cryoglobulinemia may be associated with hepatitis B virus infection. It is not clear whether viral infection is the primary etiological factor or whether infection occurs after the mixed cryoglobulinemia has been established.

Clinical and Pathologic Manifestations

About 5 percent of patients present with acute nephritic syndrome and become anuric within a short time. Extrarenal symptoms such as purpura, arthralgia, and splenomegaly are often present. Most patients, however, develop chronic progressive disease with proteinuria, nephrotic syndrome, microscopic hematuria, hypertension, and renal failure.

Light Microscopic Findings. Acute cases are characterized by an increased number of mesangial cells, endothelial cells, and polymorphonuclear leukocytes in the glomerular tufts, together with large irregularly distributed PAS-positive subendothelial and intraluminal deposits. In the chronic form there is usually either diffuse mesangiocapillary glomerulonephritis or focal and segmental glomerulonephritis. There are wire loops and sometimes crescents. Chronic inflammatory cells are present in the interstitium, and there may be necrotizing arteritis.

Electron Microscopic Findings. The glomeruli contain large subendothelial, mesangial, and capillary luminal deposits. There are occasionally subepithelial humps. The deposits commonly contain cylinders, 25 nm in diameter or larger, arranged in curved parallel arrays. Crystalline inclusions with a similar tubular structure can be found in mesangial, endothelial, and epithelial cells.

Immunomicroscopic Findings. Granular deposits of IgG, IgM, C3, C1_q, and C4 are present in the capillary walls and mesangium. Immunoglobulins and complement components are also found in the intraluminal deposits.

POLYARTERITIS NODOSA (NECROTIZING VASCULITIS)

Persistent hepatitis B infection is associated with polyarteritis. Hepatitis B surface antigen (HbsAg) and HbsAb form circulating immune complexes, and HbsAg has been demonstrated in the injured vessels. However, HbsAb has not been demonstrated in the vessel walls, and there is no proof that the circulating immune complexes cause the arterial lesions. The strongest evidence that hepatitis B has an etiological role comes from a longitudinal study of 266 hemodialysis patients who were chronic carriers of HbsAg. Necrotizing vasculitis developed in three, whereas no cases occurred among 384 similarly dialyzed patients who were not carriers.

Clinical and Pathologic Manifestations

Polyarteritis is more common in men than in women, and the incidence increases with age. Patients typically have acute illness characterized by fever, arthralgia, muscle pains, and peripheral neuropathy. Renal involvement is common. It is usually manifested by microscopic hematuria and proteinuria, but about 30% of patients present with rapidly progressing renal failure. Hypertension may be a later complication. The clinical course is characterized by remissions and exacerbations. Treatment with steroids and immunosuppressive drugs is only partially successful.

Two variants of polyarteritis are recognized: a classical form affecting predominantly arcuate and larger segmental arteries and a microscopic form affecting capillaries, arterioles, small interlobular arteries, and venules. These two broad categories overlap.

Classic Form of Polyarteritis: Pathologic Manifestations

Macroscopic Findings. The kidneys are often smaller than normal. The subcapsular surface shows evidence of infarction, with old lesions in the form of depressed scars. Thrombi may be present in the arcuate arteries, and small aneurysms are occasionally present in the segmental arteries.

Light and Electron Microscopic Findings. Changes occur focally in the larger interlobular, the arcuate, and the segmental arteries. The lesions do not all develop at the same time; and it is common to see acute, healing, and healed lesions together. In the acute stage the whole or part of the circumference of the arterial wall is destroyed and replaced by fibrin. The change usually involves the whole thickness of the vessel wall, and the internal elastic lamina is disrupted. The necrotic area is infiltrated by neutrophils, mononuclear cells, and a variable number of eosinophils. The cellular reaction often surrounds the vessel. The lumen may become obliterated by thrombosis with consequent parenchymal necrosis. Segmental damage to the vessel wall produces small aneurysms, which can rupture and hemorrhage. The necrotic muscle of the vessel wall is replaced by fibrous tissue as the lesion heals, but the disrupted internal elastic lamina does not regenerate. The intima becomes thickened and the lumen narrowed. The smaller interlobular arteries and the arterioles are normal or may show hypertensive changes. Infarcts of all ages are present. The rest of the renal tissue, particularly the proximal tubules, may have undergone ischemic atrophy. The glomeruli in these ischemic areas contain collagenous crescents and shrunken tufts.

The electron microscopic findings confirm those of light microscopy.

Immunomicroscopic Findings. Immunoglobulin deposits are infrequent and scanty. C3 is more common and fibrinogen is constantly found when lesions are recent. Small granular deposits of HbsAg have been demonstrated in the media of acutely affected vessels.

Microscopic Form of Polyarteritis: Pathologic Manifestations

Macroscopic Findings. The kidneys may be enlarged. The subcapsular surface is smooth and often speckled with petechial hemorrhages. The arteries appear normal.

Light Microscopic Findings. The glomeruli are the frequent site of damage, and anything from a few to most show segments of fibrinoid necrosis. Recent and old lesions co-exist, sometimes even within the same glomerulus. These are usually accompanied by a small amount of endocapillary proliferation and by cellular crescents; occasionally there is associated diffuse mesangial proliferative or mesangiocapillary glomerulonephritis. Fibrinoid necrosis and inflammatory change involves the entire circumference and thickness of segments of the walls of scattered small interlobular arteries, arterioles, and venules. Proximal tubular damage is common. Mononuclear cell infiltration of the interstitium may be marked. These various forms of glomerulonephritis also occur, albeit less frequently, in

classic polyarteritis nodosa, and the classic and microscopic forms may occur together.

Electron Microscopic Findings. Occasionally there are subendothelial deposits on the glomerular capillary walls; usually there are none.

Immunomicroscopic Findings. In the glomeruli and affected small blood vessels immunoglobulin deposits are uncommon and scanty. C3 is present in about a quarter of the cases and fibrinogen in most. HbsAg has been demonstrated in small vessel walls but not in glomeruli.

AIDS VIRUS (HUMAN IMMUNODEFICIENCY VIRUS)

Since its initial description in 1981, the acquired immunodeficiency syndrome has been extensively studied, with criteria modified and expanded. It has been shown to be the result of infection by the *Lentivirus* human immunodeficiency virus (HIV), previously classified as a retrovirus called human T lymphotrophic virus type III (HTLV-III) or lymphadenopathy-associated virus (LAV), with apparently selective destruction of T helper cells. There are at present individuals who possess antibodies to the agent and are asymptomatic; a group of patients with a syndrome that appears to be a prodrome ("pre-AIDS", or AIDS-related complex); and a group with the complete picture of multiple and varied opportunistic infections, Kaposi's sarcoma, lymphomas, or other less frequently observed malignancies, and altered T helper/ T suppressor cell ratios. The greatest incidence was initially reported in homosexual males; but recipients of contaminated blood or blood products, especially intravenous drug abusers and hemophiliacs, and heterosexual males and females constitute a progressively greater portion of affected patients.

Clinical and Pathologic Manifestations

Renal manifestations in AIDS patients are varied, although they most commonly include renal failure, low-grade proteinuria, and nephrotic syndrome. In patients with nephrotic syndrome, only about 50 percent are intravenous drug abusers, so that "heroin nephropathy" is not the only explanation for the glomerulopathy. The glomerular lesions associated with AIDS may rapidly evolve to chronic azotemia or end-stage renal failure in as little as 6 months. Focal and segmental glomerulosclerosis, the major form of glomerular injury, may be the initial manifestation of AIDS and may antedate the complete syndrome by 3 to 18 months. In patients without glomerular disease, renal insufficiency is often a terminal or preterminal event and is usually related to sepsis and shock, direct renal infection, and/or antimicrobial or antineoplastic drugs.

Light Microscopic Findings. There are two common glomerular lesions. In some patients with proteinuria, mesangial proliferative glomerulonephritis, usually with only a modest degree of hypercellularity, is observed. Capillary lumens are patent, and capillary walls and basement membranes are thin and single contoured. Most nephrotic patients have focal and segmental glomerulosclerosis, with all the features that characterize the broad spectrum of the segmental lesion in all stages of evolution. Localized enlargement, hyperplasia, and vacuolization of visceral epithelial cells that overlie the sclerotic segment are observed. "Insudative" lesions ("hyalinosis"), collapsed capillaries, increased mesangial matrix, and capsular adhesions constitute the balance of the alterations. Many distal and a few proximal tubules are filled with large and probably obstructing casts, and Bowman's spaces are often dilated. Proximal tubular cells contain numerous protein reabsorption droplets. The interstitium in affected kidneys may be mildly edematous and infiltrated with mononuclear leukocytes or focally fibrotic. There may be degenerative changes and necrosis of tubular epithelium. In addition to focal and segmental glomerulosclerosis, other glomerulopathies, usually of a post- or peri-infectious nature, have been reported. The morphologic findings are not different from these lesions in patients without AIDS.

A variety of infectious agents have been identified throughout kidneys of AIDS patients; these include Mycobacterium avium-intracellulare, Candida, Cryptococcus, and cytomegalovirus, all either with or without a cellular inflammatory component. Depending upon the preterminal and terminal events and therapies, acute tubular necrosis is present. Focal tubular and interstitial calcifications, presumably related to amphotericin B therapy, may occur.

Neoplastic involvement of the kidneys, including Kaposi's sarcoma and lymphomas, is relatively uncommon. Occasional instances of renal cell carcinoma are known.

Electron Microscopic Findings. The ultrastructure of the glomerular lesions is not unlike that in the same form of glomerular damage occurring in the absence of AIDS. Mesangial electron-dense deposits are observed in patients with either focal and segmental glomerulosclerosis or mesangial hypercellularity. In nonsclerotic portions of glomeruli, the foot processes of visceral epithelial cells are largely effaced. The sclerotic segments contain increased mesangial matrix and basement membrane or large electron-dense masses that occlude lumens. Tubuloreticular structures are present in the cytoplasm of endothelial cells, often in unusually large numbers. Their presence in focal and segmental glomerulosclerosis may indicate infection with HIV. In the other glomerular lesions (infection-associated glomerulonephritis), there may also be numerous intracellular tubuloreticular structures in addition to the expected ultrastructural abnormalities.

Immunomicroscopic Findings. The results of this procedure are variable for the glomeruli. In some nephrotic patients with normal glomeruli or with mesangial hypercellularity, there are deposits of IgM or IgG and C3 in a granular pattern and a diffuse and generalized mesangial distribution; less commonly, the immunofluorescence studies have been negative. In glomeruli with segmental sclerosis, segmental IgM and C3, corresponding to the "insudative" lesions, are noted. The standard immunofluorescence findings in infection-associated glomerulonephritides parallel those of non-AIDS patients.

LANDRY-GUILLAIN-BARRÉ-STROHL SYNDROME

Landry-Guillain-Barré-Strohl syndrome, usually referred to as Guillain-Barré syndrome is characterized by polyneuropathy that develops acutely over a few days or several weeks and follows a prodrome of a nonspecific viral type of infection by 1 to 3 weeks. There is usually an upper respiratory infection or an infection with *Enterovirus, Mycoplasma,* or *Psittacosis* and various other organisms (eg, *Campylobacter*). The pathogenesis is obscure; but it appears to be autoimmune, with antibodies to peripheral nerve tissue.

Most patients recover within weeks to months, but severely affected persons may need assisted respiration and may have residual muscle weakness. Clinical and autopsy studies have shown evidence of frequent renal involvement, which has been attributed to the deposition in the renal glomeruli of antigen-antibody complexes, formed against altered nerve constituents.

Clinical and Pathologic Manifestations

Renal involvement in Guillain-Barré syndrome is relatively common, presenting as acute glomerulonephritis with hypertension, periorbital edema, and microhematuria. Nephrotic syndrome has been rarely recorded and is not responsive to steroids and immunotherapy. Many cases may be undetected, as the clinical manifestations of renal involvement may be minimal, with microhematuria occurring 10 days later. Urinalysis shows proteinuria and abnormal urinary sediments, with granular cells and erythrocyte casts.

Light Microscopic Findings. The usual glomerular abnormality is diffuse moderate thickening of the basement membrane, with variable mesangial cell proliferation and mesangial widening due to matrix condensation. The capillary lumen may contain several polymorphonuclear neutrophils. The glomeruli may also show focal, segmental, and global sclerosis. Interstitial nephritis has been recorded; and the tubules may show foci of atrophy and focal interstitial fibrosis with heavy infiltration by lymphocytes, plasma cells and polymorphonuclear neutrophils. The blood vessels usually are not involved.

Electron Microscopic Findings. The glomerular basement membrane is thickened, with a moth-eaten appearance. There are electron-dense deposits in the subepithelium and also in the mesangium. The endothelial cells are swollen, and in some areas there is focal increase in mesangial matrix, and there is extensive obliteration of the podocytes.

Immunomicroscopic Findings. The common feature is the deposition of IgG_4, IgM, and complement in a finely granular pattern along the glomerular basement membrane. Uncommonly, a "linear" fluorescence, with both IgG and complement on the glomerular basement membrane, has been reported.

INFECTIOUS MONONUCLEOSIS (EPSTEIN-BARR VIRUS)

Infectious mononucleosis is an infection by a herpesvirus, Epstein-Barr (EB) virus, usually acquired and passed without symptoms in young children. Other patients may present with malaise, sore throat, fever, cervical lymphadenopathy, a nonitchy morbilliform skin rash, hepatomegaly with hepatitis-like findings, or thrombocytopenia. In severe cases, infarcts and rupture of the spleen with hemorrhages may occur. Recent infections show rising antibody to viral capsid antigen and to EB virus early antigen, and the appearance of EB specific IgM antibody. The Paul-Bunnel test with heterophile agglutinins for sheeps' red blood cells is diagnostic for infectious mononucleosis.

Renal involvement in the form of transient nephritis is fairly common, (reported to occur in 6 to 13 percent of cases), but severe renal disease is rare, and the prognosis is excellent.

Clinical and Pathologic Manifestations

A transient rise in blood urea and creatinine levels, with episodes of microhematuria, is common; but gross hematuria and azotemia have been reported in only a few cases. Some cases present as acute nephritis with periorbital edema and bloody urine associated with the infectious mononucleosis. The hematuria occurs at the onset or during the first week of the disease and resolves within 7 to 10 days. The urinary sediment contains red cell casts and granular casts, and there is proteinuria. The rapid disappearance of the hematuria and proteinuria, normal serum complement, and no progression to chronic nephritis are unlike the findings in poststreptococcal glomerulonephritis.

Light Microscopic Findings. The common renal abnormality is acute tubulointerstitial nephritis, with marked interstitial edema, focal aggregates of histiocytes, lymphocytes, monocytes, some plasma cells, and a few granulocytes. There are foci of tubular necrosis, with severely damaged epithelial cells and basement membranes. Some tubules are dilated, with flattened epithelium; red blood cells, hyaline, and nucleated casts can be found in the lumens of some tubules. Rarely, granulomas in the interstitium have been recorded.

Less frequently, focal mesangial proliferative glomerulonephritis with mesangial cell hyperplasia and segmental destruction with focal sclerosis may occur. The capillaries are patent, and the basement membrane is not thickened.

Blood vessel involvement is rare. One case with vasculitis showed lymphocytes surrounding, involving, and occasionally destroying the small to medium-sized arterioles.

Electron Microscopic Findings. The glomerular basement membrane is essentially normal, and no appreciable thickening is noted. No subepithelial "humps" or deposits are seen, as in poststreptococcal glomerulonephritis. Some cases show some mesangial cytoplasmic protrusions into the capillary lumens.

VARICELLA

Varicella, or chickenpox, is caused by a varicella zoster virus whose size and structure are similar to those of the herpes simplex virus. The virus damages the stratum germinativum and stratum spinosum of the epidermis to produce superficial vesicles. The incubation period is about 2 weeks. It is an infection predominantly of the young, with minimal prodromal symptoms, followed by typical rash and fever. In normal adults, the disease may occasionally mimic smallpox in severity. However, except in immunosuppressed patients, severe systemic infections with pneumonitis, hepatitis, encephalitis, hemorrhagic diathesis, or secondary bacterial infection are rare.

Varicella infection with clinical nephritis is rare. In one large study of 2,584 cases, only three (0.12%) of patients were affected. Renal lesions are more common in fatal cases.

Clinical and Pathologic Manifestations

Renal involvement in varicella infection is uncommon, presenting as acute glomerulonephritis with hematuria, hypertension, puffy face, and fever following the original signs and symptoms of varicella infection. There is no preceding streptococcal infection, no rise in antistreptolysin O titer, and no C-reactive protein. Rarely it may present as rapidly progressive glomerulonephritis. Another rare manifestation is the nephrotic syndrome with puffy face, generalized edema, and proteinuria with microhematuria. As the varicella skin lesions fade, the acute glomerulonephritis and the nephrotic syndrome resolve.

Light Microscopic Findings. There is diffuse endocapillary proliferative glomerulonephritis with polymorphonuclear and monocytic infiltrates and partial occlusion of the glomerular capillaries. The greatly enlarged hypercellular glomeruli show proliferation of both mesangial and endothelial cells. There are focal adhesions to Bowman's capsule. Some cases may show foci

of tubualr epithelial cell degeneration and interstitial mononuclear cell infiltrations.

Electron Microscopic Findings. The glomeruli show granular, electron-dense deposits in the paramesangium and occasional subendothelial deposits, which are associated with focal degeneration of the glomerular basement membrane, with obliteration of the overlying podocytes.

Immunomicroscopic Findings. The glomeruli show granular deposits of immunoglobulins IgG, IgA, and IgM and small amounts of complements C3 and C1q, mainly in the mesangium. Varicella antigen is also deposited in the same location, suggesting an immune complex deposition with C3 activation of complement via the classical and alternative pathways.

CYTOMEGALOVIRUS

Cytomegalovirus (CMV) is a member of the herpesvirus group. Frequency of infection varies from country to country, depending upon socioeconomic status. Cytomegalovirus-infected human cells are increased in size and contain prominent nuclear and cytoplasmic inclusions, especially in the salivary glands, liver, pancreas, lungs, and kidneys.

Congenital infection acquired during the first two trimesters of pregnancy is well described. Perinatal infection from the mother's genital tract or from breast milk has also been recognized as an important method of transmission. Most infections in children and adults are acquired by direct contact, as in day care centers or by sexual contact.

Clinical and Pathologic Manifestations

Congenital infection may produce severe, overwhelming disease or, more commonly, central nervous system defects such as microencephaly, cerebral palsy, and psychomotor retardation.

Infection in children and adults may be asymptomatic. Symptomatic infections often present with signs similar to those of influenza or mononucleosis: fever, lymphadenopathy, hepatosplenomegaly, and lymphocytosis. CMV infection is rarely complicated by hepatitis, pyelonephritis, and polyneuritis. Severe disseminated disease with complications such as pneumonia is quite common in immunosuppressed patients. Renal involvement with CMV may be indicated by viruria, but no renal functional derangement occurs.

The diagnosis of CMV infection can be confirmed by cultures of body fluids and tissues. Rising titers of IgG and IgM antibody can also be detected by complement fixation, immunofluorescent antibody, and enzyme-linked immunosorbent assay techniques.

Light Microscopic Findings. Cytomegalovirus infects predominantly the tubular epithelial cells, and occasionally the endothelial cells of the glomeruli. There are abundant large intranuclear and small variable intracytoplasmic inclusions in the enlarged epithelial cells. The size of these inclusions may be almost half that of the nucleus. There may be occasional foci of tubular necrosis with lymphocytic cell infiltrates.

Urine cytology studies show CMV-infected exfoliated tubular epithelial cells to be round or oval and 3 to 10 times larger than normal epithelial cells. The dense nuclear inclusion is surrounded by a clear intranuclear halo.

Electron Microscopic Findings. The nuclear inclusions comprise condensed and altered chromatin intimately associated with developing viruses. Smaller cytoplasmic inclusions, composed of dense viral particles arranged in a crystalloid pattern, are also present. The individual virus is made up of a central core with a less dense outer matrix, and the intranuclear viral particles appear to be incompletely formed.

COXSACKIEVIRUS

The coxsackieviruses types Al-A24 and B1-B6, belong to the family Enterovirus and are common infectious agents spread by the fecal-oral route. Most enterovirus infections are silent or cause only minor and transient symptoms, mainly in the upper respiratory tract. The symptoms may be accompanied by skin rashes and/or vesicular oropharyngeal lesions. Both groups of viruses cause myositis, but coxsackie B-5 is known also to produce myocarditis. Renal involvement has been reported with coxsackie B-5 and A-4 infections.

Coxsackie B-5 viral antigens isolated in exfoliated cells in the urinary sediment indicate the viruses may directly involve the kidney and induce renal disease either by multiplication within the kidney or by the formation of antigen-antibody complexes and subsequent development of immune complex glomerulonephritis.

Clinical and Pathologic Manifestations

Most patients have microhematuria and mild proteinuria with mild transient disease during the course of the illness, without apparent renal sequelae. Several children have presented with clinical features of acute glomerulonephritis, and there are isolated reports of fatal cases with deterioration in renal function. Coxsackie A-4 and B infections in children have led to the hemolytic-uremic syndrome, characterized by thrombocytopenia, hemolytic anemia, and acute renal failure.

Light Microscopic Findings. There is focal or diffuse proliferative glomerulonephritis, reflecting the severity of the disease. The glomeruli are swollen and hypercellular, with proliferation of mesangial and endothelial cells. There may also be focal interstitial nephritis with foci of tubular damage as well as interstitial edema and inflammatory infiltrates by lymphocytes and monocytes. Some tubules are dilated and lined by flattened epithelial cells, and some lumens contain eosinophilic casts.

Electron Microscopic Findings. The glomeruli show focal widening of endothelial fenestrae, edema of the lamina rara interna of the glomerular basement membrane, and obliteration of podocytes.

Immunomicroscopic Findings. Deposition of fibrin in glomerular capillaries is related to the hypercoagulable state in the pathogenesis of hemolytic-uremic syndrome. Coxsackie B-4 antigen is identified within glomeruli and the renal interstitium by immunofluorescent antibody techniques.

OTHER VIRAL INFECTIONS

A number of other viruses have been implicated in diseases of the urinary tract. The major ones are the adenoviruses, mumps virus, the myxoviruses of influenza, ECHO viruses, measles virus, and rubella virus. Viruria has been demonstrated in many cases. The usual clinical presentation is microhematuria and proteinuria, which is mild and transient during the febrile phase of the illness. In an ECHO-9 epidemic, microhematuria was observed in nearly 50 percent of patients and low-grade proteinuria in 10 percent.

Isolated cases of acute glomerulonephritis have been associated with ECHO-9 virus and measles virus infections. The glomeruli show diffuse endocapillary proliferation with hyperplasia of mesangial and endothelial cells and narrowing of the capillary lumens. Measles virus antigen immunoglobulin IgG and C3 are deposited along the glomerular basement membrane, indicating an immune complex glomerulonephritis. In fatal and severe cases of measles, giant cells and inclusions can be found in bladder mucosa and in exfoliated cells in the urine.

Goodpasture's syndrome with crescentic glomerulonephritis may be associated with influenza virus infection. Rubella virus may be isolated from kidney tissues of infants who die of congenital rubella.

ADENOVIRUS

Disseminated adenovirus infection occurs as a complication of immunosuppression in patients undergoing bone marrow transplantation. The infection is thought to result from endogenous viral reactivation, and several viral species have been identified. Virus has been cultured from urine and from renal biopsy specimens, among other sites.

Clinical manifestations include pneumonia, diarrhea, and renal failure, although particular signs and symptoms may be referable to other concomitant infections from which these patients suffer. Renal abnormalities include azotemia, hematuria, dysuria, and flank pain.

The kidneys contain focal areas of necrosis in the tubules. The lesions often look like irregularly shaped infarcts. Immunohistochemical studies with monoclonal antibodies have shown multifocal tubular involvement with glomerular sparing, even though glomeruli sometimes seem to be caught in areas of necrosis. Tubular cells appear to have undergone coagulative necrosis with variable surrounding cellular infiltration, and surviving cells often contain large intranuclear inclusions. Tubular mitotic activity at the margins of necrotic foci appears to be a response to necrosis.

Hantavirus (Bunyaviridae)

FIGURE 7.1   The kidney is edmatous, with a pale reddish cortex sharply demarcated from the congested and hemorrhagic medulla.

FIGURE 7.2   There is a hemorrhage at the cortico-medullary junction and necrosis of the papilla. (H & E × 3.5)

FIGURE 7.3   There is massive hemorrhage at the corticomedullary junction with fresh erythrocytes separating the tubules, which are necrotic and contain hyaline or blood casts. (H & E × 60)

FIGURE 7.4   The cortex near the corticomedullary junction shows tubulorrhexis and interstitial inflammation. (H & E × 235)

7.1

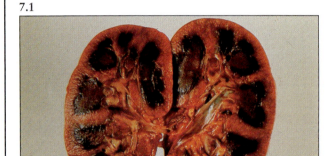

7.2

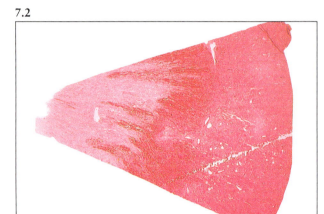

7.3

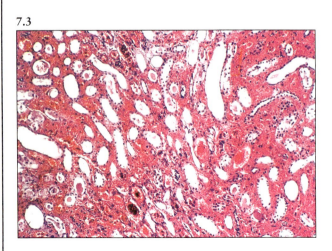

7.4

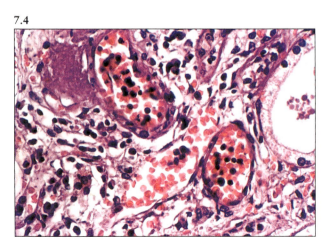

HANTAVIRUS (BUNYAVIRIDAE)

FIGURE 7.5   Nucleated cells are observed in the vasa recta of the medulla. (H & E × 235)

FIGURE 7.6   Severe form of hemorrhagic fever with renal syndrome. Interstitium is diffusely edematous and hemorrhagic; there is tubular necrosis and interstitial cell infiltration. (H & E × 50)

FIGURE 7.7   Same case as in Figure 7.6. At higher power, tubular damage, as well as interstitial edema and mononuclear cell infiltration, can be seen. (H & E × 190)

7.5

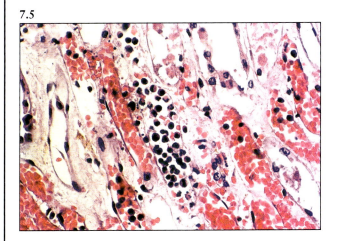

7.6

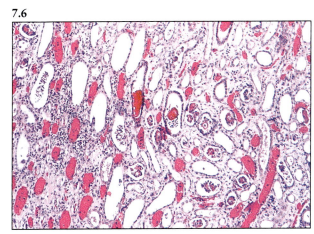

7.7

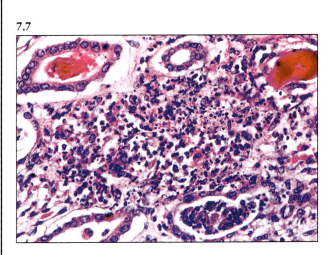

ARENAVIRIDAE

FIGURE 7.8   The kidney shows severe hemorrhage in the pyramids with papillary necrosis.

FIGURE 7.9   Bolivian hemorrhagic fever. Kidney shows arteriolar thrombosis. (H & E × 470).

FIGURE 7.10   Bolivian hemorrhagic fever. Hemoglobin casts are seen in the tubular lumens. (H & E × 165)

7.8

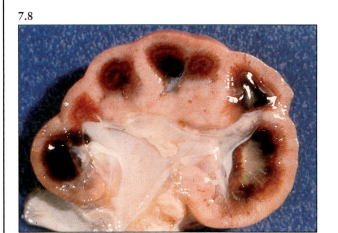

7.9

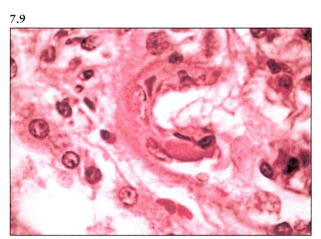

7.10

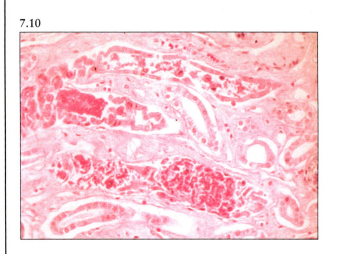

YELLOW FEVER

FIGURE 7.11   Yellow fever endemic zone in Africa, 1985. (Courtesy of World Health Organization.)

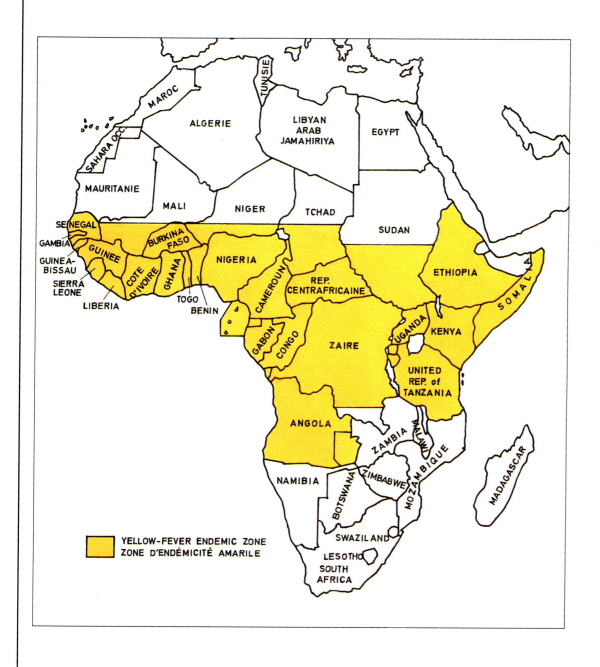

YELLOW-FEVER ENDEMIC ZONE
ZONE D'ENDÉMICITÉ AMARILE

YELLOW FEVER

FIGURE 7.12 Yellow fever endemic zone in the Americas, 1985. (Courtesy of World Health Organization.)

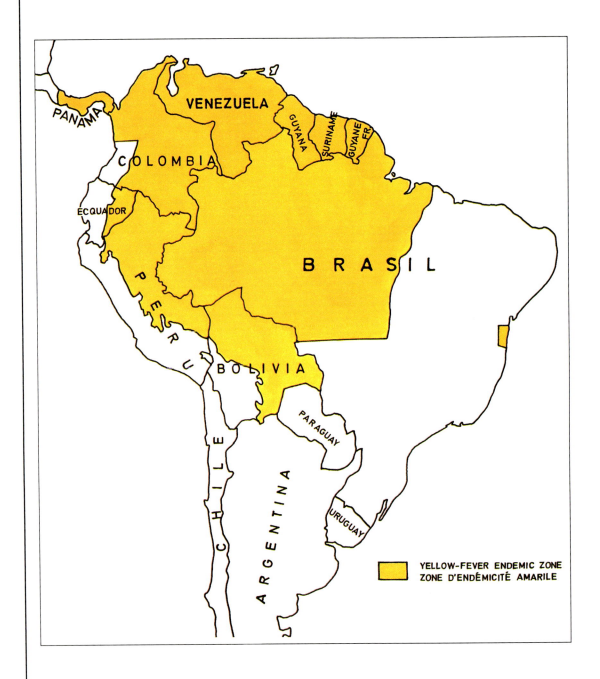

YELLOW FEVER

FIGURE 7.13   Kidney in yellow fever (fixed specimen). The parenchyma is yellowish and traversed by perpendicular yellow streaks.

FIGURE 7.14   Extensive tubular degeneration and many casts filling tubular lumina. (Russell-Movat × 95)

FIGURE 7.15   Yellow fever. Acute tubular necrosis with leucine crystals and pigment casts in tubular lumens. The tubular epithelial cells are vacuolated, and the interstitium is edematous. (H & E × 285)

FIGURE 7.16   Same case as in Figure 7.15. The leucine crystals are birefringent. (Polarized light × 235).

7.13

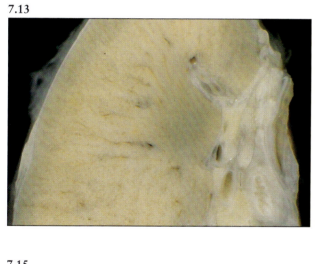

7.14

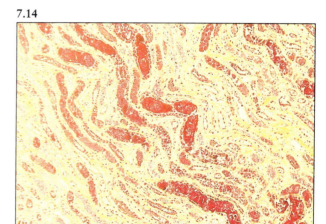

7.15

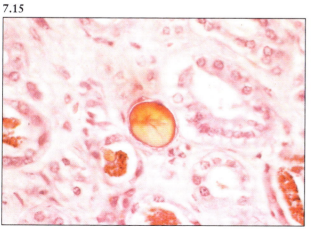

7.16

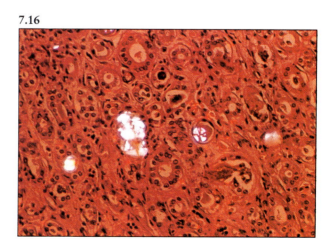

CHIKUNGUNYA FEVER

FIGURE 7.17   Severe form of chikungunya fever. Acute tubular necrosis with ruptured walls, pigment casts, interstitial edema, and moderate cellular infiltration are seen. (H & E × 50)

FIGURE 7.18   Same case as in Figure 7.17, showing an interstitial hemorrhage beneath the caliceal epithelium. (H & E × 50)

FIGURE 7.19   Same case as in Figure 7.17, showing interstitial hemorrhage in the renal papilla. (H & E × 30)

7.17

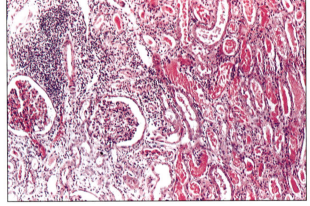

7.18

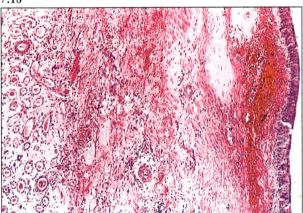

7.19

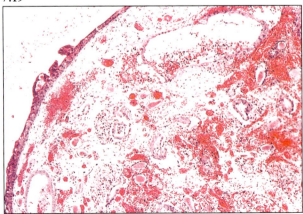

DENGUE HEMORRHAGIC FEVER

FIGURE 7.20   World distribution of dengue infections based on virus isolation from man within the past decade, or areas considered permissive to dengue because of the prevalence of urban *Aedes aegypti*, 1980. (Courtesy of World Health Organization.)

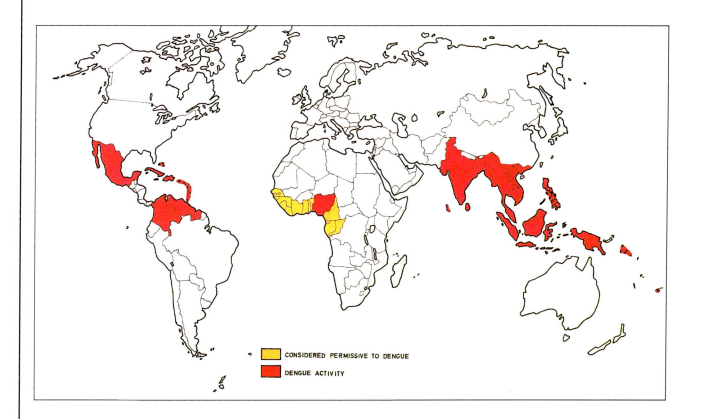

DENGUE HEMORRHAGIC FEVER

FIGURE 7.21   Dengue hemorrhagic fever. Pale renal cortex and congested medulla indicate acute vasomotor nephropathy.

FIGURE 7.22   Dengue hemorrhagic fever. Postmortem examination shows glomerulus with marked hypercellularity, especially of mesangial cells and mononuclear cell infiltrates. (H & E × 310)

FIGURE 7.23   Same case as in Figure 7.22, showing focal interstitial nephritis with mononuclear cells infiltrates, tubular necrosis, erythrocytes, and hyaline casts in the tubular lumens. (H & E × 235)

7.21

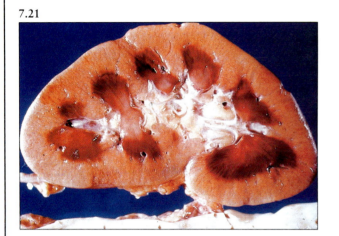

7.22

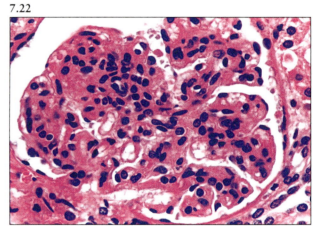

7.23

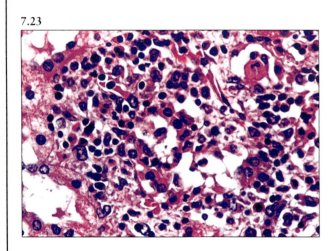

DENGUE HEMORRHAGIC FEVER

FIGURE 7.24   Immunofluorescence microscopy showing deposits of IgG in the glomerular mesangial areas. (× 235)

VIRAL HEPATITIS

FIGURE 7.25   Chronic infection with hepatitis B virus. Membranous glomerulonephritis with marked thickening of capillary walls and some increase in mesangial matrix. (PAS × 295)

FIGURE 7.26   Hepatitis B and nephrotic syndrome in an 11-year-old girl from Cameroon, Africa. This glomerulus shows moderate mesangial expansion and slight capillary wall thickening. (PAS stain of an Epon section × 235)

7.24

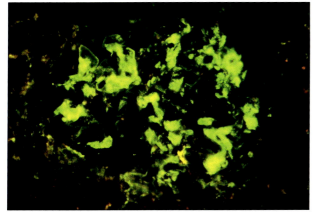

7.25

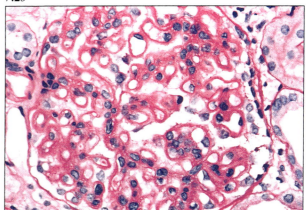

7.26

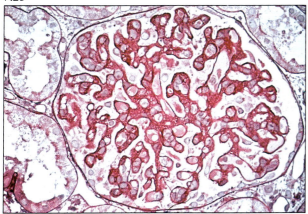

VIRAL HEPATITIS

FIGURE 7.27 Hepatitis B associated with membranous glomerulonephritis. There are diffuse thickening of basement membrane and subepithelial spikes. (PASM × 470)

FIGURE 7.28 Immunofluorescence microscopy. Same case as in Figure 7.25. There are extensive granular deposits of HBeAg, mainly along the glomerular capillary walls. (× 235)

FIGURE 7.29 Immunofluorescence microscopy. Same case as in Figure 7.27. Extensive granular deposits of HBeAg, mainly along the glomerular capillary walls. (× 235)

7.27

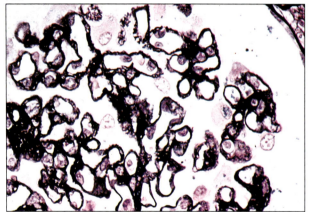

7.28

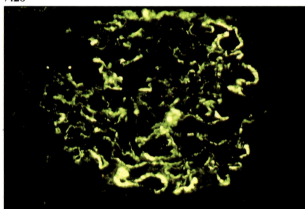

7.29

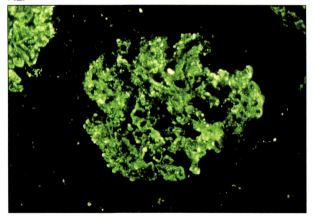

FIGURE 7.30 Electron micrograph. Same case as in Figure 7.25. Many subepithelial deposits, "spikes" of basement membrane, and widespread loss of epithelial foot processes. (× 5,000)

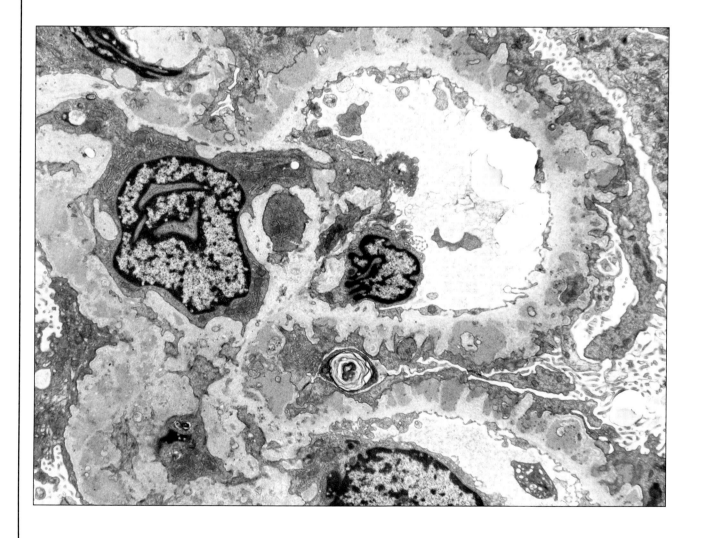

VIRAL HEPATITIS

FIGURE 7.31   Electron micrograph. Viral hepatitis. Multiple subepithelial, intramembranous, and mesangial deposits together with mesangial interposition (arrowhead). Red blood cells and a platelet are seen in the capillary lumen. (× 5,000)

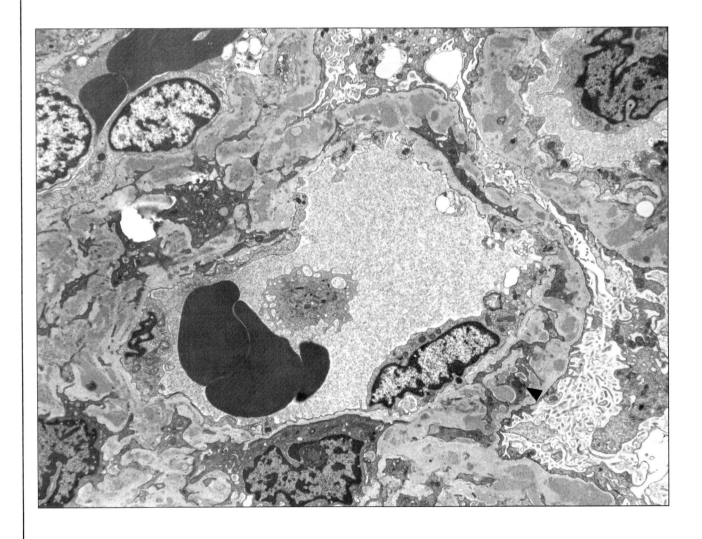

MIXED CRYOGLOBULINEMIA

FIGURE 7.32 Electron micrograph. Viral hepatitis associated with chronic mixed cryoglobulinemia. Glomerular capillary wall with subendothelial and mesangial deposits, apparently consisting of fibrils or "tubules." (× 32,800) *Inset*: Cryoglobulin deposit from another case of viral hepatitis, stained with lead only. The "tubular" structure is more distinct. (× 47,000)

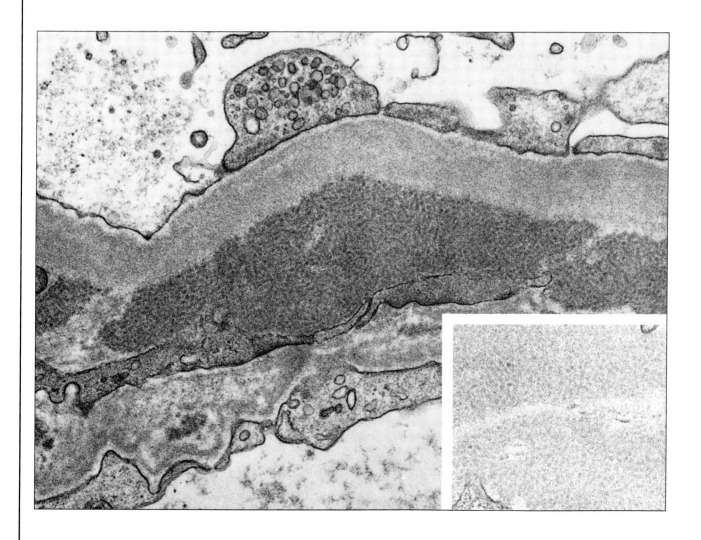

POLYARTERITIS NODOSA

FIGURE 7.33 Viral hepatitis associated with microscopic polyarteritis. Acute stage. Glomerular tuft is partly destroyed by fibrinoid necrosis. (H & E × 190)

FIGURE 7.34 Viral hepatitis associated with classic polyarteritis nodosa. Acute stage. Whole circumference of an interlobular artery is destroyed and replaced by "fibrinoid." The vessel is surrounded by chronic inflammatory cells. (H & E × 50)

FIGURE 7.35 Same case as in Figure 7.34, showing interruption of internal elastic lamina and mural thrombus in part of wall of interlobular artery destroyed by polyarteritis. (Elastica × 190)

7.33

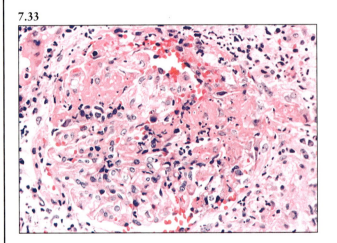

7.34

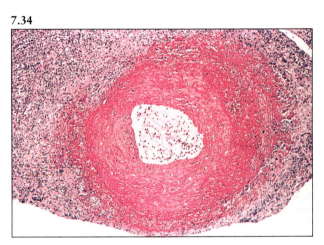

7.35

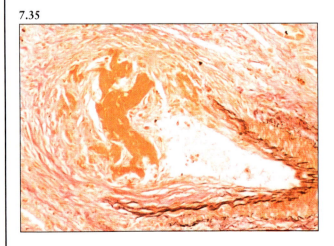

Polyarteritis Nodosa

FIGURE 7.36 Immunofluorescence microscopy. Viral hepatitis associated with classic polyarteritis. Granular deposits of HBs antibody in the wall of an artery. (× 190)

FIGURE 7.37 Immunofluorescence microscopy. Same case as in Figure 7.36. Deposits of immunoglobin (IgM) in the wall of an artery. (× 190)

AIDS Virus (HIV-3)

FIGURE 7.38 Portion of kidney showing massive cast formation in dilated tubules. (PAS × 95)

7.36

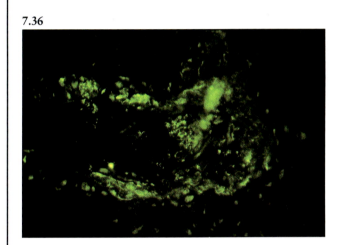

7.37

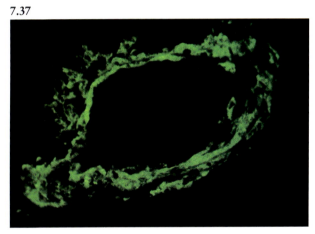

7.38

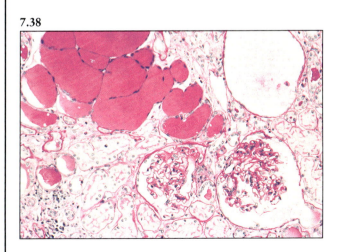

AIDS Virus (HIV-3)

FIGURE 7.39 Glomerulus with segmental sclerosis. There are several clearly defined sclerotic segments with overlying enlarged visceral epithelial cells. (Masson's trichrome × 190)

FIGURE 7.40 Several clusters of *Mycobacterium avium* within interstitial cells. (Ziehl-Neelsen × 380)

FIGURE 7.41 Immunofluorescence microscopy. IgM in a segmental, mesangial, and capillary wall distribution in glomerulus from same biopsy specimen as in Figure 7.38. (× 235)

FIGURE 7.42 Numerous reabsorption droplets within tubular epithelial cells and within a single glomerular visceral epithelial cell. (Anti-albumin antiserum × 140)

7.39

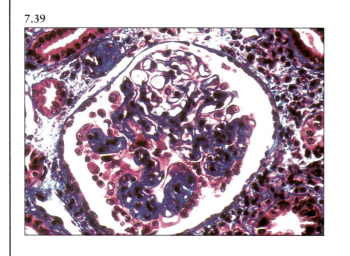

7.40

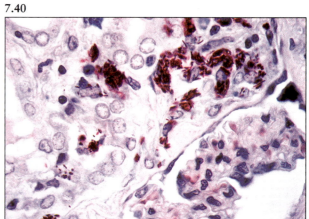

7.41

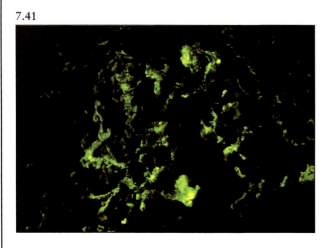

7.42

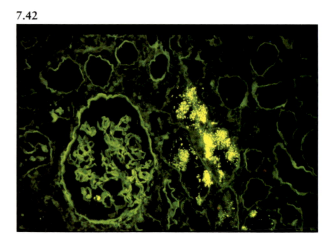

AIDS Virus (HIV-3)

FIGURE 7.43 Electron micrograph. Portion of glomerulus with complete effacement of foot processes of epithelial cells. A small electron-dense deposit is present within the mesangium (arrow). (× 5,000). Inset: Higher magnification of a part of the endothelial cell, disclosing a cluster of tubuloreticular structures (arrowhead). (× 20,000)

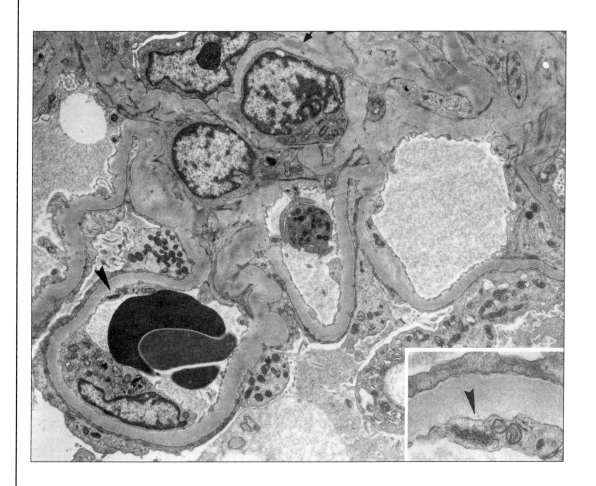

Varicella

FIGURE 7.44   Varicella. There is diffuse endocapillary proliferative glomerulonephritis with polymorphs and monocytes, and partial occlusion of glomerular capillaries. (H & E × 235)

Cytomegalovirus

FIGURE 7.45   Cytomegalovirus infection. Infection of the tubular epithelial cells is indicated by abundant large intranuclear and intracytoplasmic inclusions. (H & E × 310)

FIGURE 7.46   A focus of interstitial inflammation and a large cell with intranuclear and intracytoplasmic inclusions. (H & E × 760)

7.44

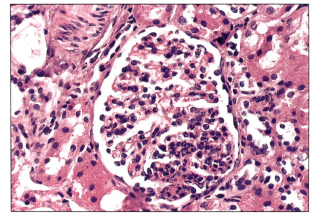

7.45

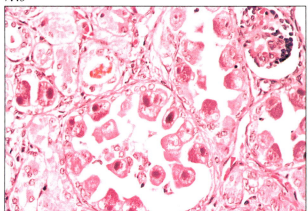

7.46

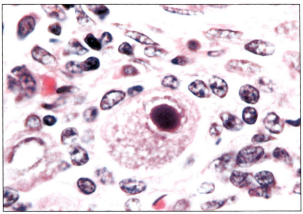

ADENOVIRUS

FIGURE 7.47 Disseminated adenovirus infection in a bone marrow transplant recipient. The kidney shows foci of tubular necrosis and interstitial inflammation. Some of the surviving cells contain large intranuclear inclusions. (H & E × 235)

FIGURE 7.48 Indirect immunofluorescence microscopy, showing tubular localization of viral antigen (adenovirus 35) as bright-green particles that can be differentiated from yellow-orange autofluorescence of necrotic epithelium. (FITC × 120)

7.47

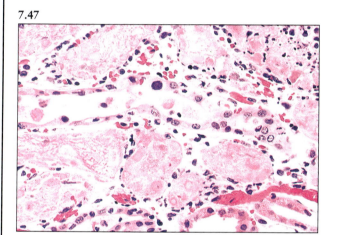

7.48

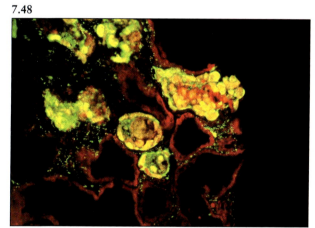

RICKETTSIAL INFECTIONS

ROCKY MOUNTAIN SPOTTED FEVER

Rocky mountain spotted fever (RMSF) is a tick-borne infection caused by *Rickettsia rickettsii*. A number of place names have been given to these diseases in North and South America.

Clinical and Pathologic Manifestations

The incubation period is 10 to 14 days and is followed by severe headaches, generalized aching, and pyrexia of up to 40°C (104°F), lasting for 10 to 14 days before subsiding in patients who recover. The highest incidence of RMSF is in children, but it occurs in all age groups. The characteristic rash develops first on the wrists and ankles; later spreads to the back, arms, legs, chest, and abdomen; and often involves the face, palms, and soles. A history of tick contact or tick bite may be obtained in about 75 percent of cases. Untreated cases have a 20 to 30 percent mortality; when patients are treated with antibiotics, the mortality is relatively low (3%–10%). In some cases severe renal involvement occurs.

The essential pathologic lesion in RMSF is a generalized vasculitis of small blood vessels due to multiplication of rickettsiae in endothelial cells. Thrombi develop, mainly in the capillaries of the brain, skin, subcutaneous tissues, and heart. Patients may die of encephalitis or myocarditis. Renal function may also be impaired, and patients may die of shock-like syndrome and disseminated intravascular coagulation. The blood volume reduction is due to severe dehydration and increased capillary permeability with edema and effusions into body cavities. There is marked hyponatremia and reduction in blood platelets to below 200,000/cu mm. Diagnostic tests are the Weil-Felix agglutination test, demonstration of antirickettsial IgG antibody titers, and localization of *R. rickettsii* in skin and blood vessels, using specific antiserum against the pathogen.

Light Microscopic Findings. Predominantly, there is nonglomerular injury in RMSF. The abnormalities involve the vessels, interstitium, glomeruli, or renal tubules. The renal vessels show vasculitis and fibrinoid necrosis. The perivascular infiltrates are lymphocytes or mixed inflammatory infiltrates. The renal arterial vessels may show "flotillas" of several *R. rickettsii* arranged parallel along the long axis of the endothelial cells; these are best demonstrated by the Brown-Hopps stain. The glomeruli may show polymorphonuclear neutrophil infiltrations and focal or segmental necrosis of glomerular capillary loops. Some cases may show extensive fibrin deposition in glomerular capillary loops consistent with disseminated intravascular coagulation. There are foci of interstitial edema and interstitial lymphocytic cellular infiltrations; there may also be foci of acute tubular necrosis and hemoglobinuric casts.

Electron Microscopic Findings. There is segmental

swelling of the lamina rara interna of the glomerular basement membrane. Fibrin deposits within glomerular capillary loops nearly occlude the lumen. There is some increase in mesangial matrix; the visceral epithelial cells may be enlarged and the foot processes effaced. No electron-dense deposits are seen in the capillary loops or in the mesangium.

Immunomicroscopic Findings. There are no glomerular or vascular deposits of immunoglobulins, complement, or fibrin-fibrinogen, except in patients with disseminated intravascular coagulation, who show fibrin in the capillary lumen and mesangium. The renal lesion in RMSF is apparently due to direct action of the organism on the vessel wall, not to immune complex–mediated disease.

EPIDEMIC TYPHUS

Epidemic typhus is a louse-borne fever caused by *Rickettsia prowazekii*. Epidemics are caused by overcrowding and cold climate, especially in the Soviet Union and eastern Europe. Between 1918 and 1922, there were three million deaths in eastern Europe. Several outbreaks occurred during World War II but were rapidly controlled by delousing with DDT and vaccination of contacts. Glomerular and tubulointerstitial renal lesions are known to occur.

Clinical and Pathologic Manifestations

The clinical picture is similar to that of Rocky Mountain spotted fever. However, in this disease the macular or maculopapular rash appears on the back and chest; then spreads to the abdomen but spares the face, palms, and soles. Patients may die of encephalitis, myocarditis, or pneumonitis; and renal function may be impaired. Those who recover have no serious sequelae. Early treatment with tetracycline drugs or chloramphenicol is effective, and those who have been vaccinated have mild infection.

Light Microscopic Findings. Glomerular injury and focal interstitial nephritis are severe in those who die from renal failure. There is vasculitis of renal vessels,

which contain *R. prowazekii* in the endothelial cells. Fibrinous thrombi are present in the capillaries, with necrosis of glomerular lobular tufts. Focal collections of mononuclear cells in the interstitium often form nodules around small blood vessels; these are called typhus nodules.

SCRUB TYPHUS

This mite-borne infectious disease is caused by *Rickettsia tsutsugamushi*. The disease is characterized by fever, a primary lesion, rash, and lymphadenopathy. Proteinuria and renal failure may occur.

Clinical and Pathologic Manifestations

Following an incubation period of 6 to 20 days, the onset of the disease is usually abrupt, with fever, chills, headache, and generalized lymphadenopathy. An eschar lesion is seen at the site of the chigger bite. A macular rash develops on the trunk 5 to 8 days after the beginning of fever. Splenomegaly may be present, and myocarditis may occur. The fever lasts for 2 weeks. Mild proteinuria with urinary sediment changes can be observed during the febrile period. Mild renal failure may occur. Intravascular hemolysis has been noted in patients with G6PD deficiency.

Light Microscopic Findings. In most cases the glomerular changes are mild, with slight mesangial hypertrophy. However, diffuse proliferative glomerulonephritis has occasionally been reported. Platelet thrombi in the glomeruli and focal thickening of the basement membrane have been seen. In patients with acute renal failure, tubulointerstitial changes are observed. There are tubular degeneration and necrosis, especially in the proximal tubules, with focal interstitial infiltration with mononuclear cells. The interlobar veins may be inflamed.

Immunomicroscopic Findings. There are fine, granular deposits of IgM and C3 in mesangial areas of the glomeruli.

ROCKY MOUNTAIN SPOTTED FEVER

FIGURE 8.1   Transmission cycle of spotted fever Rickettsiae.

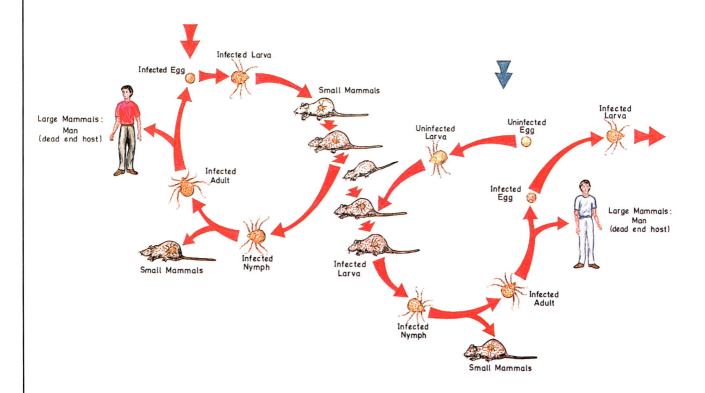

ROCKY MOUNTAIN SPOTTED FEVER

FIGURE 8.2   Rocky mountain spotted fever. Vasculitis involves an interlobular artery, with surrounding tubulointerstitial nephritis. (H & E × 140)

FIGURE 8.3   There are extensive fibrin thrombi within the capillary lumens and segmental necrosis of the glomerular tuft. (H & E × 380)

FIGURE 8.4   Rocky mountain spotted fever. Hemoglobinuric nephrosis. Hemoglobin cast in the tubular lumen. (H & E × 105)

FIGURE 8.5   High-power view of endothelial cells, with "flotilla" of *Rickettsia rickettsii* parallel to the long axis of the cell. (Brown-Hopps × 685)

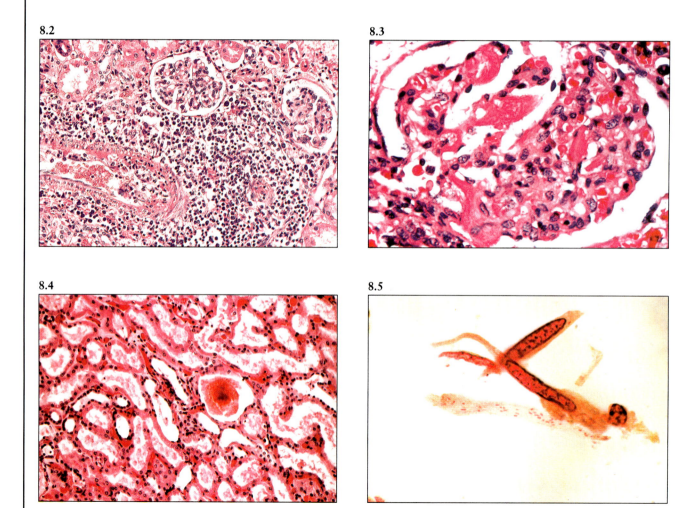

ROCKY MOUNTAIN SPOTTED FEVER

FIGURE 8.6   Electron micrograph of rickettsiae in the cytoplasm of cultured endothelial cells (to the right of the nucleus). (× 6,100)

FIGURE 8.7   Rickettsiae in the nucleus of endothelial cells. Same specimen as in Figure 8.6. (× 10,800)

8.6

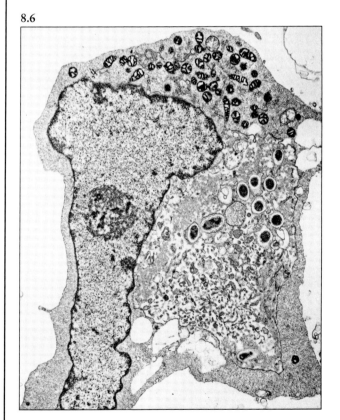

8.7

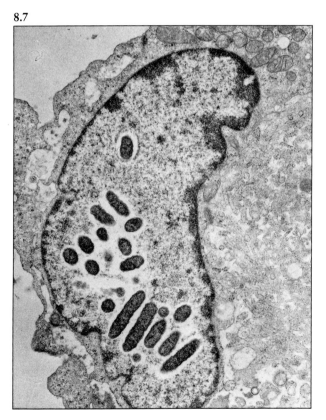

Rocky Mountain Spotted Fever

FIGURE 8.8 Electron micrograph. The glomerular capillary loop is nearly occluded by fibrin deposits and swollen cells. (× 8,000)

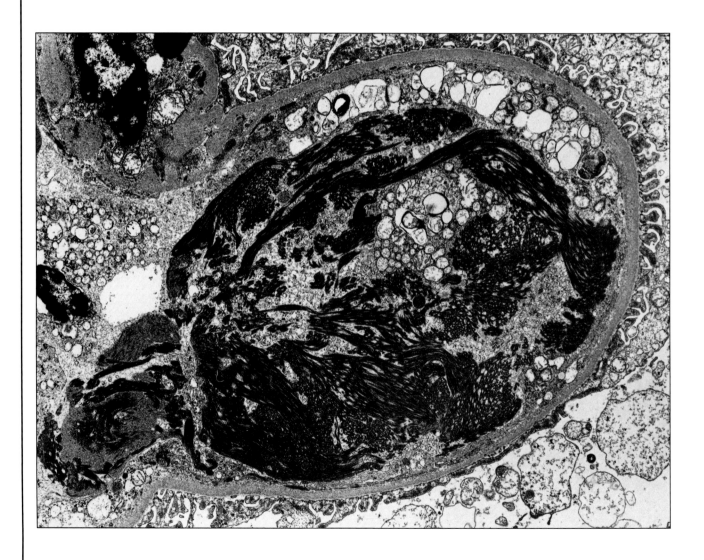

SPIROCHETE INFECTIONS

LEPTOSPIROSIS

Leptospirosis is an infectious disease caused by the pathogenic species called *Leptospira interrogans*. These organisms comprise over 100 subspecies, including *L. icterohemorrhagiae, L. canicola, L. pomona, L. batavia*. The disease is characterized by fever, chills, muscular pains, conjuctivitis, and jaundice. The kidney is invariably involved, and renal failure may occur. Weil's disease is characterized by renal failure and jaundice.

Leptospira enter the host through abrasions in the skin or through the intact mucous membrane. Infection can also occur through the intestinal mucosa when food contaminated with leptospira is ingested. The leptospira are transported through the bloodstream to various organs, and after 48 hours the organisms can be detected in any tissue. Leptospira disappear from the blood after the rise in serum agglutinin. Leptospiruria is present for 1 to 4 weeks.

Clinical and Pathologic Manifestations

The common symptoms are fever, chills, conjunctivitis, headache, muscular pains, and jaundice. The onset is sudden following an incubation period of 7 to 12 days. The symptoms vary with the number of organisms and with host factors. In mild form the disease may present with fever and can be diagnosed only by serologic tests.

Urinary sediment changes are often observed, and mild proteinuria may be present. Granular casts, micro-hematuria, and leucocyturia are usually seen; and bile and heme casts may be demonstrable. These urinary changes clear up when the disease is under control. Leptospira can be found by dark-field microscopy, and fluorescent techniques can be used to detect leptospira in the urine and tissues.

Renal failure in various forms is present in 20 to 67 percent of cases. In most patients it is anicteric, mild in degree, often nonoliguric, of short duration, and may be prerenal. Renal failure with jaundice is a severe form of infection, generally known as Weil's disease. Any serotype of leptospira with severe infection can cause this syndrome. Renal failure is often catabolic in type, with a rapid rise of serum creatinine and blood urea nitrogen levels. Hyperkalemia, hyperphosphatemia, and hyperuricemia may be observed. Renal failure can be very severe when associated with hyperbilirubinemia over 25 mg/dL. Rarely, hemolytic-uremic syndrome may be observed.

Macroscopic Findings. The kidneys are grossly enlarged and tense. Hemorrhages may be present in the subcapsular and intraparenchymal tissues.

Light Microscopic Findings. The striking renal lesions in the biopsy specimens obtained during the second, third, and fourth weeks of disease are the tubulointerstitial changes, which are diffuse in both cortical and medullary tissues. The interstitial infiltrates consist of mononuclear cells, mostly lymphocytes, plasma cells, macrophages, and eosinophils. These inflammatory cells may destroy the tubular basement membrane and penetrate into the tubules. Some short segments of tubules show epithelial degeneration, necrosis, and desquamation. Heme and bile casts may be seen in the tubular lumens. Inflammatory cell infiltration into a few sclerotic and nonsclerotic glomeruli is occasionally observed. Otherwise, most of the glomeruli show no specific alteration except for mild irregular mesangial cell proliferation.

Electron Microscopic Findings.   Focal widening of foot processes and focal thickening of glomerular basement membranes are noted. Pseudovilli, representing the long projections of the visceral epithelial cells into the urinary spaces, are seen. Fibrin deposits may be noted occasionally in the paramesangial areas.

The most common ultrastructural changes in the tubules are loosening and disruption of the folded basement membrane, with occasional separation of the epithelial lining of proximal, distal, and collecting tubules. Among such changes are necrosis of some epithelial cells. Intact leptospira may be detected in tubular lumens and peritubular capillaries. Severe interstitial edema with lymphocyte, plasma cell, and mononuclear phagocytic cell infiltration is usually observed.

Vascular changes include swelling and vacuolation of the endothelial cells. Endothelial necrosis is observed in the peritubular capillaries.

Immunomicroscopic Findings.   Granular antigens of leptospira are seen in the interstitium around the tubules. Immunoglobulins are usually not detected in the glomeruli or tubules, although occasionally glomerular deposition of IgM may be noted. Trace amounts of C3 appear as fine, granular deposits in some glomeruli and/or arteriolar walls.

RELAPSING FEVER

Glomerular and tubulointerstitial changes are associated with a louse-borne and tick-borne acute febrile illness caused by diverse strains of spirochaetes of the *Borrelia* genus.

Borrelia spirochetes are thicker and less regularly curved than the treponemes. The louse-borne form of the disease is caused by *Borrelia recurrentis*, and the tick-transmitted form by any of eight different spirochetes of the *Borrelia* genus, including *Borrelia duttoni*. Relapsing fever due to *B. recurrentis* is transmitted from man to man by the body louse *Pediculus humanus* var. *corporis*. The organisms are taken up when the louse feeds on the host's blood, pass through the louse stomach wall, and multiply in the tissues. They infect man only when the louse is crushed on the skin. The organism can penetrate intact skin and mucous membranes.

The tick-borne form is different. It is transmitted by bites of various species of soft ticks of the genus *Ornithodorus*. *Borrelia* multiply in the salivary glands of the soft ticks, and infected saliva enters the host when the tick is feeding. In central, eastern, and southern Africa, man is the reservoir of tick-borne relapsing fever; elsewhere it is primarily a disease of animals, transmitted only incidentally to man. Animal hosts include monkeys, squirrels, chipmunks, rats, and hedgehogs.

Clinical and Pathologic Manifestations

Louse-borne relapsing fever is largely a disease of people living in squalor. It is particularly prevalent in Ethiopia but occurs in many parts of the world and may become epidemic in conditions of famine when people crowd together in search of food. Tick-borne relapsing fever tends to be sporadic and is found in the Near East, the southern Soviet Union, Spain, northern Africa, Israel, Africa south of the Sahara, western and southern United States, and Central and South America. After an incubation period of 2 to 10 days the onset is sudden, with high fever and severe malaise. Jaundice, splenomegaly, and petechiae are common. In the tick-borne form, there may be serious central nervous system complications. Proteinuria and mild impairment of renal function are common but usually transient. Microscopic hematuria is found in some patients, and massive hematuria in a few. The attack commonly lasts 5 to 7 days, and the temperature then drops dramatically. Relapse often occurs 5 to 9 days later and is less severe. There are often five to eight relapses of diminishing severity. About 10 percent of patients die in the first attack of hemorrhage, hepatic coma, myocarditis, and disseminated intravascular coagulation. During acute attacks, the organism can be found in the blood and cerebrospinal fluid by direct staining methods.

Macroscopic Findings.   In about half the cases, the kidneys are enlarged. Petechial hemorrhages are common. Complicating septicemia, particularly salmonella infection, may cause abscesses in the cortex.

Light Microscopic Findings. The glomeruli often appear normal. Sometimes there is an increase in the number of mesangial cells and swelling of the endothelial cells. Fibrin thrombi are often seen in a few capillary loops. In untreated patients, spirochetes can be demonstrated in the capillary lumens. The tubules contain occasional protein and red cell casts. Spirochetes are often present in these casts. More severe cases are associated with the changes of acute tubular necrosis and focal interstitial inflammation. The extent and distribution of tubular damage and regeneration depends upon the time the tissue was taken in relation to the onset of shock.

Electron Microscopic Findings. Spirochetes may be seen in the glomerular capillary lumens or in tubular casts. Other changes are nonspecific.

Immunomicroscopic Findings. No deposits of immunoglobulins or complement components have been seen. Fibrinogen is often detected in glomerular capillary loops.

Treponematoses

These infections include syphilis, yaws, and pinta. Renal lesions have been described only in syphilis. Accurate data concerning the incidence of syphilis is hard to come by, but this disease is clearly a persistent problem.

Glomerular disease accompanies syphilis in its congenital, secondary, and latent forms. It occurs in a minority of patients and is reversed by treatment of the *Treponema pallidum* infection. The main histologic change is diffuse membranous glomerulonephritis. Interstitial nephritis and gummata are not commonly found.

T. pallidum is a small, thin, tightly coiled spirochete with 8 to 14 close, regular spirals and ends that are drawn out into extremely fine fibrils. The organism moves slowly and flexes slightly. Silver impregnation methods render the organism thick and black against a yellowish background. The spirochete dies quickly outside the body because it is very sensitive to drying, cooling, changes in osmotic pressure, pH levels, and standard disinfectants. Soap and other detergents quickly destroy it. *T. pallidum* enters the body through the skin or mucous membranes. Most often it is acquired vener-

ally, but any close contact between an infected lesion and a break in the skin may lead to transmission of the disease. It can also be transmitted by blood transfusions when the blood has been refrigerated for less than 3 days, and a woman may transmit syphilis to her child if she has the disease at the time of conception or acquires it during pregnancy.

Clinical and Pathologic Manifestations

Syphilis progresses through primary, secondary, and latent phases. In about two thirds of untreated patients no other manifestations develop; but in about one third lesions of tertiary syphilis occur, usually after many years. Fetal infections are referred to as congenital syphilis. The protean manifestations of syphilis are legendary, and the kidney may be affected in all these stages. Renal involvement usually presents as proteinuria with or without nephrotic syndrome, usually in the secondary stage or in congenital infection. The proteinuria is often accompanied by microscopic hematuria. Rarely, the first manifestation is acute nephritic syndrome. Renal function is generally normal. Complement components of the classical pathway are often depressed in congenital syphilis but rarely in the other stages. Circulating immune complexes are present.

Macroscopic Findings. The kidneys may be enlarged and pale in nephrotic patients, and gummata have occasionally been found in late cases.

Light Microscopic Findings. In some cases there are very few changes. In others there may be proliferative lesions with an increased number of mesangial cells, endothelial swelling, and infiltration by polymorphs. Cellular crescents may occur in some cases, and rarely as an extensive lesion of the glomeruli. The common lesion in both adults and infants is thickening of the glomerular capillary walls, with characteristics of membranous nephropathy. In babies with congenital syphilis, membranous nephropathy and tubulointerstitial nephritis may occur together. The interstitium is edematous and contains mononuclear cells and polymorphs when the glomeruli show proliferative activity. The tubules and blood vessels are generally normal. Stillborn fetuses usually manifest interstitial nephritis and miliary gummata. Large numbers of spirochetes are present in the interstitium, tubular cells, and tubular lumens. In the tertiary stage, tubular damage and focal infiltration of the interstitium by predominantly plasma cells is found in about 17 percent of cases at necropsy. Spirochetes have not been demonstrated in these lesions.

Electron Microscopic Findings. Scattered electron dense-deposits are present on the subepithelial aspects of the glomerular capillary basement membranes. The deposits are usually small and discrete (ie, stage I). Rarely, there are also subendothelial deposits.

Immunomicroscopic Findings. Fine granular deposits of IgG, C3, and, occasionally, IgM are usually present on all the glomerular capillary membranes and often in the mesangium. Treponemal antigen and antibodies against this antigen have been demonstrated in several cases. The deposits disappear after antisyphilitic therapy, but sometimes some distortion of the lamina densa persists.

LEPTOSPIROSIS

FIGURE 9.1   The kidney is grossly enlarged and tense, and shows intraparenchymal hemorrhages (fixed specimen).

FIGURE 9.2   Low magnification of medulla showing diffuse interstitial inflammation. (H & E × 60)

FIGURE 9.3   There is marked interstitial, predominantly mononuclear inflammation. Some tubules are dilated and show epithelial degeneration and necrosis, with heme and bile casts in the lumens. (H & E × 235)

FIGURE 9.4   Immunofluorescence microscopy, showing interstitial cells that bear leptospira antigen. Antileptospiral (serovar bataviae) antibody. (× 590)

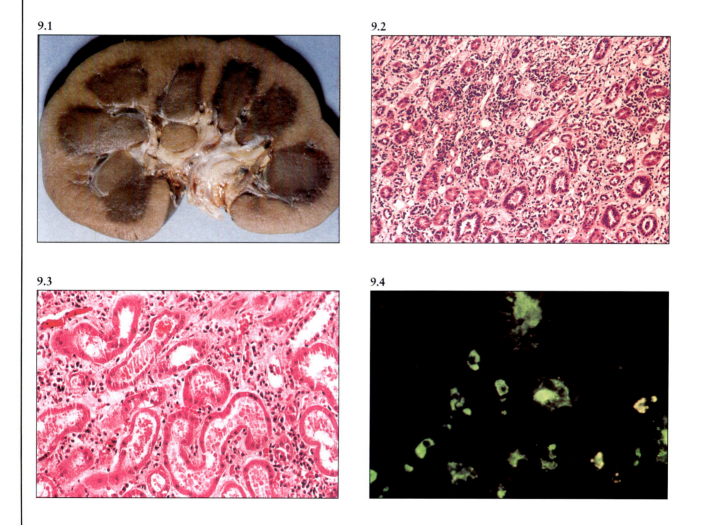

9.1

9.2

9.3

9.4

LEPTOSPIROSIS

FIGURE 9.5   Electron micrograph of proximal tubule, showing disruption of the in-folded basilar membrane and detachment of cell from the tubular basement membrane. Cross-section of a leptospira is in the lumen of a peritubular capillary (arrow). (× 4,100)

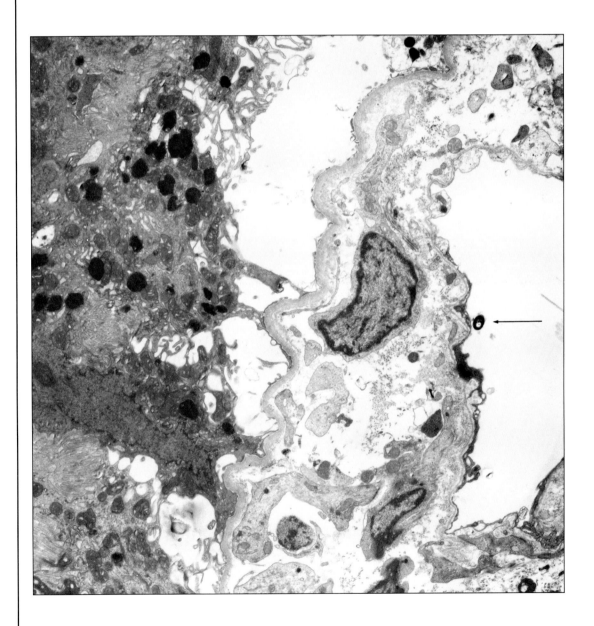

LEPTOSPIROSIS

FIGURE 9.6 Leptospira in a tubular lumen. ($\times$ 34,000)

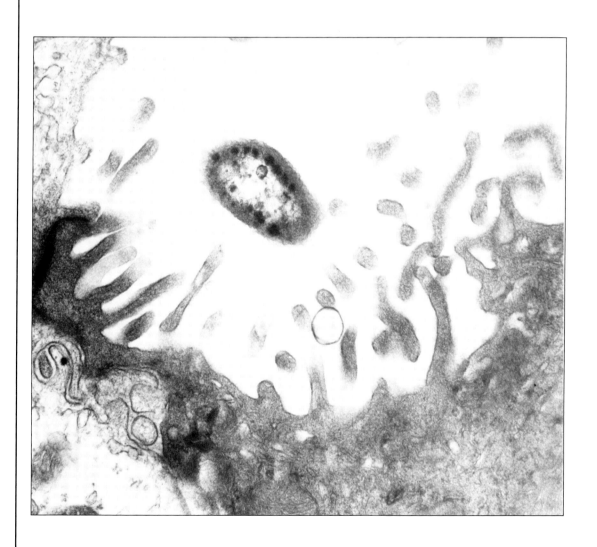

RELAPSING FEVER

FIGURE 9.7 Relapsing fever. Borrelia spirochetes can be seen in the blood film, which was taken before treatment was started. The renal biopsy came later and the organisms were not demonstrable in this tissue. (Giemsa × 825)

FIGURE 9.8 Relapsing fever. Marked acute tubular damage with widespread edema, inflammation, and congestion of peritubular capillaries. (H & E × 120)

FIGURE 9.9 Dilatation of the tubules, with epithelial damage and regeneration. Many of the tubular lumens contain protein and red cell casts. (H & E × 120)

9.7

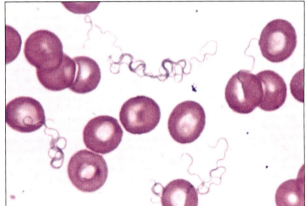

9.8

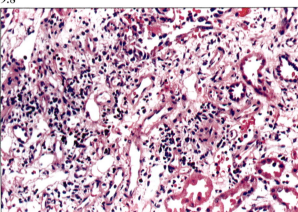

9.9

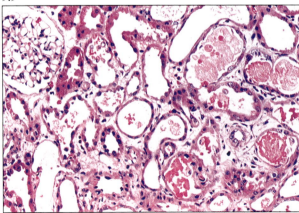

TREPONEMATOSES

FIGURE 9.10 Syphilis in young adult. Membranous glomerulonephritis with diffuse thickening of glomerular capillary walls and normal tuft cellularity. (H & E × 295)

FIGURE 9.11 Nephrotic syndrome in an infant with congenital syphilis. The glomerulus shows a very slight increase in the number of mesangial cells. The podocytes are prominent but perhaps no more so than in any infant of similar age. (H & E × 235)

FIGURE 9.12 Congenital syphilis in a child with nephrotic syndrome. The capillary loops show subepithelial spikes and widening of the mesangium by matrix and mild mesangial hypercellularity. (PASM × 380)

FIGURE 9.13 Congenital syphilis. There is interstitial nephritis with mononuclear, predominantly plasma cell, infiltrates. (H & E × 120)

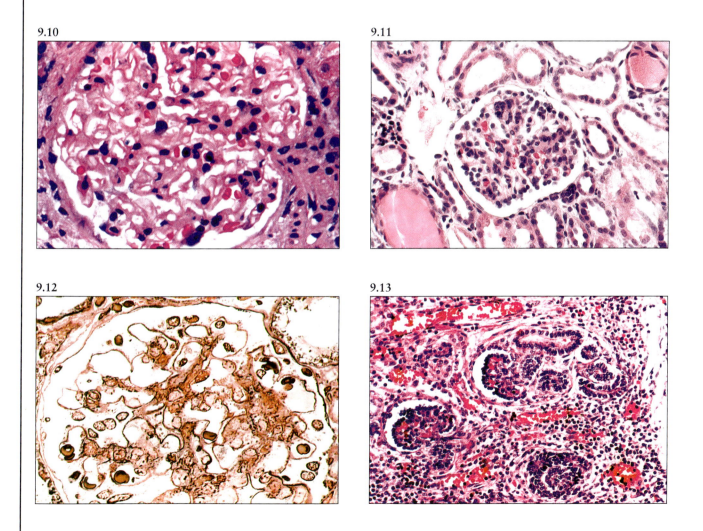

TREPONEMATOSES

FIGURE 9.14   Syphilis. Gumma in the kidney. (H & E × 30)

FIGURE 9.15   Syphilis. Same case as in Figure 9.14, showing heavy plasma cell infiltrates in the wall of the gumma. (H & E stain × 190)

FIGURE 9.16   Same case as in Figure 9.10, showing fine granular IgG deposits in capillary walls and mesangium. (Immunoperoxidase × 235)

9.14

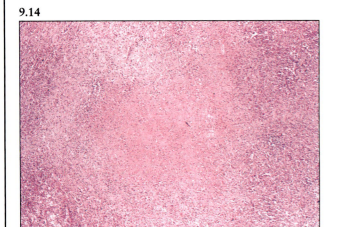

9.15

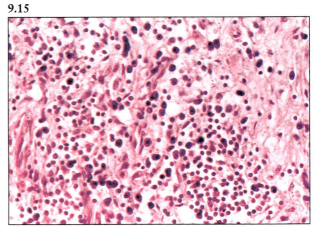

9.16

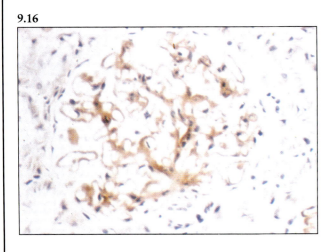

Treponematoses

FIGURE 9.17   Electron micrograph. Same case as in Figure 9.10. Numerous subepithelial deposits.
(× 16,200)

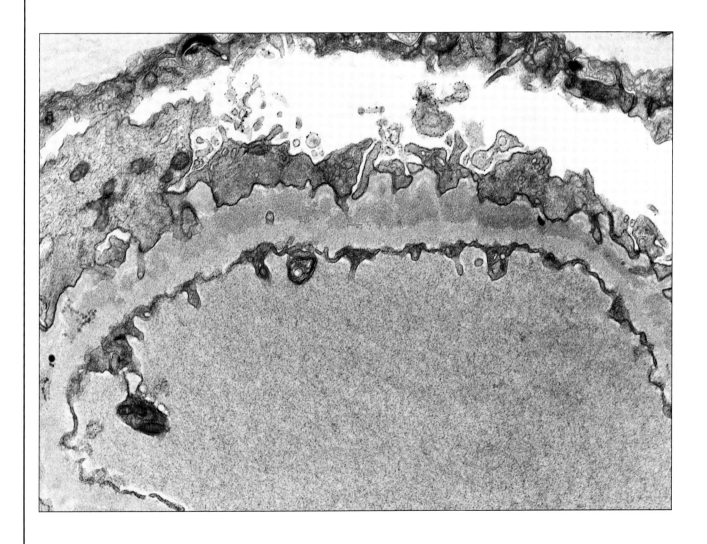

BACTERIAL INFECTIONS

ENTERIC INFECTIONS

A wide range of Gram-negative bacilli (Enterobacteraciae) normally inhabit the gut. Enteric fever and gastroenteritis syndromes are caused by pathogens such as Salmonella, Shigella, Campylobacter, Yersinia, Vibrio, and pathogenic *Escherichia coli*. Renal involvement may be seen with some of these organisms.

SALMONELLOSIS

Salmonellae are motile, Gram-negative, non–spore-forming straight bacilli that are aerobic and facultative anaerobes.

Salmonella may be classified into three primary species based upon their clinical presentation. These include the enteric fever group (*S. typhi, S. paratyphi* A, *S. schottmuelleri* (paratyphi B), *S. hirschfeldi* (paratyphi C); *S. choleraesuis*, which causes mainly bacteremia or focal infection; and the gastroenteritis group designated *S. enteritidis* subspecies *typhimurium, enteritidis*, etc, which encompasses most of the more than 1,800 species and serotypes described to date. The organisms multiply in the gut and invade the intestinal mucosa of the ileum and colon, causing localized gastroenteritis and bacteremia. The most important animal reservoirs are poultry, pigs, cows, rats, and various pets such as dogs, cats, and budgerigars. Consuming contaminated food or water is the usual method of infection. In severe extraintestinal

salmonellosis, acute tubular necrosis may occur; and less frequently microabscesses may form within the renal parenchyma.

TYPHOID FEVER

Clinical and Pathologic Manifestations

After the incubation period of 1 to 2 weeks, the disease manifests as fever with headache and abdominal pain, malaise, and either constipation or diarrhea. Fever accompanied by signs of toxemia lasts for 4 weeks in untreated cases. The spleen is often enlarged.

Renal manifestations consist of mild urinary sediment changes with proteinuria, erythrocyturia, and leukocyturia. These changes are transient and disappear when the disease is under control. The patient may be hyponatremic but without any evidence of hypovolemia. Classic signs of acute glomerulonephritis are usually absent. Acute renal failure may be observed with severe infection. Jaundice usually accompanies renal failure, which may be catabolic in nature, with a rapid rise in serum creatinine and blood urea nitrogen levels. Yet renal failure may be nonoliguric. Hemoglobinuria may be observed, especially when associated with intravascular hemolysis due to glucose-6-phosphate dehydrogenase deficiency. Rarely, myoglobinuria may occur. Disseminated intravascular coagulation has been reported. Recovery of renal function is usually complete, except in patients with severe renal failure.

Light Microscopic Findings. In biopsy specimens, all glomeruli are enlarged. Mesangial matrix and mesangial cells are focally increased. The glomerular capillary walls are normal. In severe infection, there are focal tubulointerstitial lesions in cortical tissue, which appear as short segments of tubules showing degeneration, necrosis, and regeneration. These tubules are surrounded by lymphocytes, plasma cells, and mononuclear phagocytes. Some of these cells infiltrate into the necrotic tubules. In cases of acute renal failure, there are acute tubular necrosis with interstitial edema and cellular infiltrations. In some patients, bacterial pyelonephritis may occur in the septicemic phase. Abscess may be present in the cortex.

Electron Microscopic Findings. The characteristic feature is enlargement of the mesangium due mainly to increased mesangial matrix. Electron-dense deposits in paramesangial areas are more prominent in patients with IgA deposition. Mesangial cell proliferation is rare. Some capillaries may contain mononuclear phagocytes and debris of necrotic cells of unknown origin. Occasionally, thickened lamina rara interna due to deposits of granular material is seen. In other salmonelloses, there may be secondary lesions due to dehydration, electrolyte loss, and shock. In septicemic conditions, there may be multiple small abscesses.

Immunomicroscopic Findings. Typically, there are granular deposits of IgM and traces of IgG and C3 in the mesangial areas and along some capillary walls. Salmonella Vi antigen is detectable in certain glomeruli. There are no deposits of immune complexes in the tubules.

Interestingly, in a smaller group of patients there is dense granular IgA in mesangial areas, usually accompanied by lesser amounts of IgM and C3. Vi antigen may be demonstrated in some cases.

SHIGELLOSIS

The shigellae are a group of Gram-negative enteric bacilli producing a clinical syndrome known as bacillary dysentery. The hemolytic-uremic syndrome following dysentery caused by *Shigella dysenteriae* type 1 has been reported. The prominent glomerular change is thrombotic microangiopathy.

Clinical and Pathologic Manifestations

In a study of a large patient group from Bangladesh, there were four types of clinical presentations in shigellosis. The first type, uncomplicated shigellosis, occurred in both children and adults who had only mild to moderately severe colitis. The second type was shigellosis with leukemoid reaction, with white cell counts over 50,000 per cu mm. This type was found only in children. The third type occurred in children who developed hemolysis and renal insufficiency. The fourth type had complications of hemolytic-uremic syndrome (HUS). Circulating endotoxin was detected in all HUS cases tested.

Light Microscopic Findings. Necropsy renal specimens from children with shigellosis who died of HUS showed cortical necrosis and extensive glomerular thrombosis with or without arterial thrombosis. Patients without HUS showed only widening of mesangial areas with a trace of fibrin thrombi in the glomeruli. Mononuclear leukocytes in glomerular capillary and arterial lumens were prominent in some cases.

Electron Microscopic Findings. Some capillary lumens contain fibrin, distorted erythrocytes, platelets, and neutrophils. Electron-dense deposits in mesangial areas were occasionally seen.

Immunomicroscopic Findings. Fibrin deposits of varying intensity were present in both HUS and non-HUS cases. Traces of IgM, IgG, or IgA with or without C3 deposits were seen in the glomeruli in some cases.

CHOLERA

Cholera is an enterotoxin-mediated disease of the small intestine caused by *Vibrio cholera*. It is characterized by profuse watery diarrhea, vomiting, muscle cramps, and fluid volume depletion. Acute renal failure may occur.

Clinical and Pathologic Manifestations

In cholera, the clinical manifestations result from rapid loss of fluid and electrolytes from the intestine. Isotonic fluid is secreted from all segments of the small intestine. Bicarbonate and potassium are lost in large quantity.

Fluid volume depletion is thus the main pathophysiologic change. Collapse, severe muscular cramps, prostration, and tachypnea are among the common symptoms. The disease may last from 12 hours to 7 days.

Renal manifestations may not be apparent, although oliguria due to volume depletion is common. Prerenal azotemia, metabolic acidosis, and hypokalemia are frequently observed. In extreme cases acute renal failure occurs. In rare cases renal failure may be very severe because of cortical necrosis.

Light Microscopic Findings. Tubular vacuoles occur in cases with hypokalemia. In some cases acute tubular necrosis may be found; rarely, there is acute cortical necrosis.

BACTERIAL NEPHRITIS

PYELONEPHRITIS

Bacterial infection of the kidney may cause acute or chronic renal disease. Chronic pyelonephritis is caused by repeated or sustained episodes of bacterial infection in association with vesicoureteric reflux, urinary obstruction, nephrolithiasis, and other predisposing renal and urinary tract abnormalities. Chronic pyelonephritis, even when accompanied by lower urinary tract obstruction, carries a strong association with concomitant reflux; and the intrarenal reflux and renal infection are additional causes of renal scarring. Chronic pyelonephritis is more common in women than in men because urinary tract infection is more common in young girls than in young boys. Renal damage occurs predominantly during the first 6 years of life, and the inception of renal scarring after early childhood is uncommon. The designation *chronic pyelonephritis* includes renal scarring, and what used to be called chronic atrophic pyelonephritis, with gross scars, is now commonly called reflux nephropathy. The most frequent offending organism is *Escherichia coli*, but many other bacteria also cause this syndrome.

Renal and urinary tract infections are discussed and illustrated in Volume 2 of this series, *Renal Disease: Classification and Atlas of Tubulointerstitial Diseases.* Examples of acute pyelonephritis are also given in the present volume. The pathology is similar in all age groups and in both sexes, but the disease is particularly severe in newborn boys.

ACUTE BACTERIAL PYELONEPHRITIS

Acute infection occurs during the course of septicemia ("descending" infection) or more often as a sequela of lower urinary tract infection ("ascending" infection). Acute pyelonephritis, secondary to hematogenous localization of bacteria in the kidney, may complicate bacteremia of any type, especially in immunocompromised patients. *Escherichia coli* and other members of the family Enterobacteriaceae cause acute suppurative pyelonephritis in apparently normal very young infants, almost always boys, during the first 2 months of life. A few of them have urinary tract malformations (eg, posterior urethral valves), but most have anatomically normal urinary tracts. The disease is ordinarily of very acute onset, frequently heralded by diarrhea and dehydration, and accompanied by conjugated hyperbilirubinemia. The condition responds to prompt and vigorous therapy, with complete recovery and no renal sequelae.

Macroscopic Findings. The kidneys are enlarged with swollen, bile-stained cortices.

Light Microscopic Findings. Tubules are distended with pus cells; the interstitium contains a heavy infiltrate of neutrophils. Bacteria are present within tubules and abscesses.

BRUCELLOSIS (UNDULANT FEVER, MALTA FEVER, MEDITERRANEAN FEVER)

Urinary tract changes are associated with infections by several species of Brucella that are transmitted to humans from domestic animals. In the acute stages of infection, acute interstitial nephritis may sometimes be accompanied by focal glomerulonephritis. The chronic stages are characterized by granulomatous lesions throughout the urinary tract and can be confused with tuberculosis.

Brucella is a Gram-negative coccobacillus or short rod. There are four species that can cause disease in man, and each primarily infects a particular domestic animal: *B. abortus* (cows), *B. suis* (pigs), *B. melitensis* (goats), *B. canis* (dogs). Brucellosis occurs in many temperate and tropical parts of the world. Infection with *B. abortus* is commonest in countries where cattle are raised for beef or milk, especially North and South America. Disease caused by *B. suis* is largely confined to North America. *B. melitensis* infection is common in countries where goats are extensively reared, such as the Mediterranean countries and the drier parts of Africa and India. *B. canis* sometimes causes disease in kennel workers. Brucella infection is transmitted to humans from animals by ingestion, through cuts and scratches on the skin, and by inhalation. *B. melitensis* is acquired mainly from goat's milk or fresh cheese, *B. abortus* from drinking raw cow's milk, and *B. suis* from direct contact with infected blood and tissues in slaughterhouses, on farms, and in veterinary practice.

Clinical and Pathologic Manifestations

Brucellosis is predominantly a disease of adult males because of their increased exposure to this microorganism in the workplace. Signs and symptoms of renal involvement are uncommon but may occur in three situations. The first is during the acute stage of brucellosis, when there may be heavy proteinuria, hematuria, pyuria, pain in the back or over the bladder, dysuria, and frequency of urination. Most of these patients recover promptly. The second is in Brucella endocarditis, when some pain in the back and abdomen may occur together with proteinuria and hematuria. The third is during a chronic stage of the disease, when predominantly lower urinary tract signs and symptoms suggestive of renal tuberculosis, chronic nonspecific pyelonephritis, or even neoplasm may appear. Dysuria, strangury, hematuria, nocturia, and pyuria are common. The diagnosis usually depends upon demonstration of specific agglutinins or complement fixation tests. Blood cultures may disclose the organism during the height of the fever. Mortality is about 2 percent.

Macroscopic Findings. The kidneys are usually enlarged in patients in the acute stage of the disease or in those with Brucella endocarditis. The subcapsular surface is smooth, and there are often abundant petechiae. On the cut surface there are often small hemorrhages in the cortex.

In the chronic stage of the disease the surface of the kidney is often irregular and nodular; the ureters and calices may be dilated and the bladder wall thickened, nodular, and ulcerated. Cut sections of the kidney may contain one or more caseating foci, 0.5 to 6 cm in diameter, with soft, yellow centers and ragged margins. The pelvis and ureter are often dilated, their lumens filled with thick yellow fluid, and their walls greatly thickened and studded with small nodules. Fine, granular calcification is common in the lesions.

Light Microscopic Findings. In acute cases there is diffuse interstitial nephritis, which may be accompanied by focal glomerular lesions. The interstitium is edematous and diffusely infiltrated with mononuclear cells, mostly lymphocytes. Sometimes there is also a segmental increase in the number of mesangial cells, with or without polymorphs, in some of the glomeruli. These changes are accompanied by protein casts and a small amount of patchy, tubular atrophy. Rarely, tubular necrosis was produced following rhabdomyolysis, which was thought to have been caused by the organism. Granulomatous lesions are not usually found. Gram stain for organisms is usually negative.

In chronic cases, focal accumulations of macrophages surrounded by a collar of lymphoid cells and fibroblasts are found in variable numbers throughout the tissues of the urinary tract. Often there are Langhans giant cells within these granulomas and central necrosis, which resembles tuberculosis. Stains usually fail to reveal bacteria, even though cultures are frequently positive. *B. suis* in the abscess can be demonstrated by MacCallum-Goodpasture stain. A few cases of glomerulonephritis have been described.

Electron Microscopic Findings. The foot processes of the visceral epithelial cells are widened, but there are no glomerular electron-dense deposits.

Immunomicroscopic Findings. No specific deposits of immunoglobulin or complement components are found.

LEGIONELLA INFECTION

The bacillus *Legionella pneumophila* causes acute respiratory infections. Legionella pneumonia (legionnaires' disease) is often community-acquired in previously healthy subjects, although a large proportion of patients smoke cigarettes or have pre-existing respiratory disorders. The pathogen, which may also be nosocomial and opportunistic, is an aerobic, pleomorphic, Gram-negative rod that grows on enriched media containing charcoal and yeast extract. *L. pneumophila* exists in more than 12 serogroups, and, despite speculation, none has been demonstrated to be especially or specifically nephropathic. Most reports of renal complications do not specify the serogroup.

Clinical and Pathologic Manifestations

Renal involvement in legionnaires' disease is relatively common in terms of proteinuria, microscopic hematuria, and modest elevation of BUN and creatinine levels. However, clinical renal failure is rare. The renal abnormality resolves on treatment of the infection, although short-term dialysis may be required, particularly in cases complicated by disseminated intravascular coagulation.

Macroscopic Findings. The kidneys may be mildly enlarged, with swollen cortices. A case of pyelonephritis with multiple renal abscesses has also been reported.

Light Microscopic Findings. The usual abnormality is acute interstitial nephritis with cortical edema, inflammatory cell infiltrates, and tubular damage. The inflammatory cell infiltrates are largely lymphocytic and plasmacytic. Tubular injury includes cellular necrosis and tubular disruption, and some cases have been reported only as acute tubular necrosis. Microorganisms are not usually present in the kidney in diffuse interstitial nephritis. The direct cause of the renal involvement has not been identified, and there has been speculation about a circulating bacterial toxin, abetted by the usual risk factors for acute renal failure in very ill patients.

A second type of lesion, acute suppurative pyelonephritis, has been described, however, in a small minority of cases. The kidney contains cortical abscesses in which bacilli have been demonstrated by direct immunofluorescence. Free and intracellular organisms are present in the lesions and in vessels. There is mention also of rare bacteria in mesangial and endothelial cells. This type of renal infection presumably develops during the course of systemic disease.

Immunofluorescence and electron microscopic studies have not been contributory, except as above.

BOTRYOMYCOSIS

Botryomycosis is a chronic progressive bacterial infection of the skin, soft tissues, and viscera, including the lungs, liver, kidneys, and heart. However, it may involve the kidney primarily. Clinically similar to actinomycotic and eumycotic mycetoma, botryomycosis produces indurated inflammatory masses with draining sinuses, which spread locally to involve adjacent structures. The lesions and the purulent exudate that drains from sinus tracts contain bacterial granules (grains). The pathogenesis of granule formation is poorly understood.

The most common agent of botryomycosis is *Staphylococcus aureus*. Other documented agents include *Pseudomonas aeruginosa*, *Escherichia coli*, *Actinobacillus lignieresi*, and species belonging to the genera *Proteus*, *Streptococcus*, *Bacteroides*, and *Bacillus*.

Clinical and Pathologic Manifestations
There has usually been a severe, persistent, and refractory infection of the urinary tract. A bacterium can usually be cultured from the urine and sometimes from the blood.

Localized draining and indurated inflammatory masses involve the skin and soft tissues of exposed surfaces such as the head, hands, and feet. Infection may spread to adjacent skeletal muscle and bone. Visceral infection is rare and usually occurs without concomitant cutaneous involvement. Patients with renal involvement may have dysuria, hematuria, pyuria, and positive urine cultures but are not clinically distinguishable from patients with ordinary bacterial pyelonephritis.

Macroscopic Findings. Renal lesions consist of abscesses surrounded by firm, fibrous tissue. Larger abscesses may burrow into perinephric fat. Involvement of ureters and bladder is rare.

Microscopic Findings. In abscesses and lesional exudate, the bacteria form soft, yellow, or white aggregates (granules or grains) that represent macrocolonies up to 1 to 2 mm in size. The bacterial granules are embedded in an eosinophilic ground substance and are surrounded by amorphous eosinophilic radiating clubs (Splendore-Hoeppli phenomenon). The granules are similar to those found in the lesions of actinomycosis and mycetoma. Although the bacteria in botryomycotic granules are usually basophilic, they are best demonstrated and differentiated from the agents of mycetoma and actinomycosis with tissue Gram stains, such as Brown-Hopps or Brown and Brenn.

The abscesses are surrounded by granulomatous inflammation with considerable fibrous scarring.

Immunofluorescence and electron microscopic studies do not contribute to diagnosis.

MALACOPLAKIA

Malacoplakia is a type of chronic granulomatous inflammation characterized by numerous histiocytes containing basophilic inclusions, the Michaelis-Gutmann bodies. Although malacoplakia is not restricted to the urinary tract, its most common location is in the urinary bladder. Renal involvement occurs occasionally. The inflammation seems to result from an altered response to bacterial infection.

Malacoplakia is most commonly caused by infection with *Escherichia coli*, although other bacterial species, including *Klebsiella*, *Staphylococcus*, and *Mycobacterium*, have been implicated. Renal infection develops in association with urinary tract abnormalities, perhaps also as the result of blood-borne infection.

Clinical and Pathologic Manifestations

Renal malacoplakia is a disease predominantly of middle-aged women with urinary tract infection. Patients present with fever, flank pain, and flank masses. Urinary findings include pyuria and positive bacterial cultures. Renal functional impairment is proportional to the severity of renal involvement; bilateral disease is associated with renal insufficiency.

Renal malacoplakia also occurs in the absence of urinary tract infection, perhaps from hematogenous bacterial dissemination, especially in patients with involvement of organs outside the urinary tract. Malacoplakia can be found in the vertebrae, intestinal tract, liver, lungs, and other organs, presumably as a result of the same abnormal response to bacterial infection. That abnormal reaction may be caused by a defect in lysosomal activity following the phagocytosis of bacteria; phagocytosis appears to be unimpaired, but the ability of cells to kill and eliminate bacteria may be impaired. The defect seems to be aggravated by altered immunologic states, so that there is a high incidence of malacoplakia in immunocompromised patients.

Macroscopic Findings. The disease may be bilateral and disseminated, occasionally unilateral and limited to a single focus. Multifocality is associated with renal enlargement. The masses are yellow and usually well demarcated, containing foci of suppuration and hemorrhage. They are predominantly cortical in distribution, occasionally affecting the medulla with necrotizing papillitis. A single focus can present as a large tumorous mass with central necrosis. Complications include perirenal extension and renal vein thrombosis.

In the bladder they are common in the trigone, around the ureteric orifices, and on the interureteral crest. Sometimes the lesions lead to stenosis of the ureters or the urethra, which in turn leads to unilateral or bilateral hydronephrosis with or without dilatation of the bladder. When malacoplakia directly affects the kidney,

multiple yellowish areas may be visible on the subcapsular and cut surface, and the organ may be enlarged. Sometimes the lesions extend down into the papillae or look like abscesses.

Light Microscopic Findings. The characteristic microscopic feature is the von Hansemann histiocyte, a large rounded macrophage with eosinophilic cytoplasm. The cytoplasm contains periodic acid-Schiff (PAS)–positive granules, corresponding to large phagolysosomes. The cells also contain cytoplasmic basophilic inclusions, the Michaelis-Gutmann bodies. They have a lamellated structure and can be demonstrated by stains for calcium and for iron. Extruded Michaelis-Gutmann bodies are also present among the cells. The Michaelis-Gutmann body develops from the calcification of lipoprotein membranes surrounding incompletely degraded bacteria within phagolysosomes. The macrophages contain alpha-1-antitrypsin, which can be used as a marker to differentiate these cells from carcinoma cells in aspiration biopsy specimens from the lesions. Cellular infiltrates in the absence of Michaelis-Gutmann bodies are sometimes referred to as megalocytic interstitial nephritis, a condition that is otherwise similar but not identical to malacoplakia; the cells in the former are often only weakly PAS-positive.

Electron Microscopic Findings. All the macrophages in the lesion contain numerous phagolysosomes of various sizes, and it is these structures that account for the PAS-positive granularity of the cytoplasm of the cells in malacoplakia. Some of the larger phagolysosomes show central calcification. Typical Michaelis-Gutmann bodies are larger and have crystalline centers; an adjacent, less-dense, crystal-free zone; and one or more surrounding rings of crystals. X-ray diffraction suggests that the crystals are hydroxyapatite. Bacilli have been described within phagolysosomes in about 40 percent of the lesions that have been examined ultrastructurally.

Immunofluoresence studies do not contribute to the diagnosis.

Radiologic Findings. Radiologic studies show the kidneys to be enlarged and to contain sonolucent masses that can be confirmed by renal arteriography. Sonograms sometimes have a hyperechoic pattern resembling cystic disease. Angiograms occasionally show neovascularity suggestive of neoplasia.

Pyelography often reveals dilation of the ureters and the pelvicaliceal system.

XANTHOGRANULOMATOUS PYELONEPHRITIS

Xanthogranulomatous inflammation of the kidney is a form of chronic bacterial tubulointerstitial nephritis characterized by large collections of lipid-filled, foamy macrophages. There may be a localized intrarenal mass, an abscess cavity containing stones, or a diffuse replacement of most of the kidney by firm, yellow tissue. The condition is usually unilateral and results in a nonfunctioning kidney. The pattern of inflammatory cell infiltration may represent an altered response to bacterial invasion, as intracellular degenerating bacteria are present within the lesions. The conditions have a very strong association with obstructive uropathy, particularly stone disease.

Xanthogranulomatous inflammation results from infection with Gram-negative enteric bacteria, the most common agents being *Proteus* spp. and *Escherichia coli*. These two microorganisms account for 70 percent of bacterial isolates; other agents include members of the genera *Aeromonas*, *Klebsiella*, and *Pseudomonas*.

Clinical and Pathologic Manifestations

Xanthogranulomatous pyelonephritis is a disease predominantly of the sixth and seventh decades of life, although people of all ages, including children, are affected. Female patients predominate, with a ratio in some series as high as 5:1. The usual signs and symptoms reflect chronic infection and the underlying obstructive urinary tract abnormality. Initial complaints include fever, chills, malaise, weight loss, urinary frequency, and pain in the flank and abdomen. Patients give histories of urinary tract infection and sometimes of stone disease. They often have tender abdominal masses. Some patients are hypertensive. Laboratory evaluation demonstrates anemia, leukocytosis, hematuria, pyuria, and proteinuria. Liver function tests are often abnormal, perhaps as a response to chronic infection.

The abnormality most often associated with xanthogranulomatous pyelonephritis is a large staghorn renal calculus. Other causes of obstruction include ureteropelvic lesions and carcinoma of the pelvis, ureter, or bladder.

Macroscopic Findings. The kidneys are enlarged, sometimes massively. In diffuse disease the calices are dilated, although the pelvis is relatively small, and are surrounded by mantles of shaggy, orange-yellow tissue that extends into the renal parenchyma. The medullary papillae are commonly necrotic and lost, resulting in a gross appearance like that of renal tuberculosis. The parenchyma, which may be greatly reduced in amount, contains abscesses surrounded by yellow nodules, and the xanthomatous tissue extends into the adjacent parenchyma. The capsules are typically thickened, sometimes ruptured, and perinephric inflammation may extend into the retroperitoneum to involve adjacent organs. Localized, tumorous lesions unassociated with pelvic inflammation appear to be encapsulated by fibrous tissue and have purulent centers; they may, however, be associated with diffuse pyelonephritis.

Light Microscopic Findings. Microscopic examination demonstrates the foamy macrophages to be admixed with neutrophils, lymphocytes, and plasmacytes. Many macrophages contain multiple nuclei, and the lesions can look like giant cell granulomas. Microscopic examination also shows central suppuration occasionally surrounded by a palisading granulomatous reaction, within the lesions.

The lesions typically contain large amounts of hemosiderin, and the foamy macrophages contain PAS-positive granules. Organisms can be identified within the abscesses and within the macrophages in sections stained by the Dieterle method.

The specific pathogenesis of the abnormality is not known, although the association with urinary tract and bacterial infection is clear enough. The presence of so many phagolysosomes and residual bodies suggests a lysosomal defect. Other suggestions have included vascular obstruction with renal ischemia, massive infection and necrosis, and lymphatic obstruction.

Electron Microscopic Findings. Ultrastructural studies show that numerous lysosomes, residual bodies, and engulfed and degenerating bacteria are present within the macrophages. Bacteria can usually be cultured from the lesions. Vascular changes include arterial intimal fibrosis and, sometimes, organizing venous thrombi, the latter in occlusive endophlebitis.

Radiologic Findings. Radiologic studies characteristically show renal enlargement, a large calculus, and excretory nonfunction. Sonography and computerized tomography reveal caliectasis and parenchymal cavitation. The pelvis is frequently contracted because of peripelvic fibrosis around the calculus. Renal arteriography, no longer frequently performed, shows hypervascularity and neovascularity around relatively avascular parenchymal masses, which have sometimes led to the erroneous diagnosis of a tumor.

GLOMERULONEPHRITIS IN CHRONIC SEPSIS

Gram-positive and Gram-negative, aerobic and anaerobic organisms can cause visceral infections, and these organisms have been shown to be responsible for the renal changes of glomerulonephritis. Subphrenic abscess, peritonitis, sustained bacteremia, osteomyelitis, septic abortions, respiratory infections—particularly lung abscesses—endocarditis, and infected ventriculoperitoneal and ventriculoatrial shunts are the common conditions.

Clinical and Pathologic Manifestations

The clinical picture is that of slowly progressive oliguria with hematuria, hypertension, and, sometimes, pulmonary edema.

Light Microscopic Findings. The changes predominate in the mesangium and show the features of mesangiocapillary glomerulonephritis, sometimes with superimposed crescents.

Electron Microscopic Findings. Electron microscopy shows granular, electron-dense deposits along the glomerular basement membrane.

Long-standing cases show focal glomerular scarring, although eradication of the offending focus of infection is followed by resolution with a good prognosis.

Immunomicroscopic Findings. Fluorescent microscopy shows IgG and C3 as granular deposits along the glomerular basement membrane.

SALMONELLOSIS

FIGURE 10.1   Severe infection with *Salmonella typhimurium*. Abscess in renal parenchyma. (H & E × 50)

FIGURE 10.2   Higher magnification of Figure 10.1, showing inflammatory necrosis of renal parenchyma. (H & E × 295)

TYPHOID FEVER

FIGURE 10.3   Typhoid fever. The glomeruli show only mild mesangial cell hyperplasia. There is focal tubulointerstitial inflammation. (H & E × 140)

FIGURE 10.4   The glomerulus shows mild mesangial cell proliferation with slightly increased matrix. (H & E × 350)

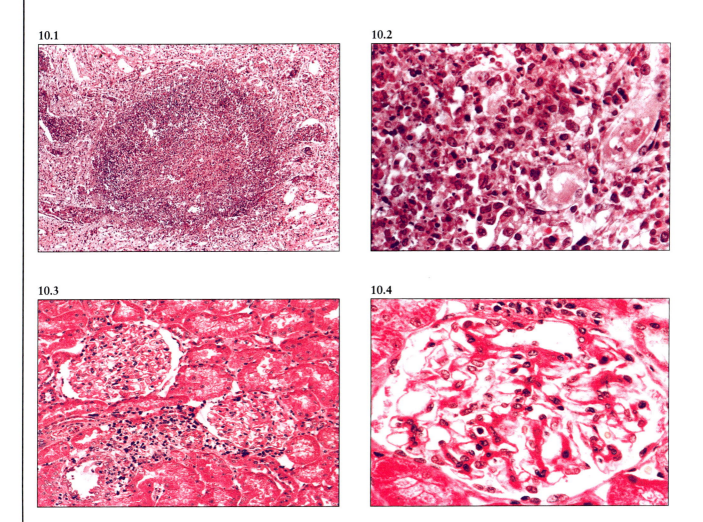

10.1

10.2

10.3

10.4

Typhoid Fever

FIGURE 10.5   Immunofluorescence microscopy shows granular deposits of IgA in mesangial areas. IgM is seen in a similar distribution but in a greater proportion of patients. (× 380)

Shigellosis

FIGURE 10.6   Shigellosis. Glomerulus showing mesangial cell proliferation, with heavy infiltrate of mononuclear leukocytes in the glomerular capillaries and in an artery. (H & E × 235)

FIGURE 10.7   There are numerous fibrin thrombi in the lumens of glomerular capillaries. (H & E × 350)

FIGURE 10.8   Immunofluorescence microscopy, showing deposition of fibrin in glomerular capillary lumens, in mesangial areas, and along the capillary walls. (× 350)

10.5

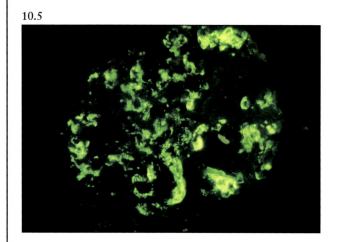

10.6

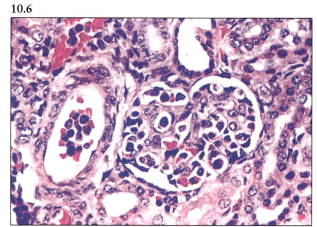

10.7

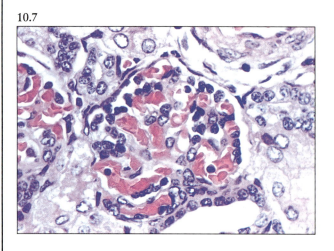

10.8

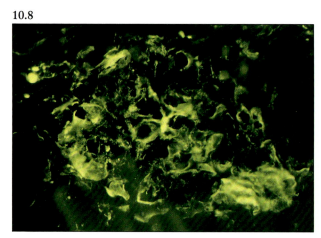

CHOLERA

FIGURE 10.9   Cholera. There is vacuolation of the epithelial cells of proximal and distal convoluted tubules. Note that the tubules in the medullary ray (left) are normal. (H & E × 190)

ESCHERICHIA COLI PYELONEPHRITIS

FIGURE 10.10   Neonatal *Escherichia coli* pyelonephritis in a 3-week-old boy. There are tubular suppuration, interstitial inflammation, necrosis, and large numbers of macrophages. The child had no obstructive abnormality of the urinary tract, and the infection is very likely to have been an ascending one associated with reflux. (H & E × 95)

STAPHYLOCOCCAL PYELONEPHRITIS

FIGURE 10.11   Staphylococcol pyelonephritis in an 8-year-old boy. The tubular suppuration and interstitial inflammation are similar to that shown in Figure 10.10. (H & E × 150)

10.9

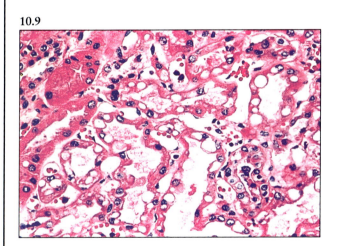

10.10

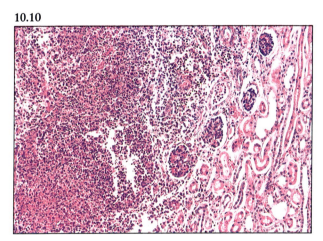

10.11

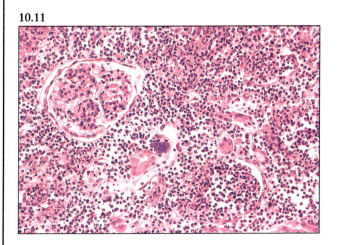

Staphylococcal Pyelonephritis

FIGURE 10.12   Staphylococcal pyelonephritis in another child. The features are similar to those in Figure 10.11, except for the masses of cocci. The extensive necrosis has the features of a renal carbuncle. (H & E × 95)

Brucellosis

FIGURE 10.13   Brucellosis in acute stage. Diffuse interstitial nephritis. (H & E × 120)

FIGURE 10.14   Brucellosis in chronic stage. Granulomata with giant cells in interstitium. (H & E × 120)

FIGURE 10.15   Brucellosis in chronic stage. Graulomatous tissue and caseation. (H & E × 30)

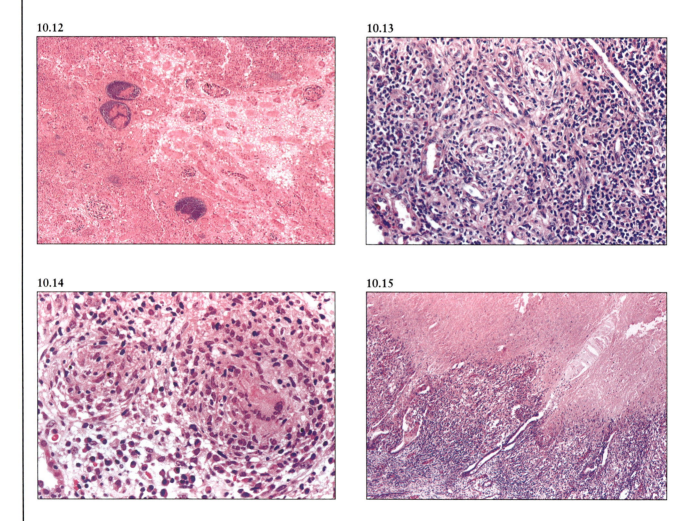

LEGIONELLA INFECTION

FIGURE 10.16 Legionella infection. There is acute interstitial inflammation with cellular infiltrates of lymphocytes and plasma cells. Tubular lumens contain similar cells. (H & E × 235)

FIGURE 10.17 Section shows acute suppurative pyelonephritis with cortical abscess formation. (H & E × 150)

BOTRYOMYCOSIS

FIGURE 10.18 Botryomycosis caused by Gram-positive cocci, probably *Staphylococcus aureus*. Microabscess bordered by granulation tissue contains bacterial granules. (H & E × 95)

10.16

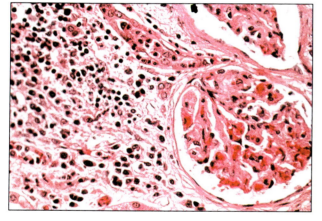

10.17

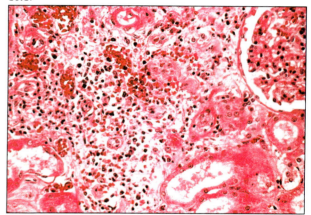

10.18

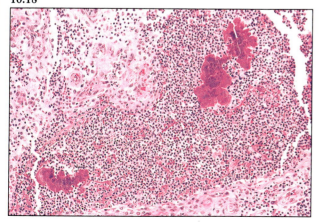

BOTRYOMYCOSIS

FIGURE 10.19   Bacterial granule of botryomycosis, probably caused by *Staphylococcus aureus*. Most of the granule is composed of Gram-positive cocci. Radiating eosinophilic clubs (Splendore-Hoeppli material) and nonviable cocci are Gram-negative. (Brown and Brenn × 380)

MALACOPLAKIA

FIGURE 10.20   The kidney is involved severely, with numerous yellow nodules on the surface. The hemisected specimen shows a lobar distribution of cortical and medullary involvement. The parenchyma in the affected area is replaced by yellow inflammatory tissue.

FIGURE 10.21   The cortex contains an accumulation of large histiocytes, with slightly foamy eosinophilic cytoplasm and vesicular nuclei. Many of the cells contain basophilic inclusions, Michaelis-Gutmann bodies. (H & E × 380)

10.19

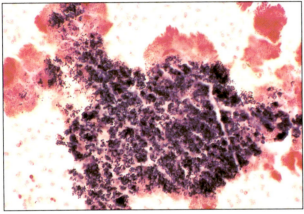

10.20

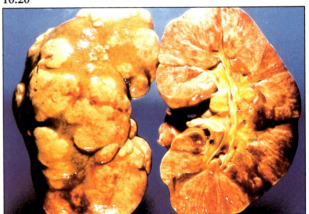

10.21

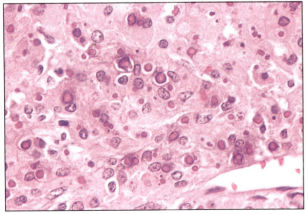

MALACOPLAKIA

FIGURE 10.22   The cortical infiltrate includes inflammatory cells, with infiltration and destruction of tubules. (H & E × 380)

FIGURE 10.23   The histiocytes are filled with PAS-positive material. (PAS × 235)

FIGURE 10.24   The Michaelis-Gutmann bodies contain calcium. (von Kossa × 380)

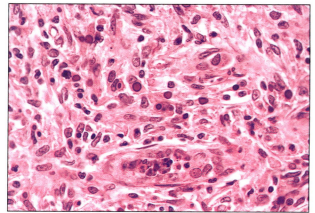

10.22

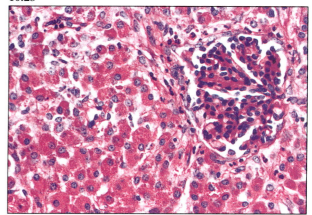

10.23

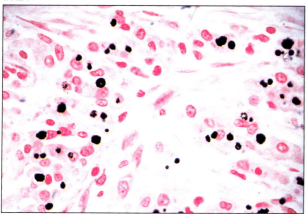

10.24

MALACOPLAKIA

FIGURE 10.25 Electron micrograph, showing well-developed calcified Michaelis-Gutmann body, lying within a membrane-bound vesicle. (× 16,100)

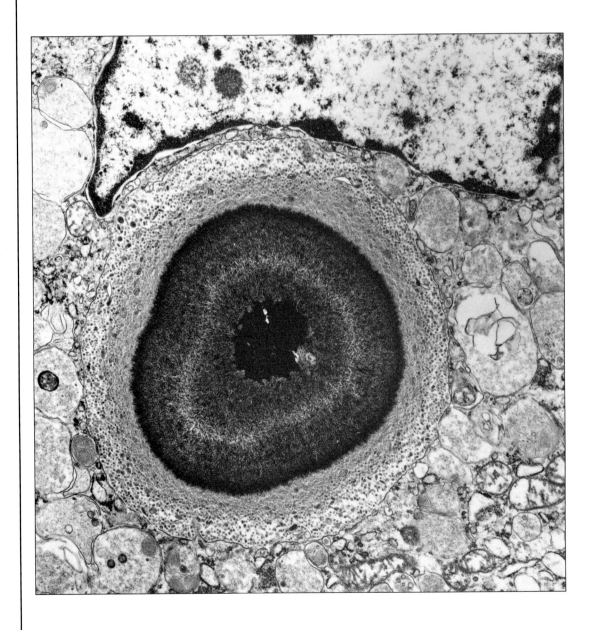

MALACOPLAKIA

FIGURE 10.26 Electron micrograph. Bacteria can be identified within membrane-bound vesicles in a partially disrupted macrophage. ($\times$ 16,100)

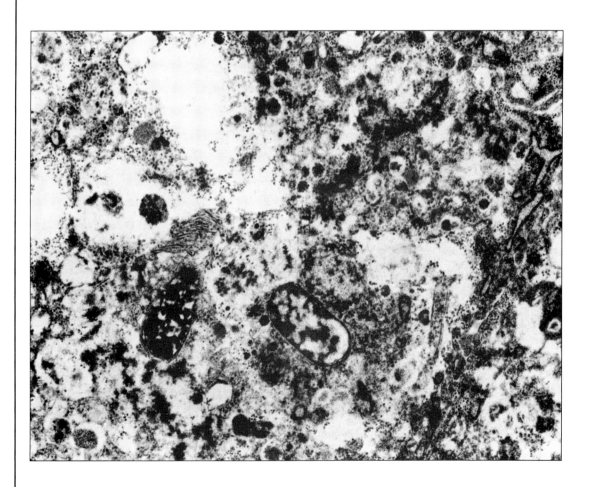

Xanthogranulomatous Pyelonephritis

FIGURE 10.27   Enlarged kidney with a staghorn calculus from an 80-year-old woman with chronic pyelonephritis with extrarenal extension and empyema. Hemisection shows a dilated pelvis and dilated calices with pyonephrosis; a portion of calculus is impacted in the pelvis (arrow). The renal parenchyma is reduced to a thin rim of tissue surrounding the dilated calices, which are lined with bright-yellow tissue. The process, with bright-yellow xanthogranulomatous inflammation, extends into the surrounding fat.

FIGURE 10.28   Kidney from a 73-year-old woman with pyonephrosis shows a dilated pelvis and dilated calices containing exudate and pasty, necrotic material. A rim of bulging, yellowish-gray material surrounds the dilated calices.

FIGURE 10.29   A cavity, possibly a dilated duct, contains exudate and is surrounded by a dense infiltrate of chronic inflammatory cells. The cavity itself is lined with large, finely vacuolated macrophages. (H & E × 150)

FIGURE 10.30   The infiltrate in xanthogranulomatous pyelonephritis characteristically includes enlarged, foamy macrophages with finely granular cytoplasm. (H & E × 380)

10.27
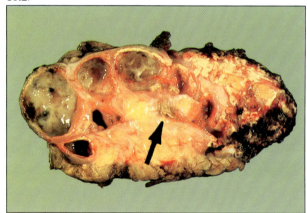

10.28
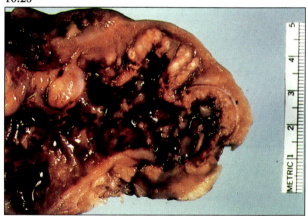

10.29
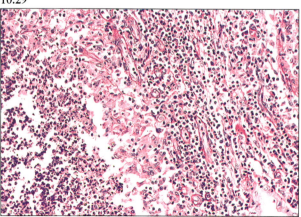

10.30
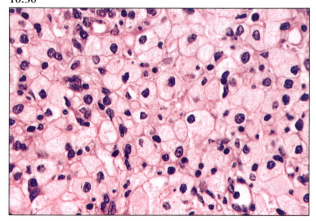

Xanthogranulomatous Pyelonephritis

FIGURE 10.31 The macrophages contain ingested material and numerous PAS-positive granules. (PAS × 380)

FIGURE 10.32 The macrophages form multinucleated giant cells. (H & E × 235)

FIGURE 10.33 The macrophages contain debris and ingested bacteria. (Dieterle's stain × 950)

FIGURE 10.34 Venous occlusion by inflammation and thrombosis in xanthogranulomatous pyelonephritis. (H & E × 60)

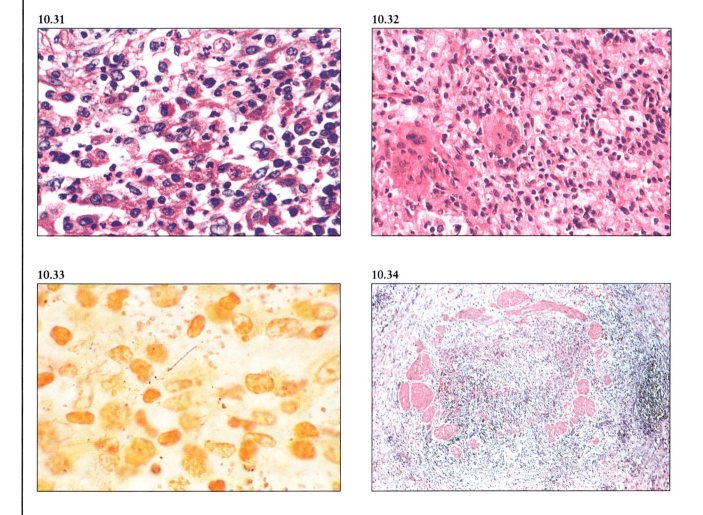

10.31

10.32

10.33

10.34

Xanthogranulomatous Pyelonephritis

FIGURE 10.35   Electron micrograph, showing xanthogranulomatous pyelonephritis and bacteria in cell cytoplasm (dark bodies). (× 21,500)

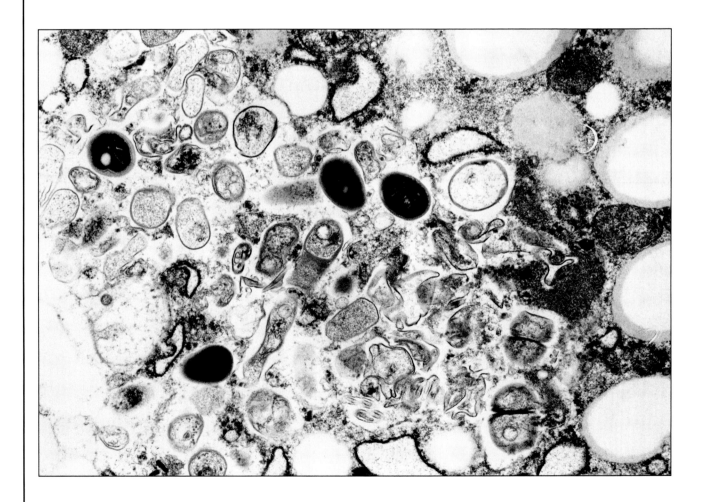

Xanthogranulomatous Pyelonephritis

FIGURE 10.36 Computerized tomogram from same case as in Figure 10.27. The calices of the left kidney are distended; and the pelvis and upper ureter contain an impacted, staghorn calculus.

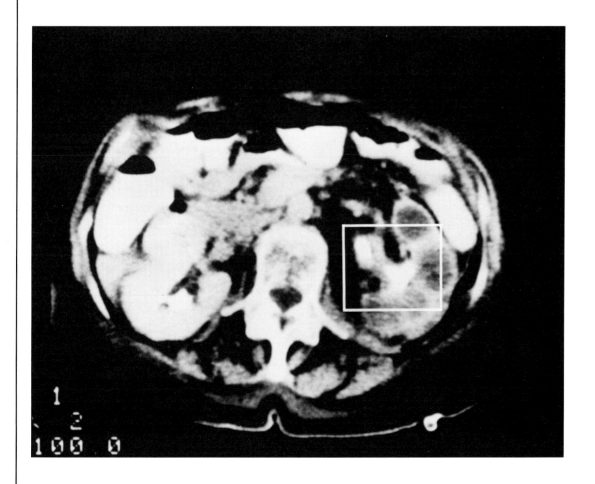

GLOMERULONEPHRITIS IN CHRONIC SEPSIS

FIGURE 10.37   Chronic sepsis. The glomerulus shows mesangial cell proliferation and segmental lobulation, as well as a small crescent. (PASM × 235)

FIGURE 10.38   Mesangiocapillary glomerulonephritis accompanied by an almost circumferential crescent in a patient with chronic sepsis. (silver trichome × 235)

FIGURE 10.39   Immunofluorescence microscopy, showing granular deposits of IgG along the glomerular basement membrane. (× 235)

10.37

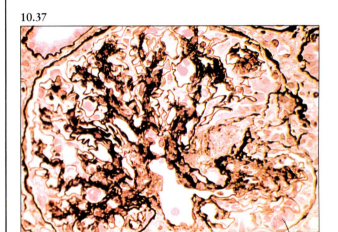

10.38

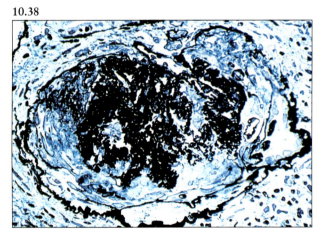

10.39

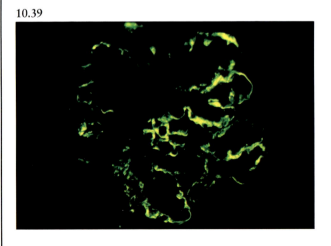

MYCOBACTERIAL INFECTIONS

LEPROSY

Leprosy is a widespread chronic inflammatory disease that is prevalent in Africa, India, Brazil, China, and many other countries of Southeast Asia and South America. There are about 12 million cases of leprosy (10.6 million according to WHO figures of 1975) all over the world, of which 3 million are in India. A variety of renal lesions including immune complex glomerulonephritis, amyloidosis, and, occasionally, leproma have been reported in association with leprosy. Interstitial nephritis has also been described. A few patients exhibit only functional renal tubular defects. Glomerulonephritis occurs more frequently in lepromatous leprosy.

The disease is caused by *Mycobacterium leprae*, or Hansen's bacillus. The incubation period is usually 2 to 4 years. Although prolonged and intimate contact is considered necessary for infection to develop, cases of infection acquired after a brief or passing contact with a person suffering from leprosy have been documented. Renal involvement often occurs during erythema nodosum leprosum reaction, although it has also been reported in patients without reaction. The antigens involved in the causation of immune complex glomerulonephritis may be mycobacterial and specific for leprosy, or they may be nonmycobacterial exogenous antigens, which could also cause glomerulonephritis in patients without leprosy.

Clinical and Pathologic Manifestations

The clinical syndrome observed in patients with proved renal involvement includes acute nephritic syndrome, nephrotic syndrome, and asymptomatic proteinuria or hematuria. Nephrotic syndrome is often seen in patients with renal amyloidosis but may be a manifestation also of glomerulonephritis. Hypertension is uncommon.

Distal tubular dysfunction, in the form of a concentrating or acidification defect or both, may be demonstrated in some patients but may not be associated with any overt clinical manifestation. Tubular defects are unrelated to the type of leprosy, the nature of treatment, and the presence or absence of hyperglobulinemia. No specific lesions to account for these functional abnormalities have been demonstrated.

Chronic renal failure resulting from amyloidosis is the leading cause of death. Only on rare occasions does rapidly progressive or proliferative glomerulonephritis progress to end-stage failure.

Light Microscopic Findings. The two most common morphologic types of glomerulonephritis observed in leprosy are diffuse endocapillary proliferative and mesangial proliferative glomerulonephritis. Focal proliferative, crescentic, mesangiocapillary, and diffuse sclerosing glomerulonephritis have also been reported in a small number of cases; mesangial sclerosis is uncommon. Secondary amyloidosis involves the glomerulus, tubulointerstitium, and blood vessels (see Secondary Amyloidosis, chap. 16).

Electron Microscopic Findings. Electron-dense deposits have been seen mainly in the subendothelium or the subepithelium, but intramembranous and mesangial deposits have also been recorded. Other alterations include focal foot process widening; areas of reduplication, with mesangial interposition; thickening and rarefaction in the glomerular capillary basement membranes; and endothelial swelling with vacuolation of the cytoplasm.

Immunomicroscopic Findings. Granular deposits of IgM or IgA and fibrin in the mesangium and/or along the capillary walls have been seen on immunofluorescent microscopy.

Interstitial Nephritis. Chronic interstitial nephritis has been observed at autopsy in some patients with lepromatous or nonlepromatous leprosy. The lesions appear to be associated with advanced disease of long duration. The relationship between leprosy and chronic interstitial nephritis is not clear, and it has been suggested that prolonged chemotherapy may contribute to the development of interstitial nephritis.

Leproma. Direct invasion of the renal parenchyma by *Mycobacterium leprae,* with formation of granuloma, is a rare form of renal involvement, and only isolated instances have been reported. Bacteria have been seen in the kidney even in the absence of leproma. In an isolated case, *M. leprae* were associated with the juxtaglomerular apparatus, between the macula densa and the capsule. The leproma consists of an aggregation of lipid-laden macrophages (lepra cells) often filled with clusters of acid-fast bacilli (globi). Bacteria-laden giant cells are also interspersed among the macrophages, and the focus is surrounded by a mantle of lymphocytes.

TUBERCULOSIS

Tuberculosis is an infectious disease caused by *Mycobacterium tuberculosis.* This organism is a slender bacillus 1 to 4 μm long and 0.3 μm wide. The most common site of primary infection is the lungs. The kidneys are involved as a result of hematogenous dissemination of bacilli, usually from the lungs.

Although morbidity and mortality from tuberculosis have steadily declined in technically advanced countries, the disease continues to be a major cause of illness and death in many developing countries of Asia and Africa. Urinary tract tuberculosis constitutes 10 to 15 percent of the urologic outpatient population in India. Even in countries like the United States, about 15 percent of all new cases of tuberculosis are extrapulmonary, and one sixth of these involve the genitourinary tract. Whereas clinical and radiological evaluation reveals genitourinary involvement in 4 to 25 percent of patients with pulmonary tuberculosis without overt urologic symptoms, renal involvement in pulmonary tuberculosis at autopsy varies from 28 to 73 percent, indicating that the disease often presents no clinical symptoms.

Clinical and Pathologic Manifestations

The disease most commonly occurs between the ages of 15 and 60 years, and males are affected twice as often as females. The onset is insidious, and symptoms may precede diagnosis by several years.

Dysuria, urinary frequency and urgency, and nocturia are the most common presenting symptoms. Gross hematuria may also occur, and blood may be seen uniformly mixed with urine, or there may be only terminal hematuria. Other symptoms include flank or abdominal pain, pyuria, fever, and weight loss. Urinary tract tuberculosis can be clinically silent in up to 20 percent of patients. When symptoms occur, they are due to destructive tuberculosis.

Hypertension is observed in some cases. A palpably enlarged kidney is seldom observed and, when present, indicates hydronephrosis due to ureteric obstruction. Urinalysis in most patients reveals pyuria or hematuria or both, but findings may be entirely normal. Pyuria without the usual bacterial organisms may be the first sign of underlying tuberculosis. Urine smears are positive for acid-fast bacilli in about half the patients, and several cultures are required. Bacilluria is often intermittent; and, therefore, repeated cultures may be necessary to confirm the diagnosis.

Tuberculosis rarely causes uremia because of asymmetrical involvement of the kidneys. Renal failure is due either to (1) parenchymal destruction, which is irreversible, or (2) ureteral obstruction.

Macroscopic Findings. In miliary tuberculosis, generalized, pinhead-sized, white nodules occur in the cortical interstitium.

In destructive tuberculosis caseous and ulcerative lesions occur. The lesions often begin in the medulla and papillae, and then spread to the pelvis and cortex. There is caseation necrosis, which is soft, white, and cheesy, with large necrotic masses. This may be followed by sloughing of the pyramids and formation of cavities that communicate with the collecting system. Later, there is secondary hydronephrosis with ureteral obstruction and strictures. In advanced cases, the kidney is converted into a hollow, cavitated, sac-like organ. Calcification of the renal parenchyma is not uncommon. In patients with long-standing disease in whom spontaneous "autonephrectomy" has occurred, the lumen of the main renal artery and its major branches may be totally obliterated.

The bladder is involved in two thirds of patients with renal tuberculosis. Initially, 1–2-mm submucosal elevations, tubercles, are seen in the region of the trigone. These spread to involve the entire bladder wall, coalesce, and ulcerate, giving rise to ulcers with undermined edges. Fistulae may develop. The bladder wall is thickened and bladder capacity considerably reduced. Ureteric orifices are often widely gaping, resulting in gross vesicoureteric reflux. The genital tract (testes, epididymis, prostate) is involved in one third of male patients with urinary tract disease.

Microscopic Findings. The classic lesion is a tuberculous granuloma, the center of which shows caseation necrosis. The necrotic area is surrounded by epithelioid cells, which have abundant pale eosinophilic cytoplasm and a vesicular nucleus. Among these cells or at their periphery, giant cells containing 20 to 40 nuclei arranged in a complete or partial marginal ring may be seen. These are called Langhans giant cells. With Ziehl-Neelsen stain, the tubercle bacilli can be seen in the center of the granuloma or toward the periphery of the area of caseation as red, rod-shaped bacilli. The granuloma has a cuff of lymphocytes at its periphery and may be surrounded by fibrous tissue.

Radiologic Findings. Destructive tuberculosis of the kidney is easily diagnosed radiographically. Renal parenchymal calcification occurs in about 30 percent of patients. In early disease, irregularities of the papillae may develop, the appearances being similar to those of papillary necrosis. In more advanced cases, cavities with irregular walls are seen. These often communicate with the collecting system. Because of fibrosis, the infundibulum of a calix may be narrowed, resulting in dilatation and cutting off of that calix. The ureters may have one or more strictures, with proximal dilatation. The bladder may have a thick wall and is sometimes calcified. In the later stages of the disease, it is contracted, and vesicoureteric reflux may develop. The multiplicity of lesions and their asymmetrical distribution are the most helpful distinguishing features.

Although it takes from 8 to 40 years following pulmonary tuberculosis for destructive nephropathy to develop, 66 to 72 percent of patients presenting with urinary tract tuberculosis have abnormal chest radiographs showing healed or active pulmonary lesions.

LEPROSY

FIGURE 11.1   Prevalence of registered leprosy cases in the world, 1985. (Courtesy of World Health Organization.)

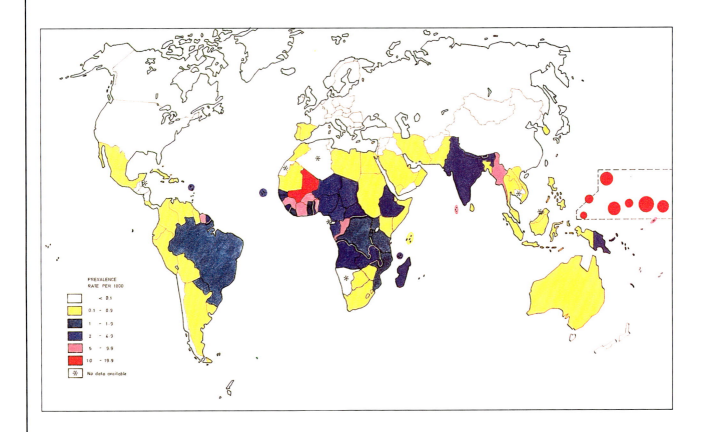

LEPROSY

FIGURE 11.2   Lepromatous leprosy, skin. There are numerous intracellular bacilli within the macrophages. (Fite-Faraco, oil × 760)

FIGURE 11.3   Leprosy. 40-year-old Indian male. Crescentic glomerulonephritis with underlying endocapillary proliferation. (H & E × 310)

FIGURE 11.4   Lepromatous leprosy, 44-year-old Indian female with heavy proteinuria. Amyloid deposition in the glomerulus and in the wall of the afferent arteriole. (Congo red × 190)

FIGURE 11.5   Immunofluorescence microscopy, showing granular deposits of IgM along the glomerular capillary loops and in the mesangium. (× 310)

11.2
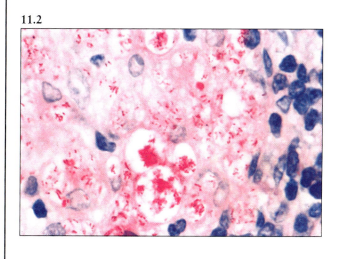

11.3
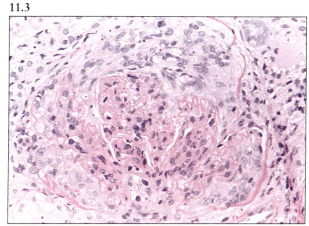

11.4
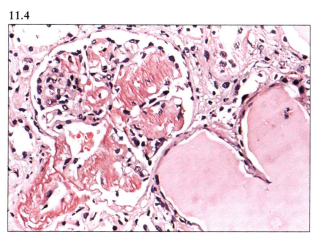

11.5
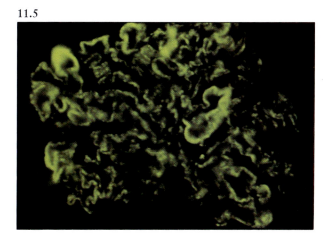

LEPROSY

FIGURE 11.6 Electron micrograph, showing electron-dense deposits along the subepithelial glomerular basement membrane (top right). There are polymorphs and monocytes in the capillary lumen, and the glomerular basement membrane is focally widened and rarefied. (× 7,600)

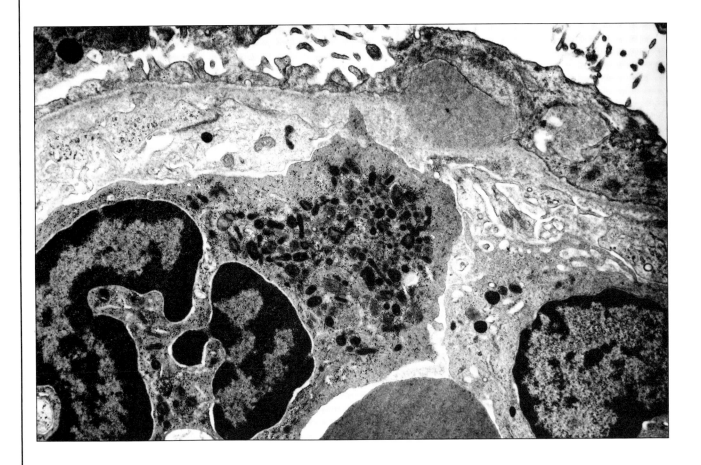

FIGURE 11.7   Electron microscopy. Same case as in Figure 11.4. Amyloid fibrils in the glomerulus. (× 43,500)

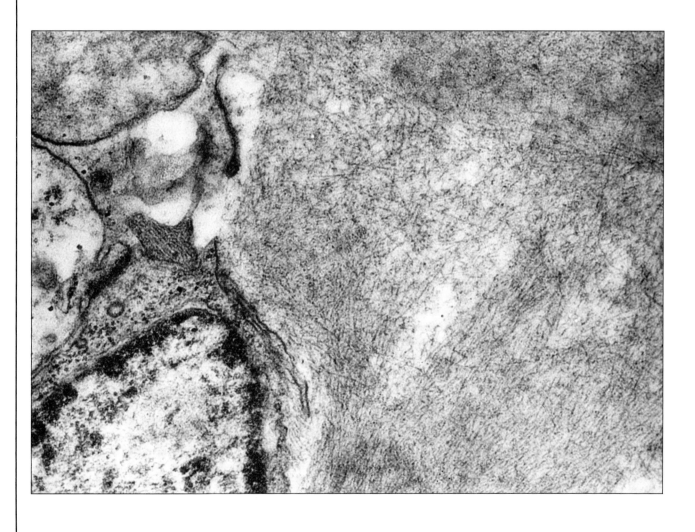

TUBERCULOSIS

FIGURE 11.8   Destructive tuberculosis of the kidney with sloughing of the pyramids and formation of cavities bordered by a mantle of soft yellow necrotic tissue.

FIGURE 11.9   Destructive renal tuberculosis. There is extensive papillary necrosis with a heavy pericaliceal mantle of yellow tissue that mimics xanthogranulomatous pyelonephritis.

FIGURE 11.10   Tuberculous granulomata with caseation necrosis in the kidney. (H & E × 95)

11.8

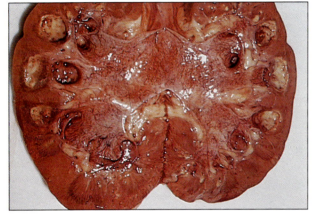

11.9

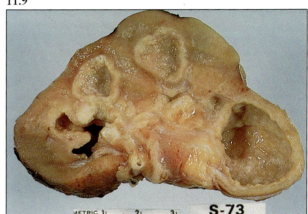

11.10

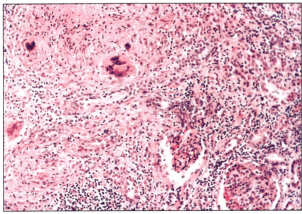

Fungal and Actinomycetal Infections

Most fungal infections of the urinary tract involve the kidneys by hematogenous dissemination from an extrarenal focus of infection, usually pulmonary, that may be clinically inapparent. Primary infections, most often caused by *Candida* spp. and *Torulopsis glabrata*, begin in the lower urinary tract and may ascend to involve the kidneys. Although fungi can often be detected in tissues stained with hematoxylin and eosin (H & E), their morphology is demonstrated better with periodic acid–Schiff (PAS) or Gomori (Grocott) methenamine silver (GMS) stains. When fresh tissues are not available for culture, histologic diagnosis can be confirmed in many cases by direct immunofluorescence, which can be performed on deparaffinized sections of formalin-fixed tissues. Infections caused by species of *Actinomyces, Nocardia,* and related genera are traditionally considered within the province of mycotic diseases and are therefore included in this chapter, although these organisms are actually filamentous bacteria rather than true fungi.

CANDIDIASIS

Candidiasis is a general term that covers opportunistic mucocutaneous and systemic infections caused by mycelial yeasts of the genus *Candida*. With the exception of *C. albicans,* the *Candida* spp. are ubiquitous saprophytes that are frequently isolated from the air and

soil. However, most infections by *C. albicans* originate from mucosal surfaces of the oral cavity, upper respiratory tract, digestive tract, and vagina, where this fungus is part of the normal microflora. These endogenous infections are usually limited to the mucosae, but hematogenous spread and systemic colonization do occur and often involve the lungs, spleen, kidneys, liver, heart, and brain. Untreated systemic candidiasis, which has an 80 percent fatality rate, is commonly seen in patients whose resistance has been severely compromised by therapy or underlying disease. Predisposing factors include abdominal or urologic surgery, indwelling venous or urethral catheters, prolonged broad-spectrum antibiotic or corticosteroid administration, leukemia and lymphoma, diabetes mellitus, obstructive uropathy, granulocytopenia, cytotoxic chemotherapy, and cell-mediated immunodeficiencies such as acquired immunodeficiency syndrome. Candidiasis occurs worldwide and is the most frequently encountered mycosis of the urinary tract.

C. albicans, the principal pathogenic species, is recovered from about 90 percent of diseased specimens. Other less common saprophytic species that are occasional pathogens include *C. parapsilosis, C. tropicalis, C. pseudotropicalis, C. guilliermondii, C. krusei,* and *C. stellatoidea.* The *Candida* spp. can be isolated on standard mycologic media at 37°C. Colonies are fast-growing, smooth or wrinkled, soft, and creamy white;

they have a distinct yeast-like odor. They are composed of short, spherical to ovoid, nonencapsulated blastoconidia, 5 to 7 μm in diameter. *C. albicans* can be differentiated from other *Candida* spp. by the formation on special media of germ tubes and mycelium with terminal, thick-walled chlamydoconidia and by its characteristic assimilation and fermentation reaction.

Clinical and Pathologic Manifestations

There are two basic clinical forms of candidiasis: mucocutaneous and systemic. Most urinary tract infections are seen in the systemic form as a result of hematogenous dissemination. Clinical findings in patients with severe renal infections, which are usually distinguishable from those of bacterial pyelonephritis, may include chronic low-grade or spiking fever with chills, hypotension, deteriorating clinical course with renal failure, persistent flank pain, costovertebral angle tenderness, hematuria, anemia, and granulocytopenia. Renal or ureteral colic can result from the passage of candidal "fungus balls," and anuria secondary to obstructing ureteropelvic "fungus balls" has been reported in adults and neonates. Candidal infections of the lower urinary tract may be primary or secondary, and they occur four times as often in women as in men. Patients with candidal cystitis usually present with complaints of urinary frequency, dysuria, and hematuria. Because *C. albicans* can be isolated from clean-voided urine of some asymptomatic persons, its mere isolation has no clinical or diagnostic significance. However, recovery of the fungus from the urine along with a positive blood culture is highly suggestive of disseminated infection. The treatment of choice in systemic candidiasis is administration of amphotericin B plus elimination or minimization of predisposing factors. In lower urinary tract infections, intrapelvic or intravesicular instillation of amphotericin B, combined with surgical resection of lesions or "fungus balls," has been effective. Another effective antifungal is 5-fluorocytosine, but resistant strains may emerge from use of this drug. Ketoconazole has shown promising results, especially in patients with renal failure.

Macroscopic Findings. In several autopsy series, renal involvement occurred in 50 to 88 percent of patients with systemic candidiasis; the urinary bladder was involved in 5 to 12 percent. About 50 percent of patients with macroscopic lesions of the kidneys have renal failure. Severe renal infections are usually seen as acute or chronic pyelonephritis with miliary abscesses or diffuse suppuration and necrosis. Pyelonephritis can be associated with papillary necrosis, and the pelves may contain sloughed or adherent necrotic papillae and candidal "fungus balls." Obstruction by the latter can also result in hydronephrosis. Lesions of the urinary bladder usually consist of hemorrhagic ulcers or whitish, thrush-like pseudomembranes. Candidal "fungus balls" can be formed in the bladder and passed in the urine.

Light Microscopic Findings. In tissue sections, the *Candida* spp. occur as a mixture of blastoconidia, pseudohyphae, and hyphae that may be difficult to delineate with H & E. However, fungal elements are readily demonstrated with GMS and PAS. The host response ranges from little or no inflammation to dispersed suppuration and necrosis with miliary abscesses and papillary necrosis. Mycotic emboli are sometimes seen in glomerular capillary loops and in intertubular arterioles in the cortex, and radiating microcolonies of *Candida* are found in the interstitium and tubules. Hyphae and pseudohyphae may invade blood vessels, but parenchymal infarction as seen in aspergillosis and zygomycosis is unusual. The renal pelves may be obstructed by sloughed necrotic papillae and masses of proliferating mycelium that aggregate to form candidal "fungus balls." Mucosal lesions of the lower urinary tract appear as superficial erosions and focal ulcerations, which are usually covered by a thrush-like pseudomembrane of fibrin, cellular debris, and abundant fungal elements.

Immunomicroscopic Findings. Specific fluorescent antibody conjugates are available for identifying the *Candida* spp. (to genus level only) in tissue sections and smears of lesional exudate.

Radiologic Findings. Renal candidiasis may not be detectable on roentgenograms. In severe infections, intravenous pyelograms may show calicectasis and poor visualization of contrast material. "Fungus balls" in the renal pelvis or bladder, but rarely in the ureter, appear as lucent intraluminal and irregularly margined filling defects in retrograde pyelograms; they may be associated with obstructive uropathy and hydronephrosis. Elongated, serpiginous, "cast-like" filling defects are sometimes found in ureteral candidiasis with fungal colonization. In candidal cystitis, a Swiss cheese appearance of the bladder mucosa with multiple rounded filling defects has been described.

TORULOPSOSIS

Torulopsosis is caused by *Torulopsis glabrata*, an opportunistic yeast-like fungus in the family Cryptococcaceae. This yeast is part of the normal microflora of the oropharynx, gastrointestinal tract, skin, urethra, and vagina of humans; but it is also found in nature. Although of low virulence, *T. glabrata* is the second most common fungal pathogen of the urinary tract. Infection can be primary (ascending) or, more commonly, associated with disseminated disease. The spectrum of disease ranges from clinically inapparent fungemia and funguria to severe life-threatening pyelonephritis, pneumonitis, endocarditis, meningitis, and wound infection. Most infections are nosocomial; common predisposing factors include contaminated intravenous lines, indwelling urethral catheters, obstructive uropathy, abdominal or urologic surgery, appendiceal abscesses, prolonged antibiotic therapy, poorly controlled diabetes mellitus, and systemic therapy with corticosteroids and cytostatic drugs. The yeast enters the circulatory system via catheters and intravenous lines, open wounds, and the gastrointestinal, urinary and respiratory tracts. In many cases, however, the source of fungemia is unexplained.

T. glabrata is a small (2 to 4 μm), budding, round to oval, nonencapsulated, yeast-like fungus, which can easily be grown on standard mycologic media. Colonies grow rapidly and are smooth, soft, shiny, and creamy white. They are composed entirely of yeast cells that are morphologically similar to those seen in tissue; hyphae and pseudohyphae are not formed.

Clinical and Pathologic Manifestations

Surveys indicate that 40 to 50 percent of *T. glabrata* infections are transient, self-limiting, clinically silent fungemias and fungurias. Infections are often superimposed on bacterial sepsis, and a positive blood culture may be the first clue to fungemia. Clinical findings in severe disseminated infection with urinary tract involvement are usually nonspecific and include low-grade or spiking fever with chills and hypotension, deteriorating clinical course with multiple organ failure, costovertebral angle tenderness, and flank pain. The treatment of choice in severe infections is parenteral, intravesical, or intrapelvic instillation of amphotericin B. Good results have also been achieved with the oral antifungal ketoconazole, especially in patients with renal failure. Elimination of predisposing factors often results in rapid improvement without treatment, but progressive localized or disseminated infections require aggressive therapy and even nephrectomy in rare instances.

Macroscopic Findings. Autopsy surveys of disseminated torulopsosis indicate that lesions most often occur in the kidneys, gastrointestinal tract, peritoneum, and heart. About 50 percent of patients with disseminated infection have renal involvement, which is often microscopic. Severe infections manifest as acute pyelonephritis with miliary abscesses or diffuse suppuration and necrosis. Pyelonephritis can be associated with papillary necrosis, and the pelves may contain sloughed or adherent necrotic papillae. Because *T. glabrata* does not produce hyphae or pseudohyphae in tissue, the formation of obstructing "fungus balls" is extremely rare. Perirenal abscesses and fibrosis rarely result from extension of infection through the capsule. Lesions of the lower urinary tract usually consist of hemorrhagic ulcers.

Light Microscopic Findings. Because of the pathogen's low virulence, tissue invasion by *T. glabrata* is minimal, except in severely debilitated patients. In the kidneys, scattered yeast cells can be seen in glomerular capillary loops, Bowman's spaces, and, occasionally, in tubules. Tissue damage and inflammation may be minimal or inapparent. In severe infections, acute pyelonephritis with miliary abscesses and necrotizing papillitis may be seen. Ulcers of the lower urinary tract are often superficially infected with *T. glabrata*, and there may be concomitant infection with bacteria or with *Candida albicans*. *T. glabrata* cells in tissue are usually amphophilic but otherwise morphologically similar to those seen in culture.

Immunomicroscopic Findings. The histologic diagnosis of torulopsosis can be confirmed by direct immunofluorescence.

Radiologic Findings. In severe renal infections, intravenous pyelograms may show calicectasis and decreased visualization of contrast material because of pyelonephritis and papillary necrosis. Retrograde pyelograms may reveal lucent filling defects like those of papillary necrosis.

CRYPTOCOCCOSIS

Cryptococcosis is an evanescent or chronic pulmonary mycosis with a proclivity for cerebromeningeal dissemination. It is a cosmopolitan disease that occurs in apparently healthy persons but more frequently and with greater virulence in immunodeficient patients, particularly those who have severe underlying diseases such as lymphoma or leukemia. In addition to the central nervous system, disseminated infection often involves the lungs, skin, bones and joints, kidneys, lymph nodes, and spleen.

The disease is caused by a single yeast-like species, *Cryptococcus neoformans*. The fungus, which is found worldwide, thrives in avian habitats, particularly those contaminated with pigeon excreta. The respiratory tract serves as the portal of entry for almost all human infections. *C. neoformans* grows in culture and in infected tissues as pleomorphic, spheroidal, thin-walled, yeast-like cells, 2 to 20 μm in diameter, which reproduce by forming blastoconidia (buds) attached to the parent cells by narrow necks. Chains of budding cells and pseudohyphae are occasionally produced. *C. neoformans* is unique among fungal pathogens in that its cells have gelatinous polysaccharide capsules, demonstrable with mucin stains such as mucicarmine and Alcian blue, which serve as convenient diagnostic markers.

Clinical and Pathologic Manifestations

Cerebromeningeal symptoms, including headache, fever, and altered consciousness, predominate in disseminated cryptococcosis. Some patients present with respiratory symptoms. Renal involvement in disseminated cryptococcosis is usually clinically silent, but patients with severe renal involvement may have costovertebral angle tenderness, pyuria, and gross hematuria. Proteinuria is negligible in the absence of underlying renal disease. Renal insufficiency occasionally develops as the result of papillary necrosis. Cryptococci can be recovered from urine in up to 40 percent of patients with disseminated cryptococcosis, and a positive urine culture may provide the first clue to dissemination. The budding yeast-form cells can be identified in urine sediment by negative staining with India ink. Disseminated infection is treated with amphotericin B and fluorocytosine.

Macroscopic Findings. Renal involvement is found in as much as 50 percent of patients who die of disseminated cryptococcosis. Lesions often are not evident on gross examination, but small parenchymal abscesses or granulomas with central liquefaction involving the cortex and medulla have been described. Papillary necrosis is occasionally found; but involvement of the pelves, ureters, and bladder has not been described.

Light Microscopic Findings. Cryptococci fill and distend glomerular capillary loops in the course of hematogenous dissemination. Focal areas of parenchymal necrosis contain cyst-like spaces filled with yeast-form cells. Interstitial microabscesses and granulomas are also seen; the latter may develop central suppurative or caseous necrosis. Yeast-form cells can be found in tubular lumens, accounting for the high prevalence of cryptococcuria in disseminated cryptococcosis. Mycotic papillary necrosis has been described in several patients treated with aspirin and corticosteroids for rheumatoid arthritis, but similar lesions have not been reported in patients with lymphoma or leukemia who have disseminated cryptococcosis.

Cryptococci can be identified with hematoxylin and eosin as budding yeast-like cells surrounded by faintly stained capsular material. The diagnosis is confirmed by demonstrating capsular polysaccharide with mucin stains.

Electron Microscopic Findings. Although not necessary for diagnosis, electron microscopy is a method to confirm the presence of capsular material. The capsule is composed of radiating filaments within a granular matrix that surrounds the cell walls of the cryptococci and can be detected even when mucin stains are negative or equivocal.

Immunomicroscopic Findings. The histologic diagnosis can be confirmed by direct immunofluorescence with a specific conjugate directed against the capsular polysaccharide of *C. neoformans*. As with mucin stains, fluorescence is weak or equivocal if the capsules are thin or have been digested by phagocytic cells.

Radiologic Findings. Intravenous and retrograde pyelograms in several symptomatic patients have shown blunted or distorted calices and delayed excretion of contrast material. Papillary necrosis was demonstrated in a group of patients with rheumatoid arthritis who had cryptococcal pyelonephritis.

BLASTOMYCOSIS

Blastomycosis is a chronic systemic infection caused by the dimorphic fungus *Blastomyces dermatitidis*. The vast majority of reported cases have originated in North

America, but the disease also occurs sporadically in Africa and the Middle East. In the United States, endemic regions include the Ohio and Mississippi River valleys and the Southeast. Most primary infections are pulmonary and result from inhalation of the conidia of the saprophytic fungus found in soil. In rare instances, cutaneous lesions result from accidental direct inoculation of the fungus into the skin and soft tissues. Blastomycosis is not a transmissible disease.

B. dermatitidis is dimorphic, existing as a budding yeast, 8 to 15 μm in diameter, in tissues and on mycologic media incubated at 37°C and as a white-to-tan, downy-to-fluffy mold when cultured at room temperature. Mycelial-form cultures bear round to oval conidia, 3 to 5 μm in diameter, on the sides of hyphae and on the ends of simple conidiophores.

Clinical and Pathologic Manifestations

Blastomycosis is seen four times as frequently in males as in females, and most cases occur in persons between 30 and 50 years of age. There are two clinical forms: systemic and cutaneous. Although both have a pulmonary inception, their presentation, clinical course, and prognosis differ. The systemic form is primarily a pulmonary disease, which may remain confined to the lungs or disseminate via the bloodstream to other organs, especially the skin, bones, joints, male genital tract, heart, lymph nodes, urinary bladder, kidneys, brain, and spinal cord. Signs and symptoms vary, depending on the organs affected and the degree of involvement. Respiratory signs, which predominate at the onset, include productive cough, dyspnea, chest pain, low-grade fever, and hemoptysis. Urinary tract involvement is usually inapparent, but in severe infections there may be costovertebral angle tenderness, flank pain, renal insufficiency, and chronic discharging sinuses or subcutaneous abscesses. Cutaneous blastomycosis presents as ulcerated or verrucous skin lesions on exposed body surfaces. Symptoms are mild, pulmonary lesions are often inapparent, and the general health of the patient is not usually impaired. Treatment for both clinical forms is amphotericin B and surgical excision of localized lesions.

Macroscopic Findings. Renal blastomycosis is usually bilateral. Lesions of the kidney range from one or more small, sharply circumscribed, firm or soft nodules to diffuse inflammation and necrosis involving the entire organ. Abscesses are usually not encapsulated. The renal cortex is more often affected than the medulla, and direct extension of infection through the capsule can produce perinephric abscesses and discharging sinuses. In several autopsy series, renal involvement was seen in about 25 percent of cases. Lesions of the ureters and urinary bladder are rare and usually consist of focal ulcers.

Light Microscopic Findings. A mixed suppurative and granulomatous inflammation is usually seen in blastomycosis. Epithelioid and giant cell granulomas, some of which have central microabscesses or caseation, are common in advanced infections and resemble those seen in chronic active tuberculosis. *B. dermatitidis* is found in both suppurative and granulomatous areas as spherical, multinucleated yeast-form cells, 8 to 15 μm in diameter, with thick, hyaline walls that give the fungal cells a double-contoured appearance. Single, broad-based buds are morphologically distinctive, and diagnosis can be made by direct microscopic examination of clinical materials.

Immunomicroscopic Findings. A histologic or cytologic diagnosis can be confirmed by direct immunofluorescence with a specific conjugate directed against cell wall polysaccharide antigens of *B. dermatitidis*.

Radiologic Findings. Roentgenograms may show many small cavities and dense but ill-defined shadows of varying sizes—findings similar to those of miliary tuberculosis. Intravenous and retrograde pyelograms are usually normal.

HISTOPLASMOSIS

Histoplasmosis is usually a mild and clinically inapparent pulmonary disease acquired by inhaling the airborne infectious conidia of the dimorphic fungus *Histoplasma capsulatum* var. *capsulatum*. The disease occurs worldwide in areas where avian and chiropteran habitats favor growth and multiplication of the fungus in soil. Highly endemic areas in the Western Hemisphere include Guatemala, Mexico, Peru, Venezuela, and the broad region of the Ohio and Mississippi River valleys in the United States. Histoplasmosis is not contagious. Surveys indicate that hematogenous dissemination from a primary pulmonary focus occurs in 2 to 5 percent of patients, in whom the yeast-form fungus disseminates via the mononuclear phagocyte system. Systemic lesions most frequently involve the lungs, spleen, liver, lymph nodes, bone marrow, gastrointestinal tract, kidneys, adrenal glands, central nervous system, oropharynx, and skin; involvement of the lower urinary tract is rare.

African histoplasmosis caused by *H. capsulatum* var. *duboisii* is confined to the African continent. This mycosis is a distinct clinical and pathologic entity in which skin and bone lesions are common, but urinary tract involvement is extremely rare. Although *H. capsulatum* var. *duboisii* in infected tissues occurs as large, spherical to oval yeasts, 8 to 15 μm in diameter, it is indistinguishable in culture from the classic or small-form *capsulatum* variety of *Histoplasma*. In this chapter, the term "histoplasmosis" refers to infection by the classic small-form variety of *H. capsulatum*.

Because *H. capsulatum* var. *capsulatum* is dimorphic, it grows as a mold in vitro at 37°C on enriched media or in infected tissues. Mycelial-form colonies on standard mycologic media are downy in texture and white to golden brown. Two types of asexual conidia are produced: large (8 to 14 μm), thick-walled macroconidia covered with digitate protuberances and small (2 to 4 μm) smooth-surfaced microconidia.

Clinical and Pathologic Manifestations

The vast majority of infections are asymptomatic and self-limiting. Localized pulmonary infections heal without antifungal therapy in most patients but may calcify and be found inadvertently on chest roentgenograms or years later at autopsy. However, about 5 percent of patients have progressive pulmonary disease or disseminated infection. Patients with disseminated infection may present with fever, chills, cough, weight loss, headache, drowsiness, malaise, diarrhea, generalized lymphadenopathy, hepatosplenomegaly, purpura, and ulcerations of the oropharynx and intestines. Symptoms can mimic those of rapidly progressive lymphoma. Involvement of the kidneys and lower urinary tract is usually inapparent, and renal function is not significantly compromised. Iatrogenic, acute disseminated histoplasmosis has been reported in patients who received kidney transplants in which the organ was not known to be infected. Most recipients died within days to weeks after transplantation, with widely disseminated lesions containing myriad yeast cells.

All degrees of disseminated infection are potentially fatal and require aggressive treatment with amphotericin B. Ketoconazole may also be effective.

Macroscopic Findings. About 40 percent of patients with progressive disseminated histoplasmosis have varying degrees of renal involvement at autopsy. The lesions resulting from hematogenous dissemination range from one or more sharply circumscribed, firm or soft nodules to severe diffuse inflammation and necrosis involving the entire organ. Papillary necrosis has been described, and there may be massive enlargement of the kidneys due to diffuse histiocytosis. Lesions of the lower urinary tract usually consist of focal ulcers.

Light Microscopic Findings. The spectrum of the inflammatory reaction in renal histoplasmosis varies from small aggregates of yeast-laden macrophages in glomerular capillary loops to epithelioid and giant cell granulomas with or without central caseation and suppuration throughout the cortex and medulla. Necrotizing papillitis and areas of caseation associated with numerous organisms may also be seen; papillitis was reported in 3 of 22 cases of disseminated histoplasmosis in one autopsy series. In about 10 percent of cases, infection is seen as diffuse histiocytosis, in which sheets of histiocytes filled with yeast forms efface the normal renal architecture. In some immunodeficient patients, myriad yeast cells multiply profusely and form "yeast lakes," with little or no apparent host response.

Immunomicroscopic Findings. A histologic or cytologic diagnosis of histoplasmosis can be confirmed by direct immunofluorescence with a conjugate directed against cell wall polysaccharide antigens of all known serotypes of *H. capsulatum* var. *capsulatum*. The conjugate used at the Centers for Disease Control, Atlanta, also stains *H. capsulatum* var. *duboisii*, but the two varieties of *H. capsulatum* are morphologically distinct in tissues and can be easily differentiated.

Radiologic Findings. Roentgenograms may show enlarged kidneys with miliary or segmental infiltrates and areas of cavitation. If there is extensive infection and papillary necrosis, intravenous pyelograms may show calicectasis and poor visualization of contrast material. Retrograde pyelograms reveal lucent filling defects.

PARACOCCIDIOIDOMYCOSIS (SOUTH AMERICAN BLASTOMYCOSIS)

Paracoccidioidomycosis is a chronic progressive pulmonary mycosis that is endemic in South America, Central America, and Mexico. Pulmonary infection is followed in most cases by limited or widespread dissemination to the mucous membranes of the mouth, pharynx, and larynx and to the skin, lymph nodes, spleen, liver, adrenal glands, and other organs. Almost all patients are adult males, many of whom have occupational contact with soil or vegetation.

The disease is caused by a single dimorphic species, *Paracoccidioides brasiliensis*. The natural habitat of this fungus is unknown, and it is not considered to be an opportunistic pathogen. The mycelial form grows slowly in culture at room temperature or at 30°C and consists of septate, branched hyphae with intercalated chlamydoconidia. The yeast form grows at 37°C and consists of pleomorphic yeast-like cells, 3 to 30 μm or more in diameter, which produce one or more blastoconidia (buds) attached by narrow necks. The multiple-budding cells, which resemble a ship's steering wheel, are diagnostic. Older cells develop thick walls, up to 1 μm in width, which may fracture and fragment.

Clinical and Pathologic Manifestations

Presenting symptoms usually include cough, dyspnea, and hemoptysis. However, some patients in whom pulmonary infection is clinically inapparent present with mucosal lesions, lymphadenopathy, hepatomegaly, fever, or weight loss. Symptoms and laboratory findings referable to the urinary tract have not been reported. Disseminated infection is treated with ketoconazole, amphotericin B, and/or sulfonamides.

Macroscopic Findings. The kidneys are involved in the course of hematogenous dissemination in 10 to 15 percent of cases. Renal lesions consist of miliary necrotic or granulomatous nodules, 1 to 2 mm in size, which are distributed throughout the cortex and may involve the medulla. Involvement of the pelves, ureters, and bladder has not been described.

Light Microscopic Findings. Systemic lesions consist of granulomas with central suppurative necrosis. Yeast-form cells of *P. brasiliensis* are found within multinucleated histiocytes and within and at the periphery of areas of necrosis. Nonbudding and single-budding cells usually predominate. They vary greatly in size, and the diagnostic cells have multiple blastoconidia. Mycotic arteritis of the renal artery has been reported in one patient. Glomerular lesions have not been described.

Immunomicroscopic Findings. The histologic diagnosis can be confirmed by direct immunofluorescence with a specific conjugate directed against *P. brasiliensis*.

COCCIDIOIDOMYCOSIS

Coccidioidomycosis is a clinically inapparent or mild pulmonary mycosis that resolves without specific therapy in most patients. The disease is endemic in the southwestern United States, northern Mexico, Central America, and South America. A few patients develop progressive pulmonary infection, but disseminated infection occurs in less than 1 percent. Factors that predispose to dissemination include pregnancy, diabetes mellitus, and immunosuppressive drug therapy. Cases of laboratory infection have been reported. Systemic lesions most frequently involve the lungs, leptomeninges, skin and subcutaneous tissue, spleen, liver, kidneys, bones, and joints.

The disease is caused by *Coccidioides immitis*, a dimorphic fungus that inhabits arid desert soils. The fungus exists in nature in a mycelial form and produces arthroconidia that enlarge to form spherules (sporangia) within the lungs following inhalation. In culture at room temperature, the mycelial form grows rapidly and produces alternating barrel-shaped arthroconidia. The fungus exists in the form of endosporulating spherules in tissues and in culture at 37° to 40°C under certain conditions of growth. Immature spherules, 5 to 30 μm in diameter, enlarge and endosporulate by progressive cytoplasmic cleavage to produce mature spherules, 30 to 100 μm or more in diameter, with refractile walls 1 to 2 μm thick. Following endosporulation, the mature spherules rupture and release their endospores into the tissues, where they enlarge to form spherules and repeat the life cycle.

Clinical and Pathologic Manifestations

Approximately 60 percent of patients who have primary pulmonary coccidioidomycosis are asymptomatic. Symptomatic patients often have fever, cough, and pleuritic chest pain. Involvement of the urinary tract occurs by hematogenous dissemination and is clinically silent. Urinalysis may show mild proteinuria and a few leukocytes and erythrocytes per high-power field. Serum creatinine and BUN are normal unless there is underlying renal disease. Almost all patients with coccidioiduria have disseminated infection, 60 percent of whom have renal involvement at autopsy. The most common cause of death in disseminated coccidioidomycosis is meningitis. The therapy of choice is amphotericin B.

Macroscopic Findings. The kidneys are involved in about one third of patients who die of disseminated coccidioidomycosis. Renal lesions consist of miliary granulomas or abscesses scattered throughout the parenchyma. Involvement of the pelves, ureters, and bladder is unusual.

Light Microscopic Findings. The granulomas are interstitial and often show central caseous or suppurative necrosis. Spherules of *C. immitis,* generally abundant in active lesions, are located within the granulomas. Specific histologic diagnosis requires identification of endosporulating spherules of the appropriate size. Glomerular and vascular lesions have not been reported.

Immunomicroscopic Findings. A histologic diagnosis can be confirmed by direct immunofluorescence with a specific conjugate directed against *C. immitis.* The conjugate stains immature spherules and endospores, but the walls of mature spherules are nonreactive.

Radiologic Findings. Intravenous pyelograms are usually normal, but ballooning of calices is occasionally seen in retrograde pyelograms. Severe involvement of the kidneys can produce infundibular constriction and caliceal ballooning that mimics tuberculosis.

ASPERGILLOSIS

The spectrum of aspergillosis includes allergic bronchopulmonary disease; colonization of preformed pulmonary cavities; indolent superficial infections of cutaneous and mucosal surfaces; and invasive, necrotizing pneumonitis, which is often accompanied by hematogenous dissemination to the central nervous system, heart, gastrointestinal tract, kidneys, and liver. Invasive and disseminated aspergillosis occur in immunocompromised patients, particularly those who have lymphoma or acute leukemia. Leukopenia and therapy with corticosteroids, cytotoxic drugs and multiple antibiotics predispose to disseminated infection.

Aspergillus fumigatus is the most common pathogenic species, but *A. flavus, A. niger,* and other species also cause disease. The aspergilli are ubiquitous in nature and are commonly encountered as contaminants in the clinical laboratory. Most species grow rapidly at room temperature or at 37°C to produce a mycelium composed of branching, septate hyphae. Speciation is based predominantly on the morphology of the conidial heads. Typical hyphae are narrow (3 to 5 μm wide) and uniform, with parallel contours. They are regularly septate and branching is progressive and dichotomous. Invasion of blood vessels, common in invasive aspergillosis, accounts for the frequency of thrombosis, infarction, and hematogenous dissemination.

Clinical and Pathologic Manifestations

Patients who have disseminated aspergillosis are acutely ill and febrile. Respiratory symptoms predominate, and involvement of the urinary tract is clinically silent. Microhematuria and pyuria are often present, but urine cultures are only rarely positive and are unreliable for diagnosis. Obstructive uropathy, caused by growth of mycelium within the calices, pelves and ureters, occurs most commonly in diabetic patients with no clinical evidence of disseminated infection. This form of renal infection, erroneously termed "mycetoma" in the literature, produces flank pain, ureteral colic, dysuria, hematuria, and pyuria and may lead to hydronephrosis with renal insufficiency. Some of these patients pass "fungus balls" in their urine. Disseminated aspergillosis is treated with amphotericin B. Pelvicaliceal obstruction is treated surgically, followed by local irrigation with amphotericin via nephrostomy or ureteral catheters.

Macroscopic Findings. Renal involvement occurs in 30 to 40 percent of patients who die of disseminated aspergillosis. Lesions consist of multiple cortical and medullary abscesses, 1 to 3 mm in diameter, which have yellow necrotic centers surrounded by hyperemic zones. Vascular invasion and obstruction lead to thrombosis and segmental infarcts, the latter occasionally accompanied by papillary necrosis. In the noninvasive form of renal aspergillosis, the renal pelvis and calices are filled with soft, grayish-tan mycelium, which may extend into and obstruct the ureter to produce hydronephrosis. The urinary bladder is involved in less than 5 percent of patients.

Light Microscopic Findings. Abscesses and infarcts contain typical septate, branching hyphae. Within infarcts, the hyphae spread diffusely through the interstitium and invade tubules. Hyphae are also found in glomerular capillary loops and Bowman's space. Papillary necrosis follows obstruction of medullary and papillary blood vessels. Invasion of larger blood vessels produces thrombosis and infarcts. Mycelial casts removed from the collecting system, ureters, or bladder consist of tangled hyphae admixed with fibrin and cellular debris. This form of infection is not usually accompanied by parenchymal or vascular invasion, but the kidney may show pyelitis with chronic interstitial inflammation and fibrosis.

Immunomicroscopic Findings. The hyphae of several other hyaline opportunistic pathogens, including members of the genera *Fusarium* and *Pseudoallescheria*, are quite similar to those of the aspergilli. Therefore, a histologic diagnosis of aspergillosis should be confirmed by direct immunofluorescence unless the fungus is isolated from cultures of tissue or urine. The fluorescent antibody conjugate is directed against Aspergillus spp. and does not provide species identification.

Radiologic Findings. In the pelvicaliceal form of renal aspergillosis, retrograde pyelograms show filling defects, with deformation of calices and papillary necrosis. Advanced changes include pyelocaliectasis and hydronephrosis.

MUCORMYCOSIS (ZYGOMYCOSIS)

Mucormycosis is an opportunistic infection caused by fungi in the Order Mucorales, Class Zygomycetes (formerly Phycomycetes). Clinical forms of mucormycosis include rhinocerebral infection in acidotic diabetic patients, pulmonary and disseminated infection in immunocompromised patients with leukemia or lymphoma, and gastrointestinal infection in the malnourished. Disseminated infection most commonly involves the lungs, central nervous system, kidneys, spleen, heart, and liver. Patients with leukopenia and those treated with corticosteroids or cytotoxic drugs are predisposed to infection.

Rhizopus oryzae is the most common pathogenic species. However, agents of mucormycosis also include species within the genera *Absidia, Apophysomyces, Mucor, Rhizomucor, Saksenaea, Cunninghamella,* and *Mortierella.* These fungi are ubiquitous in the environment and, like the aspergilli, are often encountered as contaminants in the clinical laboratory. Most species grow rapidly at room temperature or at 37°C to produce a sparsely septate mycelium. Some species produce anchoring filaments (rhizoids). The fungi replicate asex-ually by production of sporangiospores within sporangia, the latter borne upon sporangiophores that develop from the vegetative mycelium. The hyphae of the mucoraceous zygomycetes are broad (5 to 20 μm wide) and pleomorphic, with irregular contours. Septation is infrequent, and the pattern of branching is haphazard. Branches are usually oriented at right angles to parent hyphae. Like the aspergilli, the mucoraceous zygomycetes frequently invade blood vessels and disseminate via the bloodstream.

Clinical and Pathologic Manifestations

Disseminated mucormycosis is a fulminant infection that occurs in debilitated patients. Such patients have fever, malaise, and symptoms referable to the primary site of infection, most commonly the lungs or the nasal cavity and paranasal sinuses. Although involvement of the urinary tract is usually clinically silent, some patients have signs and symptoms of renal infarction, including flank pain, dysuria and gross hematuria, without clinical evidence of disseminated infection. Laboratory studies show hematuria and pyuria, but BUN and serum creatinine levels are normal unless renal involvement is bilateral. Urine cultures are usually negative. Disseminated infection is treated with amphotericin B, along with local excision or drainage of infected foci.

Macroscopic Findings. Renal involvement occurs in 50 percent of patients who die of disseminated mucormycosis. Renal artery thrombosis, which is found in most of these patients, is associated with segmental or subtotal renal infarction. In some cases, one sees papillary necrosis and erosion or ulceration of pelvic mucosa. When infection extends beyond the kidney, the perinephric fat is necrotic and indurated.

Light Microscopic Findings. Vascular invasion and permeation produce necrotizing inflammation and thrombosis of segmental, interlobar, and arcuate arteries, resulting in ischemic parenchymal necrosis with peripheral acute inflammation. Hyphal fragments are scattered throughout the infarcts in the interstitium, glomeruli, and tubules. Necrotizing inflammation may extend into perinephric soft tissues.

Immunomicroscopic Findings. The hyphae of the genera *Rhizopus* and *Absidia* can be identified by direct immunofluorescence with a fluorescent antibody conjugate. This screening conjugate does not detect other pathogens in the class Zygomycetes.

Radiologic Findings. Intravenous pyelograms usually show enlarged, nonfunctioning kidneys. Retrograde pyelograms may show caliceal distortion.

ACTINOMYCOSIS

Actinomycosis is a chronic localized and suppurative infection caused by endogenous, filamentous bacteria in the order Actinomycetales. The principal agent in humans is *Actinomyces israelii*, a common commensal of the mouth and throat of healthy individuals. Poor oral hygiene, recurrent tonsillitis, and intra-abdominal mucosal breaks predispose a person to endogenous infection. From a primary focus, infection can spread to contiguous tissues or rarely disseminate. Actinomycosis is sporadic and seen throughout the world. Unlike nocardiosis, it does not occur preferentially in immunodeficient patients. Urinary tract involvement is rare. To date, about 50 cases of renal infection have been documented.

Other than *A. israelii*, agents of actinomycosis in man include *A. naeslundii*, *A. odontolyticus*, *A. viscosus*, *Arachnia propionica*, and *Rothia dentocariosa*. All these actinomycetes are anaerobic or microaerophilic. They grow best at 37°C on enriched, antibiotic-free media, forming small, raised, whitish colonies that are either rough or smooth, depending on the degree of filamentation. Colonies are composed of delicate, Gram-positive, branched filaments 1 μm in diameter. Identification of an isolate is based on the morphologic, physiologic and biochemical characteristics in culture.

Clinical and Pathologic Manifestations

Infections are classified based on the anatomic site of involvement as either cervicofacial, thoracic, abdominal, or genital. Renal involvement results from either contiguous spread from a primary infection in the abdominal cavity or from hematogenous dissemination from another site. There has been one report of intra-abdominal actinomycosis with bladder involvement and passage of sulfur granules in the urine, but infection of the lower urinary tract is uncommon. Symptoms of renal involvement, which are usually those of abdominal actinomycosis, often suggest a malignancy; they include fever, weight loss, change in bowel habits, loss of ap-

petite, localized pain and tenderness, vomiting, and palpable abdominal masses. Sinus tracts discharging to the skin may be seen. Treatment consists of high doses of penicillin for prolonged periods combined with surgical drainage and excision of diseased tissues.

Macroscopic Findings. Renal lesions are either localized or diffuse. Localized lesions appear as pyramidal abscesses, ramifying sinus tracts, and extensive scarring. When sectioned, lesions often appear yellowish-tan and honeycombed. Severe, diffuse involvement occurs as suppurative and necrotizing pyelonephritis, with ureteral obstruction and hydronephrosis being rare complications. Infection may extend through the capsule to produce perirenal abscesses.

Light Microscopic Findings. Lesions are characterized by suppuration, fibrosis, and the formation of draining sinus tracts. Abscesses contain sulfur granules—compact masses of haphazardly arranged or radially oriented actinomycete filaments embedded in an amorphous matrix and surrounded by eosinophilic, refractile, club-like projections (Splendore-Hoeppli phenomenon). Although entire granules are easily seen with hematoxylin and eosin, individual filaments are not stained. Filaments are best seen after staining with Gram's procedures or Gomori methenamine silver. Because the agents of actinomycosis are morphologically and tinctorially indistinguishable in tissue, microbiologic or immunologic confirmation of a histologic diagnosis is essential.

Immunomicroscopic Findings. Specific fluorescent antibody conjugates are available for identifying *A. israelii*, *A. naeslundii*, *A. viscosus*, and *Arachnia propionica* in tissue sections and smears of lesional exudate.

Radiologic Findings. Multiple encapsulated abscesses appear as scattered opacities with cavitation and a soap-bubble appearance on roentgenograms has been described. In severe diffuse infections, intravenous and retrograde pyelograms may reveal distortion of calices, delayed excretion of contrast material, and ureteral obstruction and hydronephrosis.

NOCARDIOSIS

Nocardiosis is a subacute or chronic bacterial infection caused by aerobic, exogenous, filamentous actinomycetes in the genus *Nocardia*. The disease occurs world-wide and is often seen in persons with underlying medical conditions, especially lymphoreticular malignancies and pulmonary alveolar proteinosis. Primary infections, which are usually pulmonary, result from inhalation of nocardiae that live as saprophytes in nature. Hematogenous dissemination can involve almost any organ, but urinary tract lesions are rare. The term "nocardiosis" refers to the disseminated disease. When nocardiae develop in the form of grains or granules in tissue, this rare form of the disease is classified under actinomycotic mycetoma.

The three principal pathogenic species are *N. asteroides, N. brasiliensis,* and *N. caviae.* About 85 percent of disseminated infections are caused by *N. asteroides.* All three species are aerobic and easily cultured on routine laboratory media that do not contain antibacterial antibiotics. Colonies develop slowly, are heaped and folded, are cream to yellow-orange, and have a surface that is either moist and glabrous or covered with a powdery white aerial mycelium. The nocardiae are morphologically similar in cultures and clinical materials, appearing as delicate, branched filaments 1 μm in diameter. The filaments are often beaded and bacillary, and coccoid forms are occasionally seen. Organisms can be speciated in culture by studying their physiologic and biochemical properties.

Clinical and Pathologic Manifestations

Nocardiosis occurs three times as often in males as in females. Symptoms of pulmonary infection mimic those of tuberculosis, including fever, chills, dyspnea, cough, chest pain, night sweats, and weight loss. Patients with disease involving the central nervous system may have headaches, nausea, vomiting, mental confusion, convulsions, paralysis, and nuchal rigidity. Symptoms of urinary tract involvement are like those of nonfilamentous bacterial pyelonephritis. Therapy consists of surgical drainage combined with high doses of sulfonamides or penicillin.

Macroscopic Findings. Virtually any organ can be involved in nocardiosis, but the lungs, brain, subcutaneous tissue and peritoneum are most often affected. Organs usually contain multiple abscesses, 1 to 3 mm in diameter, filled with thick, greenish-yellow, odorless pus. Subcutaneous abscesses are often accompanied by draining sinus tracts. Renal infections are seen as abscesses or severe diffuse pyelonephritis. Lesions of the pelves, ureters, and urinary bladder have not been described.

Light Microscopic Findings. Inflammation is typically suppurative and necrotizing with the formation of encapsulated abscesses and sinus tracts. Interstitial microabscesses are seen in the kidneys. In chronic infections, there is pyelitis with interstitial inflammation and fibrosis. Glomerular and vascular lesions have not been described. Individual organisms are diffusely distributed in the inflammatory exudate, where they are readily demonstrated with the GMS stain and Gram's stains such as Brown and Brenn and Brown-Hopps. The nocardiae do not stain with hematoxylin-eosin, PAS and Gridley fungus procedures, but they are weakly acid-fast in tissue sections stained with modified acid-fast procedures that use an aqueous solution of a weak acid for decolorization.

Immunomicroscopic Findings. Specific fluorescent antibody conjugates are not yet available for identifying the Nocardia spp. in clinical materials. Diagnosis is confirmed by isolating the organism in culture and demonstrating typical Gram-positive and weakly acid-fast filaments in tissue sections or smears of lesional exudate.

Radiologic Findings. Roentgenographic findings are usually indistinguishable from those of pyelonephritis caused by nonfilamentous bacteria. In severe infections, numerous small opacities with cavitation can be seen in both cortex and medulla.

CANDIDIASIS

FIGURE 12.1 Kidney in disseminated candidiasis due to *Candida albicans*. External and sectioned surfaces show miliary abscesses and papillary necrosis.

FIGURE 12.2 Disseminated candidiasis. Renal abscess contains aggregate of blastoconidia and pseudohyphae of *Candida albicans*. (H & E × 95)

FIGURE 12.3 Hematogenous candidal nephritis. Proliferating hyphae and pseudohyphae occlude glomerular capillaries and penetrate Bowman's capsule, interstitium, and tubules. (PAS × 235)

FIGURE 12.4 Typical spherical-to-oval blastoconidia and narrow, frequently septate pseudohyphae of *Candida albicans* in renal abscess. (PAS, 1-μm plastic section × 380)

12.1

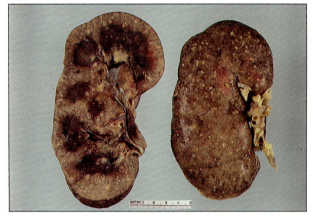

12.2

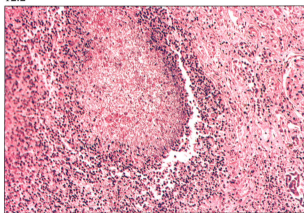

12.3

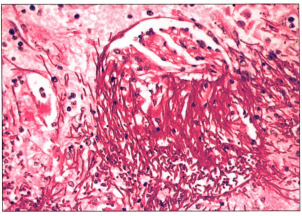

12.4

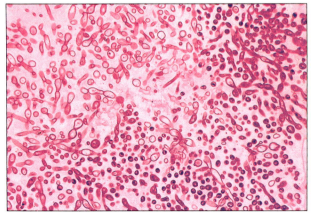

CANDIDIASIS

FIGURE 12.5 Renal candidiasis with papillary necrosis.

FIGURE 12.6 Papillary necrosis in renal candidiasis. Tubulointerstitial aggregates of *Candida albicans* are present. Sloughed papillary tip (center) contains numerous fungal elements. (H & E × 95)

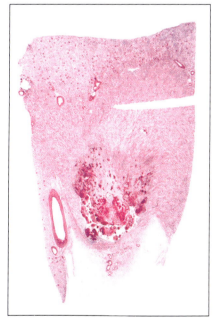

12.5

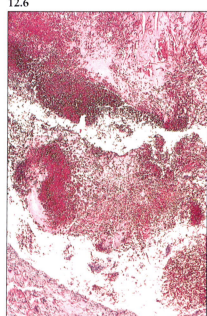

12.6

CANDIDIASIS

FIGURE 12.7 "Fungus ball" in renal pelvis contains haphazardly arranged hyphae, pseudohyphae, and blastoconidia of a *Candida* sp. (GMS × 380)

FIGURE 12.8 Mucosal candidiasis of the urinary bladder. Focal ulcer with hyphal and pseudohyphal invasion of lamina propria. (PAS × 190)

FIGURE 12.9 Direct immunofluorescence microscopy. Blastoconidia and pseudohyphae of a *Candida* sp. in renal abscess. (× 470)

12.7

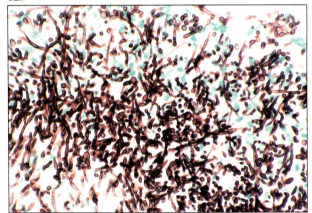

12.8

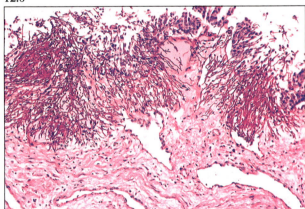

12.9

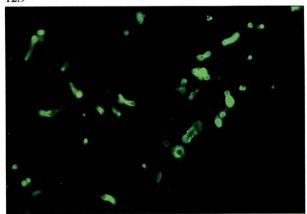

TORULOPSOSIS

FIGURE 12.10 Disseminated torulopsosis. Clustered yeast-like cells of *Torulopsis glabrata* are amphophilic and stain entirely. Host response is minimal. (H & E × 380)

FIGURE 12.11 Disseminated torulopsosis. Macrophages (center) contain amphophilic yeast-like cells of *Torulopsis glabrata*. (H & E × 590)

FIGURE 12.12 Compact aggregates of single and budding *Torulopsis glabrata* cells within arterial thrombus. Hyphae and pseudohyphae are not formed in tissue. With the GMS stain *T. glabrata* cells resemble those of *Histoplasma capsulatum* var. *capsulatum*. (GMS × 380)

12.10
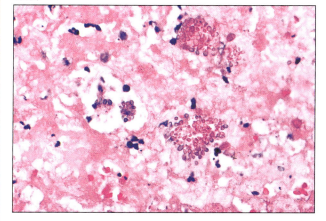

12.11
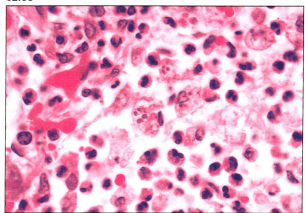

12.12
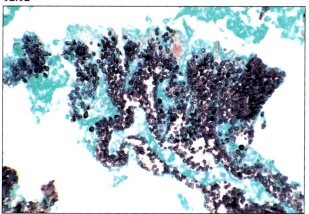

CRYPTOCOCCOSIS

FIGURE 12.13   Hematogenous cryptococcal nephritis. Tubulointerstitial granuloma. (H & E × 95)

FIGURE 12.14   Hematogenous cryptococcal nephritis. Cryptococci distend glomerular capillary lumens. Some have entered Bowman's space. (PAS × 235)

FIGURE 12.15   Cryptococcal nephritis. Tubulointerstitial microabscess with early cystic change due to accumulation of fungal capsular material. Capsules are carminophilic. (Mucicarmine × 235)

FIGURE 12.16   Direct immunofluorescence microscopy. Specific fluorescence restricted to the capsular material of *Cryptococcus neoformans*. The cell bodies of these cryptococci are autofluorescent. (× 470)

12.13

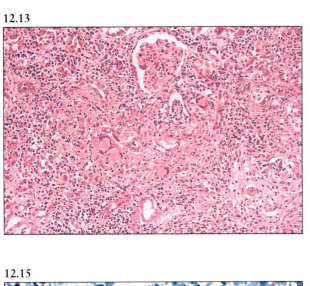

12.14

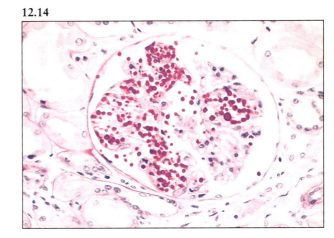

12.15

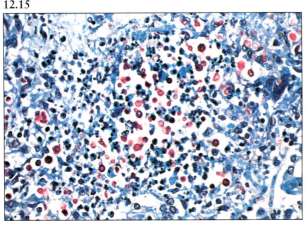

12.16

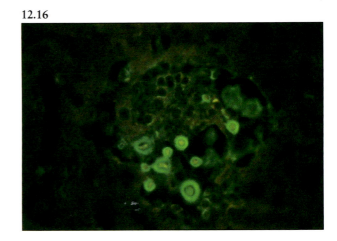

CRYPTOCOCCOSIS

FIGURE 12.17 Electron micrograph, showing *Cryptococcus neoformans* within a phagocytic vacuole. Electron-dense cell wall is surrounded by a thick capsule composed of radiating fibrils and tubules in a finely granular matrix. (× 5,800)

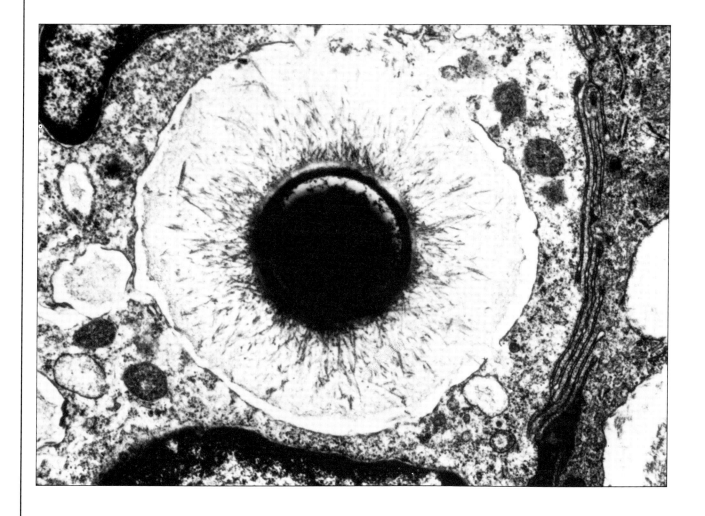

BLASTOMYCOSIS

FIGURE 12.18 Disseminated blastomycosis. Spherical yeast-form cells of *Blastomyces dermatitidis* with doubly contoured walls, in an area of suppurative and granulomatous inflammation. Multiple basophilic nuclei are seen in some of the fungal cells. (H & E × 380)

FIGURE 12.19 Typical yeast-form cells of *Blastomyces dermatitidis*. The broad-based attachment of buds to their patent cells is diagnostic for this fungus in tissue. (GMS with H & E counterstain × 380)

FIGURE 12.20 Direct immunofluorescence microscopy. The walls of single and budding *Blastomyces dermatitidis* cells are brightly fluorescent. (× 470)

12.18

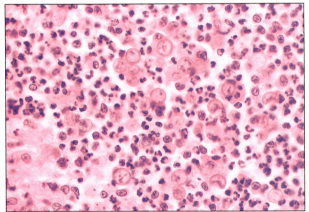

12.19

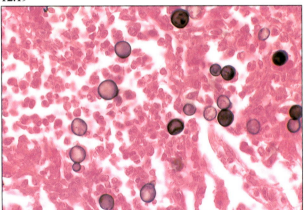

12.20

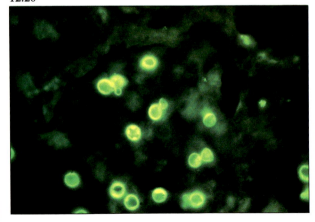

HISTOPLASMOSIS

FIGURE 12.21 Acute disseminated histoplasmosis. Histiocytes contain numerous yeast-form cells of *Histoplasma capsulatum* var. *capsulatum*. Basophilic cytoplasm of fungal cells is retracted from poorly stained cell walls, giving the false impression of an unstained capsule. (H & E × 380)

FIGURE 12.22 Diffuse histiocytosis in progressive disseminated histoplasmosis. Yeast cells are clustered because of their intracellular confinement. Because entire fungal cells are stained, there is no "capsule" effect. (GMS with H & E counterstain × 380)

FIGURE 12.23 Direct immunofluorescence microscopy. The cell walls of *Histoplasma capsulatum* var. *capsulatum* are brightly fluorescent. (× 590)

12.21

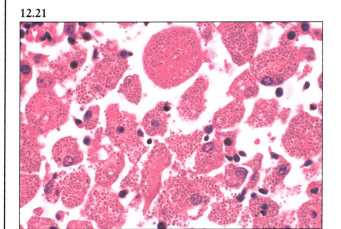

12.22

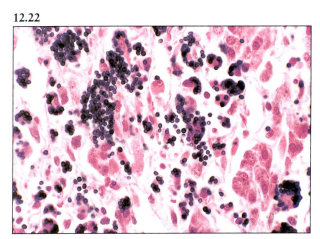

12.23

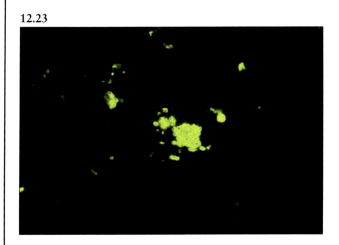

Paracoccidioidomycosis

FIGURE 12.24   Disseminated paracoccidioidomycosis. Epithelioid and giant cell granuloma. Yeast-form cells located within cytoplasm of multinucleated giant cells. One yeast-form cell (center) has multiple buds. (H & E × 380)

FIGURE 12.25   Yeast-form cells of *Paracoccidioides brasiliensis*. Note variability in size. Several typical multiple-budding cells are present. (GMS × 380)

FIGURE 12.26   Direct immunofluorescence microscopy. Nonbudding and single-budding cells of *Paracoccidioides brasiliensis*. (× 295)

Coccidioidomycosis

FIGURE 12.27   Disseminated coccidioidomycosis. Circumscribed renal medullary granuloma contains immature spherules of *Coccidioides immitis*. (H & E × 95)

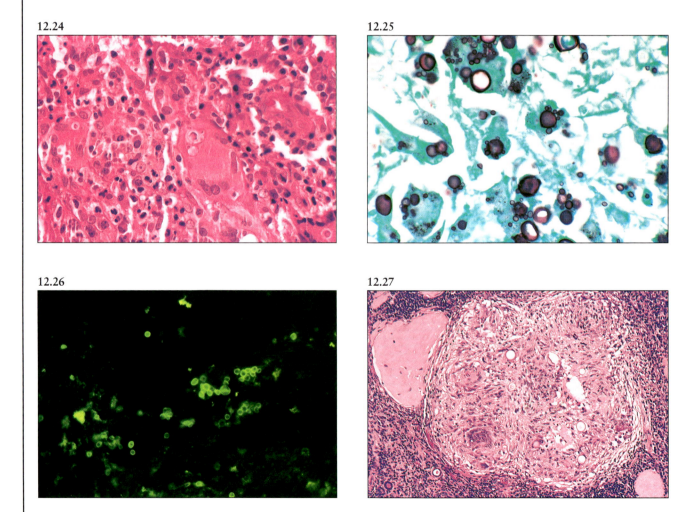

12.24

12.25

12.26

12.27

COCCIDIOIDOMYCOSIS

FIGURE 12.28   Spherules of *Coccidioides immitis*. Two mature spherules have ruptured and released endospores into surrounding tissue. (GMS × 380)

FIGURE 12.29   Direct immunofluorescence microscopy. Immature spherules and endospores of *Coccidioides immitis* are brightly fluorescent. The walls of mature spherules are weakly fluorescent or nonreactive. (× 295)

ASPERGILLOSIS

FIGURE 12.30   Kidney is disseminated aspergillosis due to *Aspergillus fumigatus*. Sectioned surfaces show abscesses with papillary necrosis.

FIGURE 12.31   Disseminated aspergillosis. Acute cortical infarct (left) has a hyperemic margin. Arcuate (not shown) and interlobular arteries are occluded by thrombi and hyphae of *Aspergillus* sp. (H & E × 40)

12.28
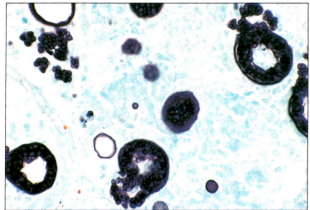

12.29
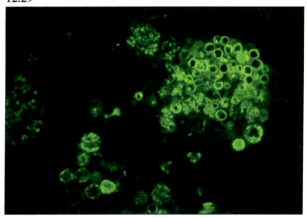

12.30
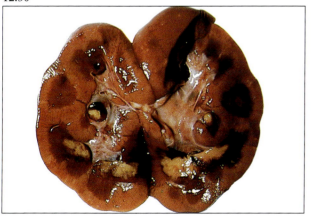

12.31
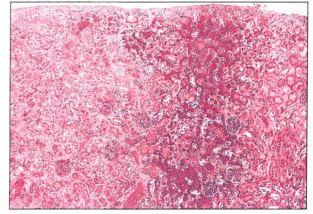

ASPERGILLOSIS

FIGURE 12.32   Hyphal fragments of *Aspergillus* sp. extend through wall of blood vessel (upper right) into interstitium, tubules, and glomerulus (upper left). (GMS × 235)

FIGURE 12.33   Typical hyphae of *Aspergillus* sp. show progressive dichotomous branching. The hyphae are narrow, uniform, and regularly septate. (GMS × 380)

FIGURE 12.34   Aspergillus. Conidiophores (fruiting bodies) characteristics of *Aspergillus fumigatus* in kidney abscess. Same case as in Figure 12.30. (GMS × 760)

FIGURE 12.35   Direct immunofluorescence microscopy. Hyphal fragments of *Aspergillus fumigatus*. One shows dichotomous branching. (× 590)

12.32

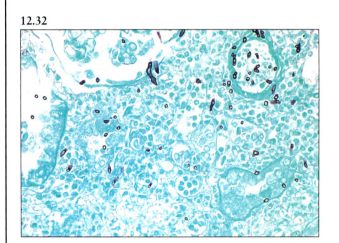

12.33

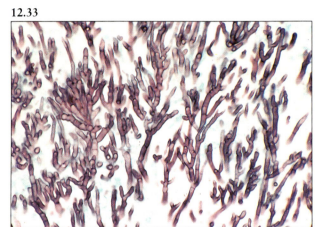

12.34

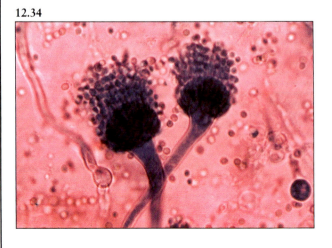

12.35

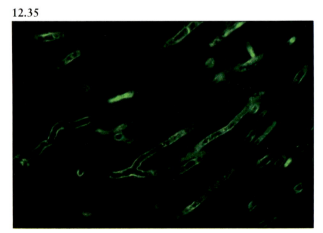

Mucormycosis (Zygomycosis)

FIGURE 12.36   Kidney in disseminated mucormycosis caused by *Rhizopus* sp. Subtotal infarction is produced by hyphal invasion and obstruction of blood vessels.

FIGURE 12.37   Thrombosis of interlobar artery. Note mucoraceous hyphae in lumen and invasion of arterial wall. (H & E × 95)

FIGURE 12.38   Disseminated mucormycosis. Hyphal fragments occlude glomerular capillaries and extend into Bowman's space, interstitium, and tubules. (GMS with H & E counterstain × 235)

FIGURE 12.39   Intravascular hyphae in disseminated mucormycosis. Mucoraceous hyphae are broad and thin-walled. Branching is haphazard, and branches are oriented at right angles to parent hyphae. Septa are not apparent. Transected hyphae appear round or oval. (GMS with H & E counterstain × 380)

12.36

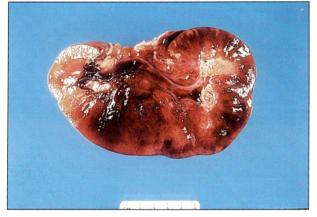

12.37

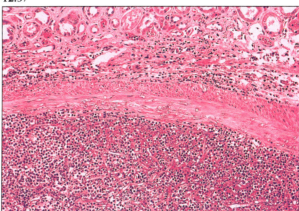

12.38

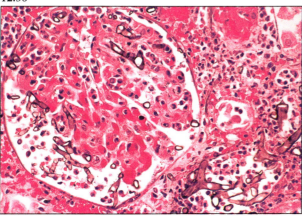

12.39

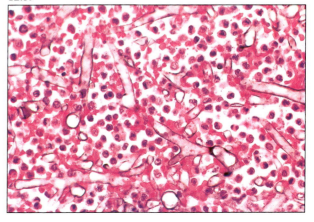

Mucormycosis (Zygomycosis)

FIGURE 12.40   Direct immunofluorescence microscopy. Twisted hyphal fragments of *Rhizopus* sp. (× 295)

Actinomycosis

FIGURE 12.41   Granule of *Actinomyces israelii* in abscess. The entire granule is well-stained, but individual filaments of the actinomycete are not visible. (H & E × 95)

FIGURE 12.42   Delicate, Gram-positive and branched filaments of *Actinomyces israelii* embedded in amorphous matrix of granule. Gram-negative Splendore-Hoeppli material borders the granule. (Brown and Brenn × 380)

FIGURE 12.43   Direct immunofluorescence microscopy of *Actinomyces israelii*. Entire filaments are brightly fluorescent. (× 470)

12.40
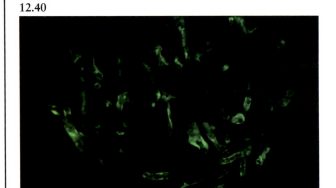

12.41
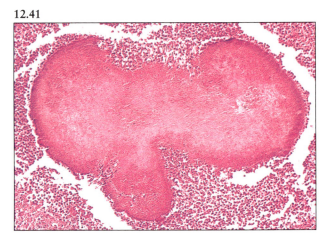

12.42
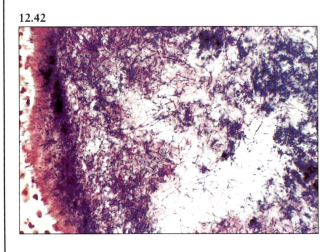

12.43
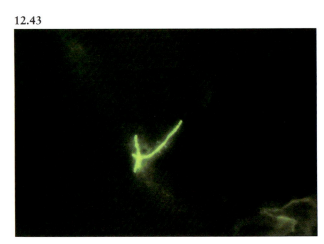

NOCARDIOSIS

FIGURE 12.44   Disseminated nocardiosis caused by *Nocardia asteroides*. Abscess contains nocardial filaments that do not stain with hematoxylin and eosin. (H & E × 95)

FIGURE 12.45   Disseminated nocardiosis. Renal abscess contains delicate, Gram-positive, branched, and beaded filaments of *Nocardia asteroides*. (Brown and Brenn × 590)

FIGURE 12.46   Nocardiosis caused by *Nocardia caviae*. A tangled mass of filaments is present in an abscess. (GMS × 590)

FIGURE 12.47   Delicate, branched, acid-fast filaments of *Nocardia asteroides*. Irregular acid-fastness gives some of the filaments a beaded appearance. (Fite-Faraco acid-fast stain × 950)

12.44

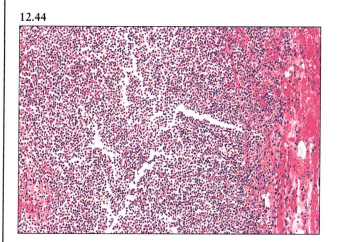

12.45

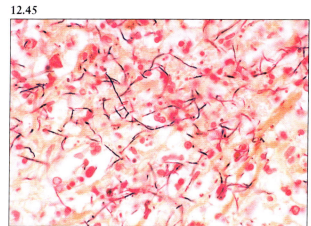

12.46

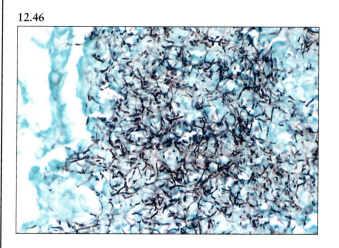

12.47

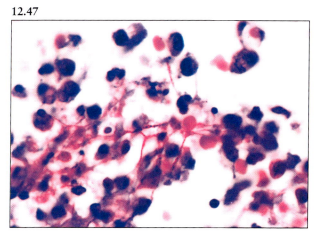

ARTHROPOD AND VENOMOUS ANIMAL BITES AND STINGS

VENOMOUS SNAKEBITES

Snakebite poses a serious health hazard to the inhabitants of tropical and subtropical regions of the world. Of the 2,700 known species of snakes, 450 are known to be poisonous. Of the more than 40,000 deaths due to snakebite each year worldwide, 15,000 occur in the Indian subcontinent. Renal involvement is a common complication contributing to death.

Renal complications have been associated with bites by Russell's viper (*Vipera russelli*), saw-scaled viper (*Echis carinatus*), puff adder (*Bitis arietans*), rattlesnake (genus *Crotalus*), other pit vipers (genus *Bothrops* and genus *Agkistrodon*), boomslang (*Dispholidus typhus*), sea snakes (family Hydrophidae), tiger snake (*Notechis scutatus occidentalis*), gwardar snake (*Demansia nuchalis*), and small-eyed black snake (*Cryptophis nigrescens*). Russell's viper is widely distributed in India, Burma, and Southeast Asia; and the saw-scaled viper in Africa north of the equator, the Middle East, India, Pakistan, and Sri Lanka. The puff adder is a widespread African species accused of inflicting more bites and deaths in man on the African continent than all other snakes put together. The South American rattlesnake (*Crotalus durissus terificus*) and the various species of Bothrops are pit vipers seen in Central and South America. Bites by pit vipers of Agkistrodon spp. occur in Japan, Korea, Hong Kong, Taiwan, Malaysia, and Indonesia. Sea snake bites have been reported mainly from Malaysia, Thailand, and

western Pacific coastal areas. The boomslang is found on the African continent. The important species prevalent along the Malaysian coast are the sea snakes, *Enhydrina schistosa*, and *Hydrophis cyanocinctus* while several species of *Hydrophis* are found along the coast of India. The tiger snake, blacksnake, and the gwardar dugite (*Demansia nuchalis affinis*) are Australian land snakes.

Pathogenesis

Acute renal failure associated with snakebite appears to be multifactorial, attributable to hypotension, hemorrhagic shock, intravascular hemolysis, and disseminated intravascular coagulation. Microangiopathic hemolytic anemia develops in human victims of gwardar and puff adder bites, and rhabdomyolysis and myoglobinuria in victims of bites by sea snakes, tiger snakes, king brown snakes, and blacksnakes. A direct cytotoxic effect of the snake venom on renal tubular cells has also been suspected.

Clinical and Pathologic Manifestations

The clinical consequences of envenomation vary from local necrosis to rapidly fatal systemic disease. The most frequent renal manifestation is acute renal failure, the frequency of which differs according to the type of snake involved.

Acute renal failure is almost invariably oliguric and

usually develops between 2 and 96 hours after the bite. Macroscopic hematuria may be associated with generalized hemorrhagic diathesis. Even in the absence of hematuria, the urine may be reddish brown because of hemoglobinuria or myoglobinuria. Acute renal failure is usually reversible, with mortality not exceeding 16 percent, except that acute cortical necrosis carries a poor prognosis.

Light Microscopic Findings.   Acute tubular necrosis predominates, with tubular dilation, casts, desquamation of necrotic cells, and tubulorrhexis. In sea snake bites especially, the tubular lumens contain myoglobin. Varying degrees of interstitial edema and hemorrhage are associated with infiltrates of lymphocytes, plasmacytes, and monocytes.

Biopsies within the first week of envenomation are likely to show hyaline tubular casts and interstitial hemorrhages, whereas later biopsies show granular and pigmented casts, inflammatory cell infiltrates, and tubular regeneration.

Russell's viper bite causes necrotizing interlobular arteritis, with occasional infarcts; no lesion has been demonstrated in the smaller vessels. Thrombophlebitis of arcuate veins and their tributaries may be present.

Most cases lack glomerular lesions, although focal or diffuse proliferative glomerulonephritis and occasional crescents have been observed.

Bilateral renal cortical necrosis also follows snakebite, particularly in victims bitten by *Agkistrodon hypnale*, *Echis carinatus*, *Vipera russelli*, and *Bothrops* species. Cortical necrosis may be diffuse or patchy. Fibrin thrombi, considered to be a hallmark of disseminated intravascular coagulation, are often present in glomerular capillaries.

The lesions differ from those seen in acute tubular necrosis due to other causes. Features unique to acute renal failure due to snakebite are the severe tubular and vascular lesions; shedding of cells in the distal tubules; and the eosinophils, mast cells, and hyperplastic fibroblasts in the interstitium.

Electron Microscopic Findings.   In the glomeruli, podocytes are enlarged, with foot-process swelling and intracytoplasmic lipid vacuoles. The urinary spaces contain cytoplasmic fragments, erythrocytes, and fibrin. Capillaries contain platelet clusters, and there are occasional subendothelial electron-dense deposits. Mesangial expansion and subendothelial mesangial interposition are frequent. Mesangiolysis and membranolysis also occur.

In patients bitten by cobras and green pit vipers, ultrastructural studies have revealed electron-dense mesangial deposits even in the absence of renal failure.

Tubular necrosis leads to denudation of the basement membrane. Cells contain degenerating organelles and protein reabsorption droplets. Collecting tubules are relatively spared.

The interstitial infiltrate contains eosinophils and mast cells, which may be degranulated. Active fibroblasts contain increased numbers of organelles and long, branching cytoplasmic processes.

Blood vessels contain swollen endothelial cells, which may be desquamated into the lumen. Fibrin tactoids are present in smaller vessels. Blood vessels are severely obstructed by swollen and necrotic endothelial cells.

BEE, WASP, AND HORNET STINGS

Renal effects are not seen in envenomation from a single bee, wasp, or hornet sting, as the volume of venom is rather small. Collective stings from swarms, such as those of the aggressive African bees, introduce massive quantities of venom sufficient to produce extensive myonecrosis and myoglobinuria. In those allergic to the venom, hemolysis may also occur and acute renal failure may supervene. The renal failure is due either to myoglobinuria or hemolysis or both. Angioneurotic edema and cardiovascular collapse may, of course, also occur and may be responsible for death.

SCORPION AND SPIDER STINGS

The effects of scorpion and spider bites are very similar. The commonest result is due to local action of 5-hydroxytryptamine. Systemic symptoms ("scorpionism") are exceptional and are due to hypoglycemia and to involvement of the central nervous system. Acute renal failure is occasionally seen. Scorpionism is by and large confined to stings from members of the genus Tityus, the most venomous member of which is *Tityus serrulatus*, which is native to Brazil.

Spider bites may be mild and may even go unnoticed, although on occasion a very painful bite and systemic symptoms may follow. These symptoms are generally similar to those of scorpionism, although disseminated intravascular coagulation and hemolysis may complicate some cases, especially in envenomation from members of the genus Loxosceles. Acute intrinsic reversible renal failure may supervene in cases of disseminated intravascular coagulation.

Although Phoneutria spp. is the most venomous spider known, *Loxosceles* and *Latrodectus* are the most important by reason of their prevalence and widespread habitus. Loxosceles is native to the American continent; *Latrodectus* is spread over the American continent, the Mediterranean region, most of Africa, the Indian subcontinent, the Soviet Union, and Southeast Asia.

Pathologic Manifestations

Loxosceles venom is both cytotoxic and hemolytic. Congestive hemorrhagic lesions occur primarily in the liver and kidneys, and extensive hemorrhagic necrosis occurs at the site of bites.

Latrodectus venom is essentially neurotoxic; but generalized lesions may also occur in the kidneys, liver, spleen, lymph glands, thymus, and adrenals.

CENTIPEDE STINGS

Centipedes are widely distributed, and their stings cause rhabdomyolysis and myoglobinuria, with secondary renal effects. (see Chap. 14).

SNAKEBITES

FIGURE 13.1   Snakebite. There are many fibrin thrombi in glomerular capillaries due to disseminated intravascular coagulation. Note glomerular damage and necrosis of tubular epithelial cells. (Phospotungstic acid-hematoxylin × 285)

FIGURE 13.2   Snakebite. Acute tubular necrosis, dilatation of tubular lumens, and casts containing myoglobin. (H & E stain × 235)

FIGURE 13.3   Acute tubulointerstitial nephritis, with infiltration by lymphocytes, plasma cells, and monocytes. (H & E stain × 235)

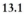
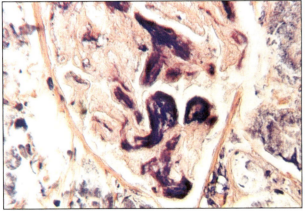

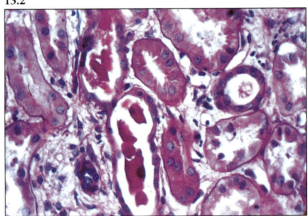

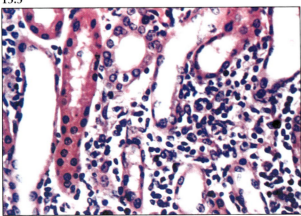

SNAKEBITES

FIGURE 13.4 Electron micrograph. Small medullary blood vessels filled with swollen and partially necrotic endothelial cells. (× 4,800)

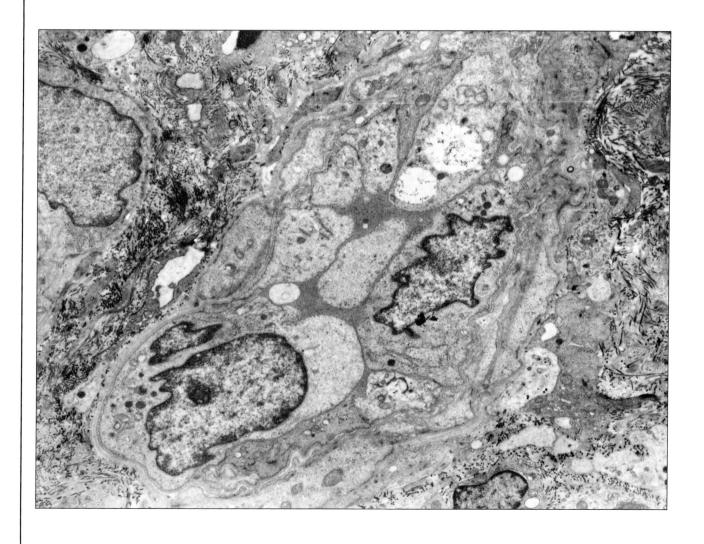

FIGURE 13.5   Electron micrograph. Distal tubule showing focal shedding of the degenerating epithelium. Interstitium contains a lymphocyte and fibroblast in contact (top left). (× 3,700)

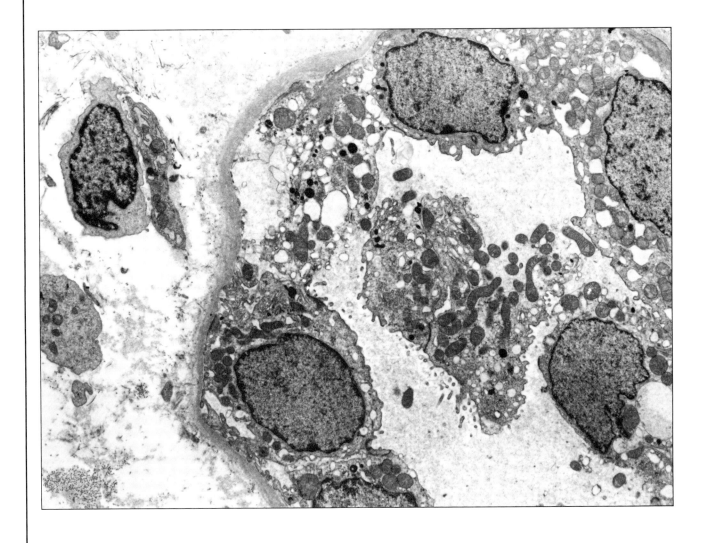

BEE-STING NEPHROSIS

FIGURE 13.6   Electron micrograph showing cellular proliferation in the mesangium, extensive effacement of foot processes, and degeneration of podocytes (upper and lower right). (× 2,800)

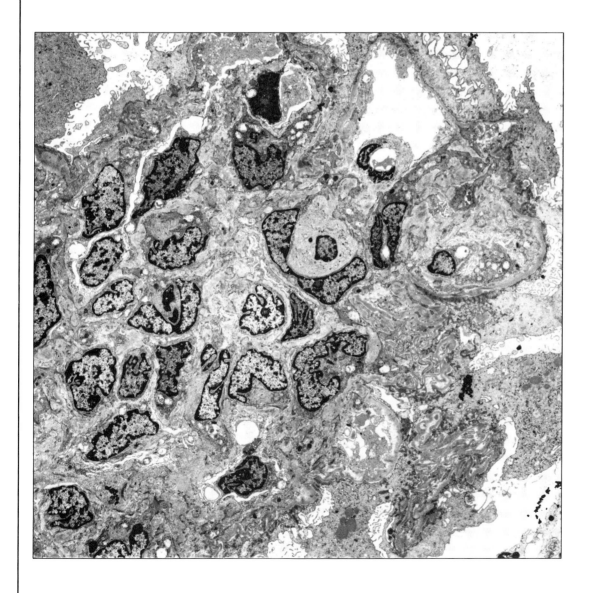

BEE-STING NEPHROSIS

FIGURE 13.7   Bee-sting nephrosis in a 51-year-old man with proteinuria, hematuria, and pyuria 6 to 8 weeks following bee sting. Urinary protein was 11 gm/24 hr. Mesangial proliferative glomerulonephritis. (Immunofluorescence negative for immunoglobulins; 1+ granular C3 along glomerular capillary walls and in mesangium). (PAS × 235)

WASP AND HORNET STINGS

FIGURE 13.8   Multiple wasp or hornet stings with patchy blackened areas of skin necrosis and angioneurotic edema.

FIGURE 13.9   Same case as in Figure 13.8. There are necrosis of tubular cells and myoglobin casts and red cells in the tubular lumens. (H & E × 190)

13.7

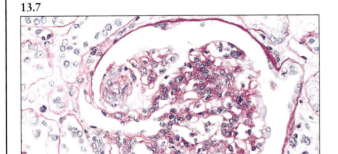

13.8

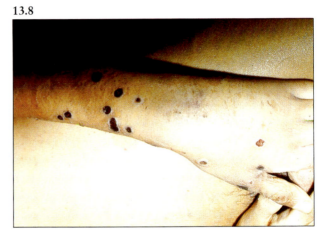

13.9

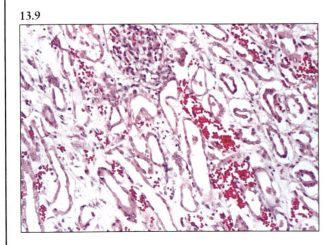

CONSEQUENCES OF METABOLIC DERANGEMENTS IN TROPICAL CLIMATES

ACUTE RHABDOMYOLYSIS AND MYOGLOBINURIA

Myoglobinuric acute renal failure is caused by the release of myoglobin from damaged skeletal muscle, with myoglobinemia and myoglobinuria. Rhabdomyolysis results from many kinds of injury to skeletal muscle: pressure and crushing, severe physical exertion, convulsions, heat stress, burns, ischemia, drug and chemical intoxication, acquired and heritable metabolic abnormalities, primary and secondary myopathies and infectious agents. Of that large list, the conditions pertinent to the tropics include tense physical activity, hyperpyrexia and heat stroke, snake and centipede envenomation, and infectious myositis. Heat stress leads to both fluid and potassium loss from the body. Hypokalemia and high body temperature contribute to the development of rhabdomyolysis caused by strenous exercise. Renal injury develops under conditions of fluid volume depletion and is exacerbated by hypotension. Despite the etiologic diversity, renal injury results from renal vasoconstriction and diminished renal perfusion and their consequences. Tubular injury and tubular obstruction by casts contribute to the renal excretory failure.

Clinical and Pathologic Manifestations

The primary clinical manifestations relate to the cause of the muscle injury, such as direct trauma (crush syndrome), coma, postural pressure, arterial thrombosis and ischemia. Muscle injury and rhabdomyolysis are associated with severe swelling and tenderness of the affected muscle, and clinical laboratory investigation reveals elevated levels of serum muscle enzymes such as creatinine phosphokinase, aspartate transaminase (AST or SGOT), and lactate dehydrogenase found on the majority of automated chemical analyzers, and adolase. Myoglobin, unlike hemoglobin, does not bind to haptoglobin and does not discolor the serum. Myoglobin is promptly excreted in the urine, which will be discolored reddish brown. Myoglobinuria, like hemoglobinuria, causes a positive benzidine or orthotolidine reaction on impregnated strips. Rapid screening of urine for the differentiation of hemoglobinuria from myoglobinuria involves precipitation of hemoglobin by 80% ammonium sulfate. Benzidine or orthotolidine reactivity in the supernatant represents myoglobin. False-negative results have been reported, however. Myoglobin can be identified and quantified accurately by immunodiffusion or radioimmunoassay. Patients with rhabdomyolysis and renal failure experience unusually rapid increases in their serum concentrations of creatinine and potassium, as those substances are released from damaged muscle. Serum creatinine concentrations rise out of proportion to urea concentrations, and a low ratio of urea nitrogen to creatinine, normally around 10, suggests rhabdomyolysis. The rapid release of purine nucleotides from damaged muscle leads to hyperuricemia.

Although concentrations of inorganic phosphate also rise and may be accompanied by hypocalcemia, patients characteristically develop hypercalcemia in the diuretic phase of the disease. The clinical findings are otherwise those of acute renal failure, and most patients respond eventually to supportive therapy. The prognosis is ordinarily good, although some patients succumb to their primary disease.

Microscopic Findings. The renal lesion is acute tubular necrosis, with necrosis of epithelial cells, disruption of tubular walls, interstitial edema, and mild interstitial inflammatory cell infiltrates. The distinctive feature is the occurrence of pigmented casts, which can be shown by immunohistochemistry to contain myoglobin. Casts are occasionally extruded from disrupted tubules into the interstitium. Recovery is associated with regeneration of tubular epithelium. The glomeruli may be collapsed and ischemic, with moderately dilated Bowman's spaces. Severe tubulointerstitial injury with cortical scarring also results in focal glomerular obsolescence. Vascular changes in the acute stage include medial swelling and edema.

HEAT STROKE

Heat stroke is the clinical syndrome produced by overheating of the body, leading to thermal injury at a cellular level. It is usually produced by prolonged physical exercise in a hot, humid environment close to or above body temperature. The exact cause is not known, and only rarely is it due to congenital anhydrosis. Factors known to lead to heat stroke include fatigue, lack of physical conditioning, failure of acclimatization, previous illness, obesity, and increased wet bulb globe temperature.

Heat stroke causes widespread damage to the heart, muscle, liver, kidneys, brain, and blood coagulation system. Damage to the vascular endothelium appears to initiate platelet aggregation, leading to disseminated intravascular coagulation. Nearly all patients die from disseminated intravascular coagulation with manifestations of bleeding diathesis and pathologic changes of widespread microthrombus formation in various organs such as the brain, lungs, kidneys, adrenals, and pituitary gland. There are massive hemorrhages into the lungs, gastrointestinal tract, kidney, brain, and other organs. Obstruction of small vessels leads to infarcts and necrosis of various organs. Damaged tissues release plasminogen activator, with resulting fibrinolysis and reduced fibrinogen levels. The incoagulability of the blood contributes to further bleeding from the damaged tissues. Renal injury may also be caused by rhabdomyolysis and myoglobinuria.

Death in heat stroke has been reported as due to renal failure, hepatic failure, hyperkalemia, cardiovascular collapse, hemorrhagic diathesis, or a combination of these.

Clinical and Pathologic Manifestations

Patients collapse after physical exercise like running or a route march. The interval from the time of collapse to time of death ranges from 45 minutes to over 90 hours. Rectal temperatures range from 40°C to 42°C, and there may be hot, dry skin or profuse sweating and diarrhea. Other manifestations are delirium, convulsions, and coma. There is evidence of disseminated intravascular coagulation with low platelet counts, and prolonged partial thromboplastin time and prothrombin time. The bleeding diathesis is manifested by frank hemoptysis, hematemesis, and melaena.

Damage to the kidney is manifested by proteinuria, raised blood urea levels, and acute renal failure.

Macroscopic Findings. The kidneys may be slightly swollen and show hemorrhages into the renal pelvis as part of the generalized bleeding diathesis.

Light Microscopic Findings. The kidneys show focal areas of hemorrhage, with microthrombi in the glomerular capillaries and arterioles. There is also sludging of red blood cells in the glomerular capillary lumens and arterioles. The tubules, especially straight tubules, show focal areas of coagulative necrosis with clumping of the proteins in the epithelial cells. Pigmented casts containing myoglobin may be found in the lumens.

The renal lesions are thought to be due partly to direct thermal injuries with coagulative necrosis of the tubular epithelium, as most patients are not hypotensive or dehydrated, and the raised blood urea nitrogen levels persist despite intravenous therapy.

Immunomicroscopic findings. There are no significant deposits. Extensive fibrin thrombi are found in the glomerular capillaries and arterioles of the kidneys.

FLUID AND ELECTROLYTE DEPLETION

Fluid and electrolyte loss resulting from acute gastroenteritis, cholera, and dysentery continue to be the commonest cause of acute oliguric renal failure in the tropics. This is due, in part, to the prevalence of these conditions and, in part, to lack of adequate and timely replacement of fluid and electrolyte losses in patients with these problems. In cholera, the initial stool volume may exceed 1,500 ml. Cholera stool is isotonic with plasma and alkaline in pH because its bicarbonate content is approximately twice that of plasma. Acute renal failure may also complicate other tropical infections such as typhoid, leptospirosis, and pyomyositis. In most instances, renal biopsy reveals acute tubular necrosis, but cortical necrosis may also rarely occur.

ACUTE RHABDOMYOLYSIS AND MYOGLOBINURIA

FIGURE 14.1   A 43-year-old woman under treatment with haloperidol and trihexyphenidyl for mental disturbance suffered acute onset of abdominal pain and oliguric renal failure. The tubules contain deeply eosinophilic casts and inflammatory cells. There is tubular necrosis with an interstitial infiltrate.
(H & E × 235)

FIGURE 14.2   A 72-year-old man with acute renal failure. The myoglobin casts are deeply acidophilic.
(Masson's trichrome × 235)

FIGURE 14.3   Same case as in Figure 14.1. The casts are strongly positive for myoglobin, although they are negative for hemoglobin. (Immunoperoxidase antimyoglobin × 235)

FIGURE 14.4   Same case as in Figure 14.1. Immunofluorescence is also positive, showing lamination of the deposits. (FITC antimyoglobin × 380)

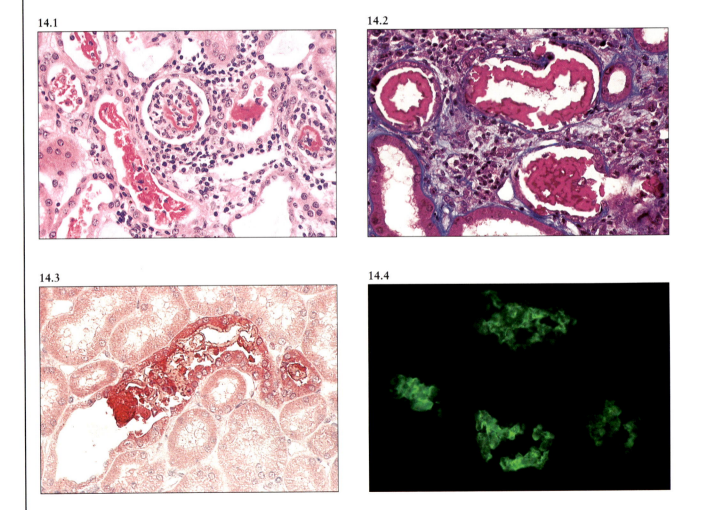

14.1

14.2

14.3

14.4

Acute Rhabdomyolysis and Myoglobinuria

FIGURE 14.5 Electron micrograph showing myoglobinuria with tubular necrosis and interstitial nephritis in a 40-year-old woman with rhabdomyolysis following hemiparesis. The lumen of the collecting duct contains an electron-dense, laminated cast of myoglobin. ($\times$ 3,900)

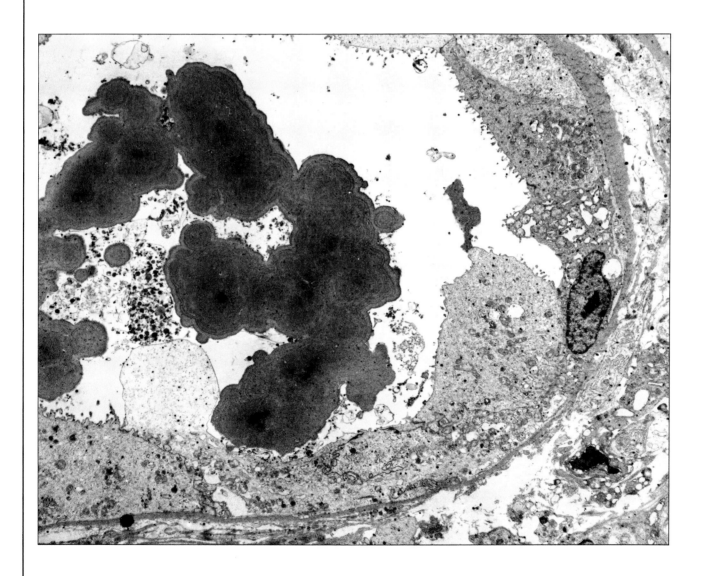

HEAT STROKE

FIGURE 14.6 A 20-year-old Chinese male soldier collapsed during a long march and died of heat stroke. The glomerulus shows sludging of red blood cells and fibrin thrombi in the capillary lumina. (H & E × 235)

FIGURE 14.7 Another young male soldier who died of heat stroke during march. The tubules, especially the straight tubules, show coagulative necrosis of the lining epithelial cells. (Masson's trichrome × 190)

FIGURE 14.8 Same case as in Figure 14.6. The intertubular arteries and arterioles show fibrin thrombi in the lumen and insudates in the walls. (MSB × 235)

14.6

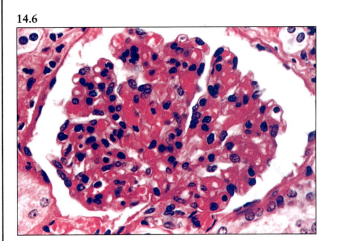

14.7

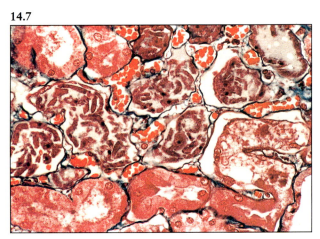

14.8

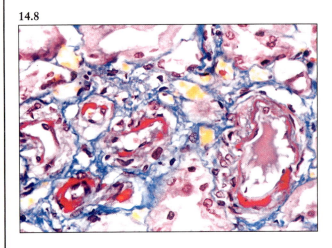

HEAT STROKE

FIGURE 14.9   Immunofluorescence microscopy shows fibrin deposition in the glomerular capillary walls and mesangium. (× 235)

FIGURE 14.10   Immunofluorescence microscopy shows extensive fibrin thrombi in the peritubular capillaries due to disseminated intravascular coagulation. (× 120)

14.9

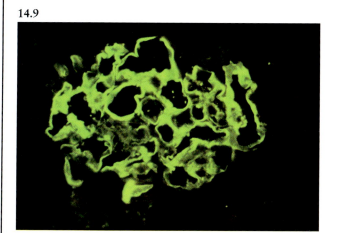

14.10

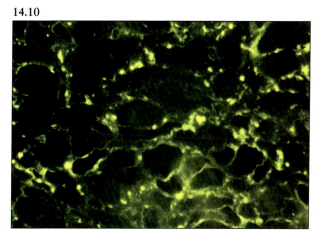

BLOOD DYSCRASIAS

SICKLE CELL DISEASE

Sickle cell trait (hemoglobin S-A) is widely distributed in equatorial Africa, varying in frequency from 0 to 40 percent (average 20%) among different tribes. This trait is also seen in the Mediterranean countries; in the Middle East, especially in the areas facing the Arabian sea; in certain indigenous peoples of India and Indochina; and in descendants of the immigrants from all these areas to South, Central, and North America.

As can be readily calculated, sickle cell disease (hemoglobin S-S) is considerably less common. However, it is a much more serious condition which frequently affects the kidneys and produces such symptoms as hematuria, proteinuria, occasionally nephrotic syndrome, progressive renal failure, and, perhaps, increased tendency to urinary infection, especially during pregnancy.

Pathogenesis

Renal damage is due essentially to sickling and sludging of red blood cells in the vascular channels, and consequent abnormal circulation through the arteries, glomeruli, peritubular capillaries, and vasa recta and capillaries of the medulla. This effect is considerably enhanced by the hypertonic medium of the medulla and papillae, which potentiates sickling due to low oxygen tension. The blood flow is generally higher than normal in the renal cortex but lower than normal in the me-

dulla. The vessels in both areas are strikingly dilated and engorged by red cells in various stages of sickling.

Clinical and Pathologic Manifestations

Renal abnormalities are purely functional ones at first. Renal concentrating ability is decreased, perhaps due to "functional ablation" of the papillae, and there is a tendency to distal tubular acidosis. In young children, the concentrating defect can be corrected by exchange transfusion. However, with time, blood vessels become damaged. Microangiography demonstrates obliteration of many channels in the medulla and abnormalities of those that remain, such as dilatation, spiraling, and formation of blunt ends.

To a large extent, the glomerular abnormalities in nephrotic syndrome represent more severe degrees of abnormalities that are observed in patients without clinical evidence of renal disease. With due regard to the differences in normal structure, changes of the glomerular capillaries can be considered analogous to those of the medullary capillaries, and both are probably caused by abnormal hemodynamic factors, especially increased viscosity of blood.

The concentrating defect becomes fixed because of the permanent impairment of circulation and its anatomic sequelae. Progressive concentrating defect is also seen in sickle cell trait and in combined hemoglobinopathies (hemoglobin S-C, hemoglobin S-thalassemia), although anatomic changes are milder and clinical abnormalities are uncommon.

Macroscopic Findings. Small shallow cortical infarcts are seen occasionally. They are due to vascular obstruction by sickled and sludged cells, often without actual thrombosis. However, there is also a tendency to thrombosis—in the renal veins, for example. Depressed scars on the surface are usually secondary to papillary necrosis and the ensuing obstruction and possible ascending inflammation.

Light Microscopic Findings. The cortical and medullary tubules often contain large amounts of iron pigment in the cytoplasm. Pigmented casts are more common in the medulla. The peritubular capillaries, especially those at the corticomedullary junction, are dilated and filled with sickled cells. This engorgement may be accompanied by capillary rupture, with formation of small interstitial extravasates. The interstitial tissue of the medulla shows edema and, later, foci of fibrosis. Because of progressive tubular atrophy, the number of functioning tubules in the medulla is considerably reduced. Occasionally, capillary aneurysms form at the tips of the papillae and serve as the source of hemorrhage. More often, bleeding probably occurs from dilated and congested vessels of the pelvic mucosa, through which the blood is shunted past the obstructed or narrowed vasa recta. Obliteration of the medullary vessels and obstruction by sludging of the sickled cells lead to papillary ischemia and occasionally to actual necrosis. The necrotic papillae may slough and appear in the urine. More often, the necrosis is limited, with preservation of the caliceal fornices ("medullary" necrosis). On intravenous pyelograms, this may manifest as ring shadows, which are caused by contrast medium surrounding the sloughed medullary tissue, and as cavities that are round or elongated.

The glomeruli become progressively and sometimes strikingly enlarged, often in proportion to the degree of anemia. At first glomerular capillaries are dilated and filled with red cells, many of which are sickled. With age, mesangial expansion and capillary wall thickening lead to narrowing of the lumens. Focal areas of glomerular sclerosis appear during the second decade of life and are sometimes followed by global sclerosis and loss of glomerular function, with eventual renal insufficiency in some patients. Uncommonly mesangiocapillary glomerulonephritis has been reported.

Electron Microscopic Findings. On electron microscopy, the thickened capillary walls may show double outlines with mesangial interposition, somewhat similar to those seen in mesangiocapillary glomerulonephritis. Proteinuria or nephrotic syndrome is often present in such cases. Occasionally, electron-dense deposits are found under the endothelium and in the interposed mesangium. Foot processes are often effaced focally or diffusely, particularly in patients with nephrotic syndrome. Granules of iron pigment can be present in the visceral and parietal epithelial cells, in the mesangium, and, occasionally, in the endothelium.

Immunomicroscopic Findings. When present, the electron-dense deposits contain immunoglobulins (IgG, IgM) and complement (C3).

THALASSEMIAS

Thalassemias include a group of familial hemolytic anemias that result from imbalanced hemoglobin synthesis due to defective production of either beta or alpha chains of globin. There are two major types with several subtypes. Alpha thalassemia is caused by retarded production of alpha (α) chains, and beta thalassemia is the result of decreased beta (β) chain production. Impaired synthesis of hemoglobin leads to anemia and microcytosis. Renal changes and alteration of renal function can occur.

Clinical and Pathologic Manifestations

There are varying degrees of clinical severity; the severe symptoms include moderate to severe hemolytic anemia, jaundice, splenomegaly, and cholelithiasis. There is impairment of growth and development, and deformity due to hyperactivity of bone marrow, with thinning of cortical bone. Cardiac enlargement may occur due to anemia and deposition of hemosiderin in the myocardium. The blood smear shows characteristic nucleated erythroblasts, target cells, and hypochromic microcytic cells with punctate and diffuse basophilic stippling.

Renal involvement, when it occurs, is usually mild, with microhematuria, slight proteinuria, and a few cells in the urine sediment. A few patients may present with acute nephritis with numerous red blood cells in the urine.

Renal functon studies in beta thalassemia have shown increased renal plasma flow and maximal tubular secretion of para-aminohippurate. Glomerular filtration is either normal or increased. Urinary tract obstruction by uric acid crystals and gross hematuria have been described. Impaired urinary concentration and increased excretion of beta aminoisobutyric acid in the urine, believed to be due to increased tissue catabolism, have been observed.

Light Microscopic Findings. The glomerular changes are not specific and, when present, consist of segmental mesangial cell hyperplasia and focal thickening of capillary loops. Red blood cells are present in glomerular capillaries, Bowman's spaces, and lumens of proximal tubules. Obsolescent glomeruli are seen in most cases. Tubular hemosiderosis is seen frequently and can be very severe in some cases. Rarely, hemoglobin pigment is seen in the epithelial cells of the proximal convoluted tubules. In the few cases, especially after splenectomy, that show diffuse endocapillary proliferative glomerulonephritis, poststreptococcal glomerulonephritis cannot be excluded.

Electron Microscopic Findings. The glomeruli show endothelial cytofolds in most of the capillary lumens, with deformed erythrocytes entrapped between these cytofolds. Focal and segmental proliferation of mesangial cells and increased matrix may be seen. Irregular thickening of the basement membrane is seen only in the lamina rara interna. Various patterns of degeneration with focal cytoplasmic degradation of podocytes are prominent.

The proximal convoluted tubular epithelial cells always contain single membrane-lined bodies with dark materials, which are presumed to be hemoglobin absorption droplets.

Immunomicroscopic Findings. There are no deposits of immunoglobulins, C3, or fibrin, except in cases with diffuse endocapillary proliferative glomerulonephritis, which may be of poststreptococcal etiology.

GLUCOSE-6-PHOSPHATE DEHYDROGENASE (G–6–PD) DEFICIENCY AND HEMOLYSIS

G–6–PD deficiency is known to cause acute intravascular hemolysis and acute renal failure. It is the commonest cause of acute renal failure in some parts of the tropics, especially western Africa. The intravascular hemolysis may be triggered by incompatible blood transfusions or ingestion of fava beans, and patients with G–6–PD deficiency are more likely to develop blackwater fever as a complication of malaria. They are also sensitive to chloroquine and other drugs given during the treatment of malaria, leading to G–6–PD hemolysis.

Hemoglobinemia is possibly not the cause of the renal damage, and a factor associated with red cell casts may be responsible. The major kidney lesion is acute tubular necrosis. Rarely, acute bilateral cortical necrosis may occur in infancy after fava bean ingestion.

SICKLE CELL DISEASE

FIGURE 15.1   Nephrectomy for massive hemorrhage in a patient with sickle cell trait. Note the blood in tip of papilla (upper right) and the small blood clot in corresponding calix.

FIGURE 15.2   Section of papilla shown in Figure 15.1. Large submucosal capillary aneurysms with sludging of red blood cells, and partial sloughing of mucosa. (H & E × 40)

FIGURE 15.3   Glomerulus in a child with sickle cell disease, showing massive congestion of capillaries. Glomerular arteriole is also dilated and congested. Sickled red blood cells can be recognized. (H & E × 235)

FIGURE 15.4   Sickle cell disease (SS hemoglobin). Patient died suddenly during exercise. Note the massive sickling of red blood cells in the glomerular capillaries. (H & E × 380)

15.1

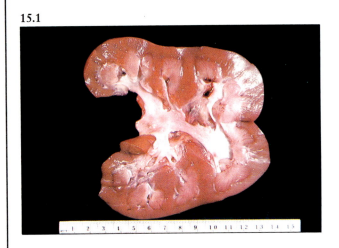

15.2

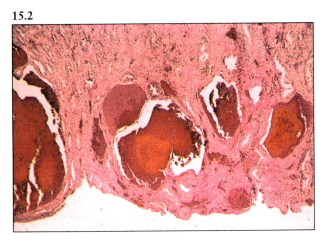

15.3

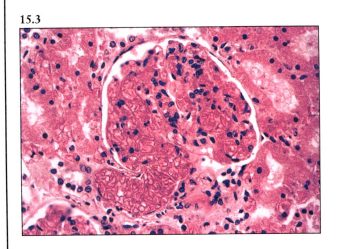

15.4

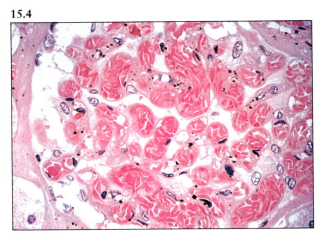

Sickle Cell Disease

FIGURE 15.5   Sickle cell disease and nephrotic syndrome. Large glomerulus shows mesangial expansion and sclerosis, and segmental thickening of capillary walls. (PAS × 235)

FIGURE 15.6   Sickle cell disease. Renal biopsy specimen shows sclerosis of many glomeruli, focal tubular atrophy, and tubular dilatation with many casts. (PAS × 40)

FIGURE 15.7   Scars of the renal medulla in a child with sickle cell disease. (H & E × 95)

FIGURE 15.8   Cavity in the renal medulla following necrosis of a papilla in a child with sickle cell disease. The cavity is lined by the ingrown pelvic epithelium. (H & E, after India ink injection × 95)

15.5
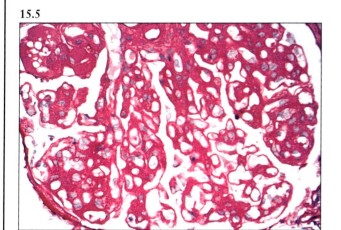

15.6
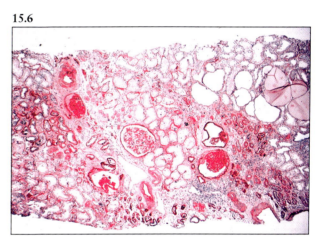

15.7
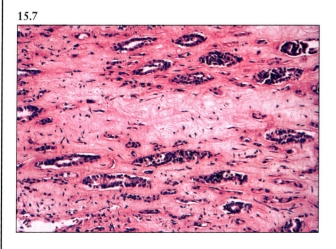

15.8
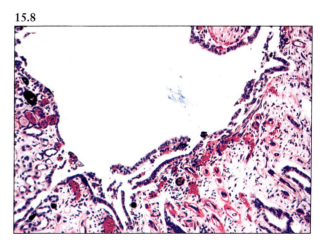

Sickle Cell Disease

FIGURE 15.9   Electron micrograph. Part of a glomerular tuft in a case of sickle cell disease and nephrotic syndrome. The capillary lumens (*L*) contain distorted red blood cells (*RBC*). There is mesangial interposition (*MI*) circling the capillary. The basement membrane (*BM*) is thin. The foot processes are extensively effaced. (× 6,250)

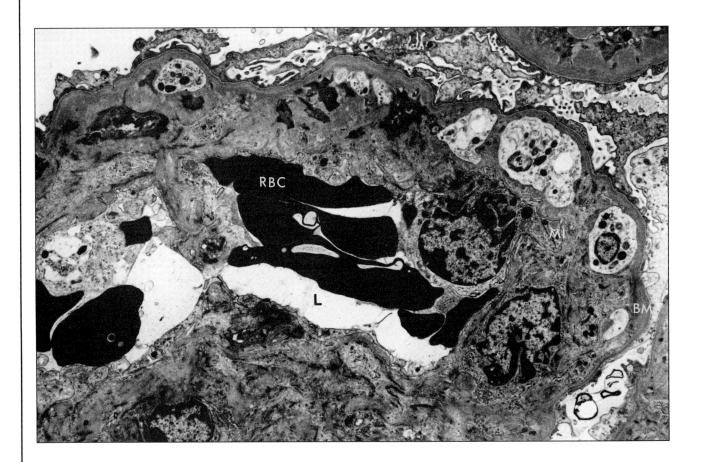

THALASSEMIA

FIGURE 15.10   Renal biopsy specimen from patient with thalassemia-hemoglobin H disease showing erythrocytes in Bowman's space and tubular lumens. (H & E × 140)

FIGURE 15.11   Another case of thalassemia-hemoglobin H disease showing heavy deposits of hemosiderin pigment in tubular epithelial cells. (Perl's stain for hemosiderin × 140)

15.10
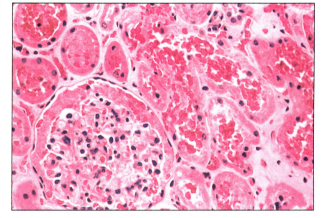

15.11
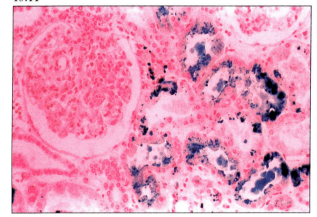

CHAPTER 16

RENAL DISEASE OF GEOGRAPHIC IMPORTANCE

TROPICAL NEPHROPATHY

In 1975, a group of 16 patients presenting with nephrotic syndrome were described under the denomination of tropical nephropathy and were studied in Dakar, Senegal.

Clinical and Pathologic Manifestations

Of these 16 patients, 10 were male, and 6 were female. Fifteen patients were children or adolescents; the one adult was 49 years old. None of the patients had had a recent attack of malaria at the time of nephrotic syndrome, nor was there any obvious triggering factor responsible for the renal disease. Seven patients had antibodies against *Plasmodium malariae*, but the titers were high in only three patients. Eight patients had antibodies against *Plasmodium falciparum*; of these, seven also had antibodies to *P. malariae*. Other infectious or parasitic diseases suspected of contributing to the renal lesions were also investigated. One patient was positive for hepatitis B antigen. In seven patients, the search for parasites and bacterial infection was entirely negative. Only one patient had a blood smear positive for *P. malariae*, ie, evidence of active infection.

None of the patients had renal insufficiency or hypertension. C3 levels were normal in 15 patients and elevated in one. Antibodies to nuclear factors and glomerular basement membrane were negative in all patients.

In all these cases the lesions were comparable, although they varied in severity and extent from patient to patient.

Light Microscopic Findings. The glomeruli showed nonproliferative changes. There was an irregular splitting of the glomerular capillary walls, giving a tramtrack appearance. These changes involved only a few lobules within the glomeruli in the less-affected patients. In the most severely affected patients, the lesions were more diffuse and affected the majority of the capillary walls. These capillary wall changes were associated with irregular foci of glomerular sclerosis and hyalinosis adhering to Bowman's capsule through fibrous synechiae. In eight cases, most glomeruli contained extensive areas of hyalinosis with large eosinophilic, PAS-positive deposits. In summary, the lesions combined a diffuse capillary abnormality with foci of glomerular sclerosis and hyalinosis.

The tubulointerstitial changes paralleled those of the glomerular lesions. Significant arterial lesions were not observed.

Electron Microscopic Findings. Electron microscopy was done in twelve biopsies. The appearance of the glomerular lesions was similar in all cases but varied in extent. Podocyte foot processes showed spreading and swelling. The basement membrane showed irregularities in thickness. Scanty electron-dense deposits were observed within the glomerular basement membranes in three cases. There was significant intrusion of basement membrane material within the capillary lumens. Conspicuous endothelial cell swelling was seen frequently. A number of lacunae containing electron-dense flecks were observed within the basement membranes.

These lesions showed many similarities to the glomerular lesions of quartan malarial nephropathy; the light microscopic lesions showed plexiform and diffuse thickening of the glomerular capillary walls associated with foci of glomerular hyalinosis, resembling those in quartan malarial nephropathy (QMN). The small lacunae have been considered specific markers for malarial nephropathy. The immunofluorescence findings, however, differ substantially from those described in QMN. That lesion is characterized by diffuse deposition of IgG along the capillary walls, whereas tropical nephropathy is unaccompanied by any diffuse deposits of immunoglobulins or complement. The pathogenesis of tropical nephropathy is unknown, but it is noteworthy that several patients did not show any immunologic stigmata suggesting *P. malariae* infestation.

Immunomicroscopic Findings. Immunofluorescence microscopy was performed in all biopsies but one and showed identical results: focal and segmental deposits of IgM were found exclusively in the areas of segmental sclerosis and hyalinosis.

TROPICAL EXTRAMEMBRANOUS (MEMBRANOUS) NEPHROPATHY

An unusual variety of membranous glomerulonephritis characterized by conspicuous cellular proliferation was initially observed in Senegal and Cameroon in seven patients. Several other cases of a comparable pathologic association were further reported in South Africa. The etiology of this tropical extramembranous (membranous) glomerulonephritis is not known.

Clinical and Pathologic Manifestations

Apart from one adult the patients were children, and all were Africans. All the patients suffered from massive nephrotic syndrome with anasarca. Microscopic hematuria was marked. Renal failure was present in the adult in this series. Serum C3 levels were measured in five patients from Senegal and in the patients from South Africa and were depressed in six. Clinical evolution was documented in four cases. In three patients from Sen-

egal, proteinuria was present; but the clinical nephrotic syndrome was in remission, with disappearance of edema. Of the two patients from South Africa who were followed regularly, one had symptomless proteinuria, while the second developed hypertension and reduced glomerular filtration.

Light Microscopic Findings. By light microscopy the lesions were diffuse and homogenous. Mesangial proliferation was constant and was associated with diffuse thickening of the glomerular basement membrane with diffuse spikes. There were no other glomerular lesions, and tubulointerstitial changes were inconspicuous.

Electron Microscopic Findings. Electron microscopy showed diffuse conspicuous extramembranous and intramembranous electron-dense deposits. At the site of the deposits there was podocyte swelling and spreading.

Immunomicroscopic Findings. IgG deposits in a granular pattern along the glomerular capillaries were found in all cases. The sites of the deposits were clearly membranous, and the mesangial regions were spared. The deposits of IgG were accompanied by C3, C1q, and C4, a finding unusual in idiopathic membranous glomerulonephritis. Moderate amounts of IgA and properdin were found in one case. Extraglomerular deposits were not observed.

POSTSTREPTOCOCCAL GLOMERULONEPHRITIS

Poststreptococcal acute glomerulonephritis (PSAGN) is characterized by the sudden appearance of hematuria, proteinuria, and cylindruria a few days to weeks after infection with β-hemolytic streptococci (usually group A). Hypertension, renal impairment, and edema develop in any combination. Most patients recover within a month, although proteinuria may persist for 6 months or more. The disease presumably results from an immune process triggered by infection with a nephritogenic strain of streptococci.

In temperate zones, pharyngitis is the most common antecedent of PSAGN, but skin infections may be involved. In tropical and subtropical areas, where children wear little clothing, sites of insect bites and traumatized skin often become colonized by streptococci, and pyoderma is the most common antecedent infection. Several large epidemics of PSAGN (350 to 1,000 cases) have been associated with skin infections in Trinidad, Israel, Venezuela, and Colombia, while somewhat smaller outbreaks have occurred in Africa, India, the United States, and islands in the Pacific Ocean.

Streptococci are present on normal skin, ready to invade any traumatized area. They are also carried by insects and transmitted by direct contact from sore to sore and from child to child. In Trinidad, gnats of the genus *Hippelates* feed on exudates and carry streptococci on their feet and proboscises. The scabies mite produces lesions in which nephritogenic streptococci flourish, and epidemics of scabies may be accompanied by epidemics of PSAGN, as occurred in Trinidad in 1971. The scabies mite also may carry streptococci from person to person and from mangy dogs to children.

Although skin infections have been related to most cases of PSAGN in the tropics, throat infection either with the skin infection strains (which may cause pharyngitis in children in the absence of skin infections) or with pharyngeal nephritogenic strains also causes PSAGN. The latter strains appear to have been responsible for the 1958 epidemic of PSAGN in Trinidad, which was associated with scarlet fever rather than skin infections. Throat infections also appeared to be responsible for an epidemic of PSAGN in Venezuela in 1974.

Etiology and Pathogenesis

Fortunately, only a handful of the nearly 100 M-types of streptococci that have been recognized are capable of causing nephritis, and only a few strains of these types are nephritogenic. M-type 12 is by far the commonest type to be isolated from the throats of nephritis patients in temperate areas. However, less than 1 percent of M-type 12 pharyngeal infections are followed by PSAGN. M-types 1 and 4 and, less often, types 8, 25, 3, and 6 have also been described as nephritogenic. M-types 2, 49, 52, 55, 57, and 60 have been recovered from skin infections in patients with PSAGN in warmer climates, but most children infected by these M-types do not develop nephritis. The largest epidemics of PSAGN in the tropics have occurred after skin infections caused by M-types 49, 55, and 57. Following each epidemic, the associated M-type has disappeared. M-type 55 recurred after an absence of 6 years in Trinidad, causing a second large M-type 55 epidemic of PSAGN. Although 22 children in the second epidemic had had PSAGN before, none of them had had PSAGN during the first M-type 55 epidemic. This observation probably reflects type-specific immunity conferred by the M-type infections experienced during the first M-type 55 epidemic.

Like PSAGN, acute rheumatic fever is a remote, non-suppurative consequence of streptococcal infections. In contrast to PSAGN, the latent period between infection and onset usually is 18 to 21 days. Furthermore, the serum complement is increased in acute rheumatic fever rather than decreased, as in PSAGN, and acute rheumatic fever has not been associated with skin infections. The M-types of pharyngeal streptococci recovered from patients with acute rheumatic fever differ from those recovered from patients with PSAGN in Trinidad, even when nephritic strains are epidemic.

Clinical and Pathologic Manifestations

Streptococcal pharyngeal infection antecedent to PSAGN may occur without symptoms; with only mild soreness; or with exudation, fever, and lymphadenitis. Antecedent streptococcal skin infections may be small and barely apparent or more obvious, with exudate and scab formation. The lesions may be multiple, and they often heal by the time PSAGN develops. Throat and skin cultures are often negative because of the latent period between the streptococcal infection and the onset of nephritis. Increased or increasing streptococcal antibodies may, however, be considered evidence of recent infection. Antistreptolysin O is usually increased after pharyngitis, and antihyaluronidase and antideoxyribonuclease B are more likely to be increased after skin infections.

PSAGN usually follows a streptococcal infection by 7 to 14 days, with the onset of proteinuria, hematuria, and hypocomplementemia. Although the nephritis may be asymptomatic, the more common onset is abrupt, characterized by hematuria (often gross), proteinuria, cylindruria, hypertension, decreased renal function, and edema of the face and extremities. The edema is due to fluid retention secondary to decreased renal function. Although proteinuria may be heavy for several days, it is rarely enough to result in nephrotic syndrome. Complications of PSAGN include oliguria, hypertension, convulsions, and circulatory failure from fluid overload.

Even in clinically inapparent attacks, total hemolytic complement and C3 are reduced from the first day through the sixth week. C4 also may be reduced in the early stages. Serum complement is reduced in only a few other renal diseases, including lupus nephropathy, mesangiocapillary glomerulonephritis, and the glomerulonephritis associated with infections like bacterial endocarditis.

Although the acute attack of PSAGN may be fatal, most patients, especially children, recover. However, in 10 to 15 percent of sporadic cases in adults, especially those who suffer severe acute attacks, the glomerular lesions fail to heal. Although the clinical symptoms disappear, continued proteinuria indicates chronic glomerulonephritis, which may progress to end-stage renal disease. These patients may have glomerular lesions other than typical postinfectious glomerulonephritis (eg, diffuse crescentic glomerulonephritis and mesangiocapillary glomerulonephritis).

Macroscopic Findings. At autopsy, the kidneys of the patients dying of PSAGN are swollen, heavy, and pale, with punctate hemorrhages and engorged glomeruli on their surfaces.

Light Microscopic Findings. Light microscopy reveals enlarged and hypercellular glomeruli, with mesangial and endocapillary proliferation and with infiltration by monocytes and neutrophils. Adhesions to Bowman's capsule and crescents occur in more severe cases. The degree of glomerular hypercellularity and crescent formation reflects quite well the clinical severity of the glomerulonephritis. In milder cases, the glomeruli are less hypercellular, with predominantly mesangial proliferation. Tubular lumens contain red blood cells and casts, and the blood vessels are normal.

As the acute phase of the glomerulonephritis passes, the glomerular hypercellularity diminishes and becomes confined to the mesangium. In patients who undergo clinical healing, some degree of mesangial hypercellularity may persist for several years. Glomerular adhesions and fibrotic crescents may remain as monuments to the acute process.

Electron Microscopic Findings. The glomerular basement membranes appear normal in patients with PSAGN. However, characteristic subepithelial electron-dense deposits, or humps, appear early in the course of the disease and diminish in a few weeks. Subendothelial and mesangial deposits are sometimes present. Capillaries and mesangium contain monocytes and leukocytes, which adhere to capillary walls.

Immunomicroscopic Findings. Immunofluorescence techniques reveal coarse granular deposits of IgG, IgM, C3, properdin, and sometimes C4 along the glomerular basement membrane. Fibrin is present in the mesangium and crescents.

MESANGIAL IgA NEPHROPATHY

IgA nephropathy is a primary glomerulonephritis characterized by diffuse deposition of immunoglobulins, predominantly IgA in the glomerular mesangium. Complement C3 is activated via the alternative pathway with utilization of properdin. The first cases were identified by Berger in Paris in 1968–1969, and the lesion is commonly referred to as Berger's disease.

A number of diseases show mesangial IgA deposits. The well-documented ones are Henoch-Schönlein purpura, systemic lupus erythematosus, liver cirrhosis, portacaval shunts, mucin-secreting cancers, celiac disease, Crohn's disease, and ankylosing spondylitis, all of which have to be excluded before idiopathic IgA nephropathy is diagnosed. As the glomerular lesions in Henoch-Schönlein purpura are similar to those of Berger's disease, it may be a systemic variant of IgA nephropathy.

IgA nephropathy is now recognized to be a widespread disease, with an especially high prevalence in the Asian-Pacific countries of Japan, Australasia, and Singapore, accounting for up to 40 percent of cases of primary glomerulonephritis. There appears also to be a high incidence in the Mediterranean countries of Europe, including Italy and Spain. Lower incidences have been reported from North America and northern Europe. These differences may be due to patient selection for biopsy, but it appears more likely to be due to real geographic variations in the disease.

Pathogenesis

The exact cause(s) and pathogenetic mechanisms in IgA nephropathy are not known. The IgA deposits are polymeric, with J-chain within the deposits and absence of the IgA secretory component. Evidence suggests that the antigen-IgA antibody complexes are probably derived from antigens in the respiratory and intestinal mucosae. The antigens may be of viral, bacterial, or dietary origin; and some cases may be associated with mucin-secreting tumor antigens evoking an IgA immune response. Much evidence points to the deposition of circulating immune complexes in the glomeruli, although the possibility in some cases of in situ immune complex formation to planted or "trapped" antigens cannot be excluded. The serum IgA level is raised in up to 50 percent of patients with IgA nephropathy, up to 25 percent of patients show deposits in the skin, and the disease recurs in renal transplant patients; all these factors are evidence in favor of a circulating immune complex nephritis.

The immune complexes activate C3 via the alternative pathway, utilizing properdin. By chemotaxis inflammatory cells, including macrophages, are attracted to the glomeruli; platelet activation and coagulation with fibrin deposition lead to glomerular damage. There may be a defect in the ability of the sera of patients with IgA nephritis to solubilize the mesangial IgA deposits. Cellular immune abnormalities with decreased IgA-specific suppressor T cell activity, and an increase in IgA-bearing lymphocytes and Tα cells have also been implicated. A genetic basis, with an increased prevalence of BW35 and/or DR4, and cases of familial IgA nephropathy have been observed, but all these have not been consistent findings.

Clinical and Pathologic Manifestations

The most common presentation is frank hematuria, usually occurring with upper respiratory infection; it may be associated with loin pain. The hematuria may recur, and the urine contains dysmorphic red blood cells and red cell casts, which help to distinguish the disease from nonglomerular causes of hematuria. A proportion of patients, variably reported up to 10%, present with acute nephritic syndrome or nephrotic syndrome with microscopic hematuria. Some patients present with renal insufficiency and hypertension with no previous history of hematuria. However, the most common means of discovery is the detection of asymptomatic microscopic hematuria and proteinuria during a regular preschool, army-induction, pre-employment, or insurance-policy medical examination.

Light Microscopic Findings. There are five major classes of glomerular lesions seen on light microscopy.

I. Minimal lesions appearing "normal" on light microscopy.

II. Minor change, with mesangial widening, and increased cellularity of up to three cells per mesangial area in the periphery of the lobular tufts.

III. Focal and segmental glomerulonephritis, usually involving less than 50 percent of glomeruli. The localized lesions are segmental areas of sclerosis, mesangial cell proliferation, and uncommonly lobular tuft necroses or segmental glomerular capillary aneurysms. The remaining glomeruli show minor changes.

IV. Diffuse mesangial cell proliferation with varying degrees of hypercellularity, graded mild, moderate, and marked. This class of basic glomerular lesions is subdivided into:

    A. Pure mesangial cell proliferation with no other superimposed glomerular lesions

    B. Diffuse mesangial cell proliferation as the basic pathology, with superimposed glomerular lesions of sclerosis, capsular adhesions, crescents; and uncommonly thrombosis, focal and segmental lobular tuft necrosis or glomerular capillary aneurysm.

V. Diffuse sclerosing glomerulonephritis with involvement of more than 80 percent of glomeruli.

In IgA nephropathy, discrete mesangial droplets can be identified in more than 30% of the cases with periodic acid–Schiff, Martius' scarlet blue, and Masson's trichrome stains.

Tubulointerstitial lesions begin as focal areas of interstitial edema and lymphocytic cellular infiltrates. Later lesions of chronic disease show varying degrees of tubular necrosis, tubular atrophy, and interstitial fibrosis, with inflammatory cellular infiltrates of lymphocytes. The changes are most marked in Class IV(b) and V lesions.

Vascular lesions are seen predominantly in the arterioles and interlobular arteries. There is arteriolosclerosis with hyalinosis, and the interlobular arteries show vascular sclerosis with medial hypertrophy and hyalinization. In later stages of chronic disease, there are clustered blood vessels due to a combination of parenchymal loss and vascular hypertrophy.

Electron Microscopic Findings. In all cases, electron-dense deposits are found in the glomerular mesangium within the matrix. Peripheral subendothelial dense deposits can be seen in more than 50 percent of cases, and less frequently subepithelial dense deposits are found. In the early acute disease, the mesangial cells are enlarged by abundant cytoplasm, with increased mitochondria and endoplasmic reticulum. The mesangial and paramesangial areas of the glomerulus show loosening of the matrix and lytic areas around and within the dense deposits, and degeneration of mesangial cells. These changes of mesangiolysis precede the later stages, which show increased mesangial matrix encroaching to obliterate the mesangial cells.

The peripheral capillaries show thinning, splitting, lamination, occasional gaps in the lamina densa, and membranolysis with aneurysmal dilatation and irregular thickening of the glomerular basement membrane. Foci of entrapped mesangial and endothelial cell components may be found within the thickened and focally reduplicated basement membrane of capillary loops. Some cases show detachment and necrosis of podocytes, widening of the foot processes, and epithelial cell hypertrophy and microvilli formation.

The changes of mesangiolysis and membranolysis associated with the deposits appear to precede the glomerular sclerosis. Later these changes may progress to glomerular sclerosis, and in chronic disease the sclerotic areas also contain collagen fibrils.

Proteinuria of more than 2.5 g/day, subendothelial deposits, and glomerular lesions of sclerosis and tubulointerstitial and vascular damage are indices of poor prognosis.

Immunomicroscopic Findings. The characteristic immunopathologic lesion is diffuse deposition of IgA in the glomerular mesangium. The deposits may be confluent masses or discrete granules. Accompanying IgG and/or IgM immunoglobulins may be observed in up to 50 percent of cases, located in the same areas as the IgA but of lesser fluorescent intensity. In up to 50 percent of cases, paramesangial-subendothelial deposits of immunoglobulins may be seen along the peripheral glomerular capillaries. The IgA deposits in all cases are IgA-$_1$ subclasses, with weaker IgA-$_2$ deposits in some of them. Complement C3 and properdin are also located in the same sites as the immunoglobulins. Rarely, extraglomerular deposits of IgA and C3 have been observed. Tubular secretions of IgA and IgA secretory component may be seen occasionally in the tubular epithelial cells, but IgA-containing tubular casts are seen frequently.

IgM Nephropathy

This is a primary glomerular disease commonly found in Southeast Asia, especially Thailand. Patients usually present with proteinuria or nephrotic syndrome. All age groups are affected, but the frequency appears to be in the second and third decades. The glomerular lesions are characterized by the constant finding of mesangial IgM deposits with relatively mild histologic changes.

Clinical and Pathologic Manifestations

The disease is male preponderant and usually occurs in young adults, constituting 35 to 40 percent of idiopathic glomerulonephritis in Thailand. It is the common cause of nephrotic syndrome and asymptomatic proteinuria. Occasionally, the disease may present with microscopic hematuria. Renal function is usually normal, and the patient is normotensive. Hypertension indicates a poor prognosis. Impaired cell-mediated immune response has been demonstrated. There is a decrease in T helper cells and an increase in T suppressor cells. Decreased platelet survival is observed in 50 percent of patients. There is good response to corticosteroids in 80 percent of cases. This is in contrast to the western experience, where more cases show steroid resistance. Patients who fail to respond to steroid therapy may do well with antiplatelet agents and cyclophosphamide. Resistant cases usually progress slowly to chronic renal failure.

Light Microscopic Findings. Glomerular lesions are similar in all biopsies. The constant finding is diffuse mesangial hypercellularity that varies in degree from one glomerulus to another, and there is increased mesangial matrix. The capillary loops are patent, and the glomerular capillary walls appear to be normal in thickness. Occasionally, mononuclear leukocytes may be seen in some capillary lumens. Some visceral epithelial cells may show hypertrophy. Focal tubulointerstitial changes with atrophic tubules surrounded by interstitial fibrous tissue and obsolescence of glomeruli are noted in 5 percent of cases.

Electron Microscopic Findings. There are increased mesangial cells and matrix of varying degrees. Well-defined, electron-dense deposits in the mesangial areas are demonstrable in some but not in all cases. Some endothelial cells show prominent cytofolds or become swollen. In most cases, the glomerular basement membranes appear normal, but occasionally the lamina densa may be irregularly thickened in the axial portion of the capillary loops.

Immunomicroscopic Findings. Deposits of IgM of

variable intensity are present in a mesangial distribution. Other immunoglobulins and complement are absent.

Secondary Amyloidosis

This disorder is characterized by the accumulation in several organs of a fibrillar protein called amyloid-AA protein, which can be identified by its distinctive affinity for certain stains. Several inflammatory, infectious, and neoplastic conditions can be complicated by the development of secondary amyloidosis. These include tuberculosis, chronic suppurative lung disease, leprosy, chronic osteomyelitis, rheumatoid arthritis, ankylosing spondylitis, ulcerative colitis, Crohn's disease, and Hodgkin's lymphoma.

In the past, the prevalence of amyloidosis in patients with tuberculosis or leprosy was up to 50 percent. With effective chemotherapy for these diseases, secondary amyloidosis is now much less prevalent. The highest prevalence of amyloidosis in the world now has been reported from Papua New Guinea, where it has been observed in more than 7 percent of all autopsies. Renal failure and goiter due to amyloid deposition were noted in children. These findings have been attributed to the high incidence of tropical splenomegaly syndrome and endemic malaria. A genetic catabolic enzyme defect in the processing of the serum amyloid-AA protein cannot be excluded. Amyloidosis is also common in Turkey, where it frequently complicates familial Mediterranean fever. In India, the commonest cause of secondary amyloidosis is tuberculosis, with 1 percent of the control autopsy population demonstrating amyloid deposits.

Clinical and Pathologic Manifestations

There is usually an interval of several years between the preceding infectious or inflammatory disorder and the development of clinically overt amyloidosis. Proteinuria, which is nonselective, is the cardinal manifestation, and nephrotic syndrome is observed in more than 60 percent of patients. Hypertension occurs in a minority of patients. Renal failure supervenes within a few years of the clinical onset of the disease. Heavy proteinuria may persist even when renal failure is far advanced. Tubular function defects, including nephrogenic diabetes insipidus, Fanconi syndrome, and distal renal tubular acidosis, may occasionally occur.

Macroscopic Findings. The kidneys are often enlarged, firm, and pale and may not be contracted even in the presence of advanced renal failure. The cut surface may appear translucent.

Light Microscopic Findings. The glomeruli are almost invariably affected. The earliest deposits of amyloid are seen in the mesangium and subendothelium, and occasionally in the subepithelial space. Although most of the glomeruli are affected, only segmental deposits are seen initially, and the degree of involvement is not uniform. With increasing deposits, the glomeruli become hypocellular and the mesangium markedly increased to form mesangial nodules. In some patients, the capillary walls may be thickened with silver-positive spikes resembling those in idiopathic membranous nephropathy. However, this occurs late in the course of the disease, and at this stage deposits can be seen on both sides of the glomerular basement membrane. Eventually, the glomerulus becomes completely obliterated.

Amyloid deposits may also be seen in the interstitium, tubular basement membranes of the loops of Henle, distal tubule and collecting ducts, and the walls of the vasa recta and the arcuate and interlobular arteries.

Amyloid can be detected on light microscopy by special stains. After Congo red staining, amyloid stains reddish pink and exhibits an apple-green birefringence in polarized light. Methyl violet stains the deposits metachromatic purple against a blue background, and, with thioflavin-T, fluorescence is observed under ultraviolet light.

Electron Microscopic Findings. The amyloid material appears as nonbranching fibrils arranged randomly and measuring 8 to 10 nm in diameter and up to 1 μm in length. They are identifiable in the glomerular mesangium and basement membranes. The foot processes are replaced by a continuous thin sheet of cytoplasm. On the subepithelial aspect of the glomerular basement membrane, the fibrils tend to lie perpendicular to the basement membrane. Similar deposits can be identified in the walls of blood vessels and tubulointerstitium.

X-ray crystallography has shown that the fibrils are composed of polypeptide chains perpendicular to the axis of the fibrils in a cross-beta-pleated sheet configuration, and therefore amyloidosis has also been called "beta-fibrillosis."

Immunomicroscopic Findings. In amyloidosis there are generally no characteristic diagnostic features on immunofluorescence. However, weak staining for immunoglobulins and C3 may be observed in the amyloid deposits. In secondary amyloidosis, the amyloid-AA protein can be identified by the peroxidase-antiperoxidase method, using monospecific antisera against the protein.

TROPICAL NEPHROPATHY

FIGURE 16.1   Tropical nephropathy. Renal biopsy specimen from a patient with moderate lesion shows splitting of the glomerular capillary walls, producing a tram-track appearance. (Wilder's silver stain × 950)

FIGURE 16.2   Tropical nephropathy. Renal biopsy specimen from another case. Only a few glomerular lobules show tram-track appearance of the capillary walls, but there is more lobular sclerosis. (Masson's trichrome × 470)

FIGURE 16.3   Renal biopsy shows extensive glomerular sclerosis and hyalinosis, with thickening of capillary walls and hypertrophy of the podocytes. (Masson's trichrome × 235)

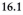
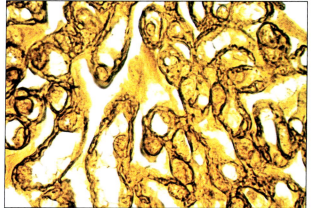

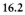
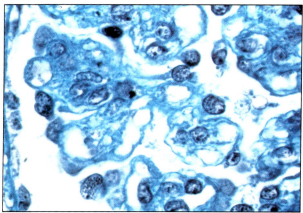

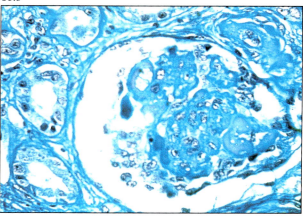

Tropical Nephropathy

FIGURE 16.4 Tropical nephropathy. Electron micrograph. Note the proliferation of cells in the mesangium, increased amount of matrix, and small electron-dense deposits in the paramesangial areas. (× 5,400)

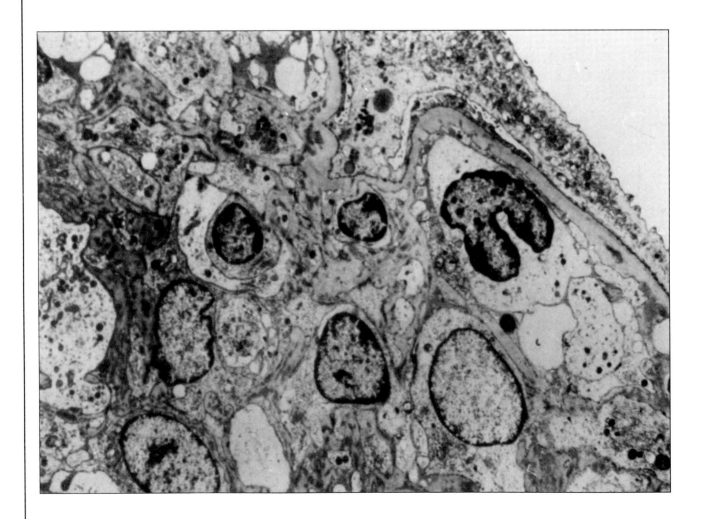

Tropical Extramembranous (Membranous) Glomerulonephritis

FIGURE 16.5   Tropical extramembranous (membranous) nephropathy. There is diffuse thickening of the glomerular basement membrane with mild mesangial cell proliferation. (Masson's trichrome stain × 235)

FIGURE 16.6   Tropical extramembranous nephropathy. There is diffuse thickening of the glomerular basement membrane with diffuse spike formation along the subepithelium. (Wilder's silver stain × 950)

FIGURE 16.7   Immunofluorescence microscopy. Diffuse granular deposits of IgG along the glomerular capillary walls. (× 235)

Poststreptococcal Glomerulonephritis

FIGURE 16.8   Scabies lesions from which group A streptococci were isolated.

16.5

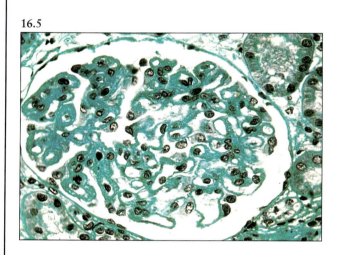

16.6

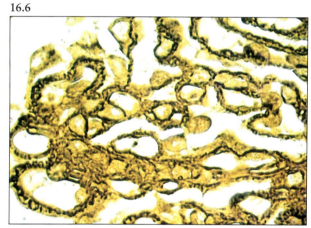

16.7

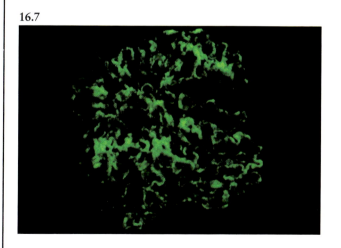

16.8

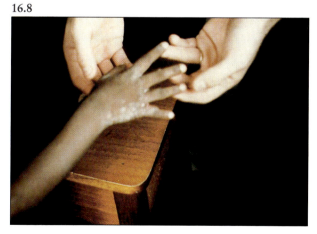

POSTSTREPTOCOCCAL GLOMERULONEPHRITIS

FIGURE 16.9   Kidneys from a fatal case of poststreptococcal glomerulonephritis. The kidneys are swollen and congested, with punctate red areas that represent engorged glomeruli.

FIGURE 16.10   Light microscopy of a renal biopsy specimen of moderately severe case showing endocapillary glomerulonephritis with many polymorphonuclear leukocytes. (H & E × 380)

FIGURE 16.11   Light microscopy of a glomerulus from a more severe case, showing crescent formation. (Trichrome × 235)

FIGURE 16.12   Immunofluorescent stain of a glomerulus, showing granular deposits of IgG along basement membranes. (× 235)

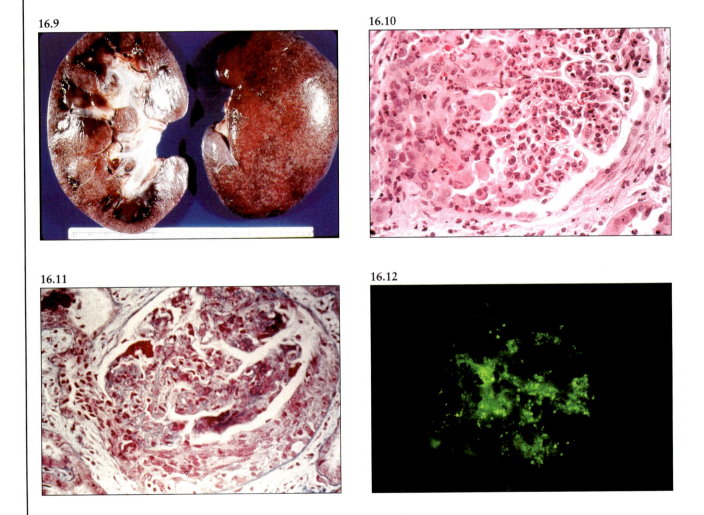

16.9

16.10

16.11

16.12

Poststreptococcal Glomerulonephritis

FIGURE 16.13   Electron microscopy of a glomerular capillary showing two subepithelial "humps" (indicated by arrows) characteristic of poststreptococcal glomerulonephritis. (× 9,000)

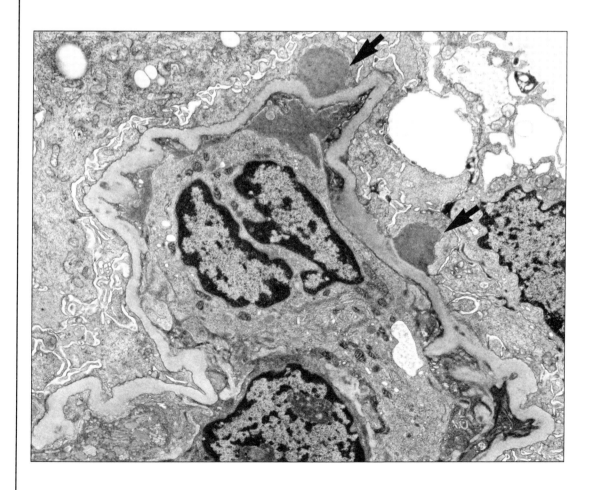

MESANGIAL IgA NEPHROPATHY

FIGURE 16.14   IgA nephropathy (Berger's disease). Immunofluorescence microscopy shows deposits of IgA predominantly in the mesangium and along some glomerular capillary loops. (× 235)

FIGURE 16.15   Berger's disease. Glomerulus shows mesangial widening with mild cellular proliferation, and mesangial deposits (class II lesion). (PAS × 310)

FIGURE 16.16   Glomerulus with segmental sclerosis and hyalinosis, adhesion to Bowman's capsule, and mild segmental mesangial cell proliferation (class III lesion). (PAS × 235)

FIGURE 16.17   Diffuse mesangial cell proliferation of moderate degree with discrete mesangial droplets (red) (class IVa lesion). (MSB × 380)

16.14

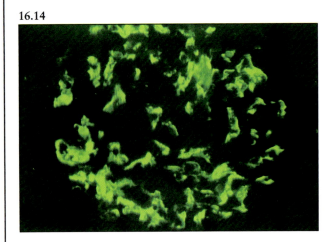

16.15

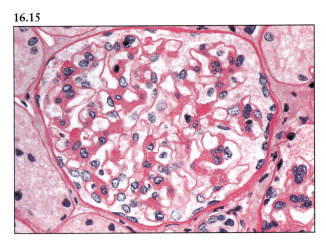

16.16

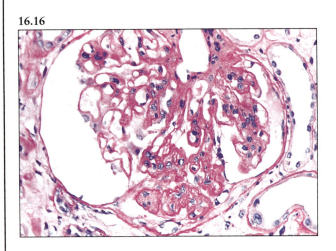

16.17

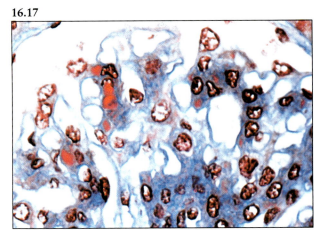

MESANGIAL IgA NEPHROPATHY

FIGURE 16.18   Diffuse mesangial cell proliferation (severe), with adhesions and crescent formation in Bowman's space (class IVb lesion). (MSB × 235)

FIGURE 16.19   The biopsy shows focal segmental glomerulosclerosis and a capillary aneurysm filled with red blood cells (class III lesion). (Masson's trichrome × 190)

FIGURE 16.20   Biopsy specimen from a patient with end-stage Berger's disease shows diffuse glomerulosclerosis, marked tubular atrophy, interstitial fibrosis, and vascular sclerosis. (Masson's trichrome × 50)

16.18
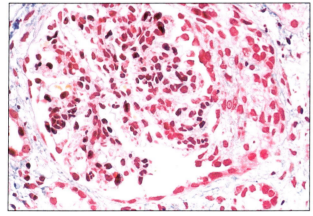

16.19
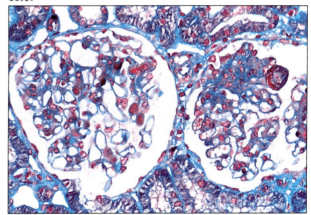

16.20
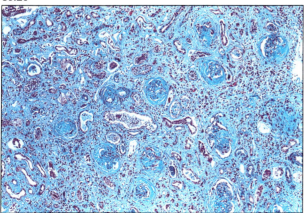

FIGURE 16.21   Electron micrograph. There are massive electron-dense deposits in the mesangium, without involvement of the peripheral capillaries. (× 6,850)

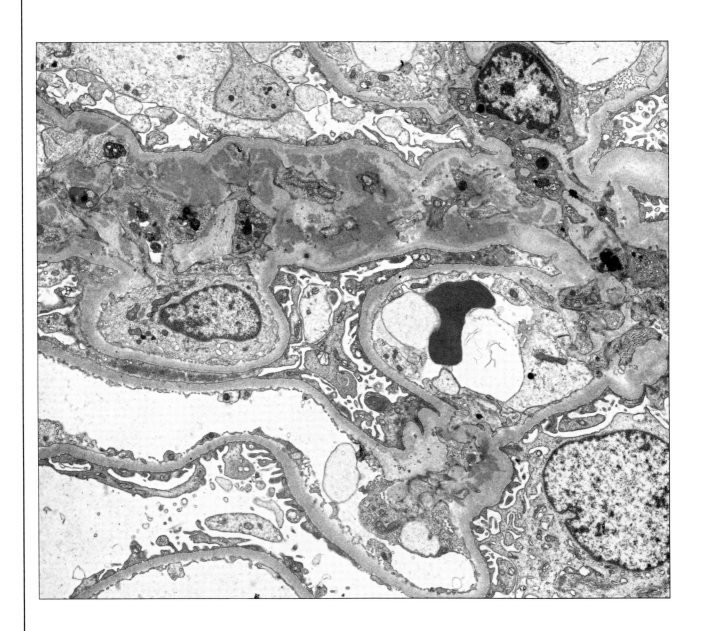

MESANGIAL IgA NEPHROPATHY

FIGURE 16.22 Electron micrograph. There are massive electron-dense deposits in the mesangium (arrows), a subepithelial deposit forming a "hump" (arrowhead), and a few discrete subendothelial deposits near the paramesangium. (× 5,500)

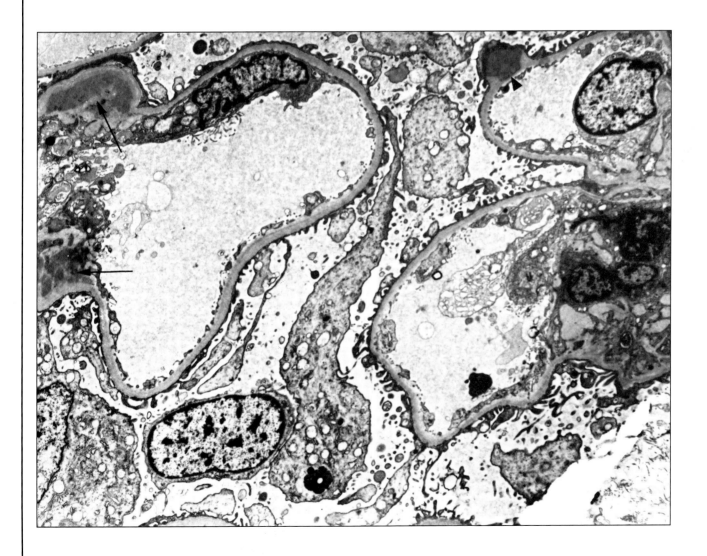

Mesangial IgA Nephropathy

FIGURE 16.23   Electron micrograph. The glomerular peripheral capillaries show extensive damage, with segmental reduplication, membranolysis, and a capillary aneurysm. These changes are related to the electron-dense deposits, which are partially lysed. The overlying podocytes are effaced. (× 11,500)

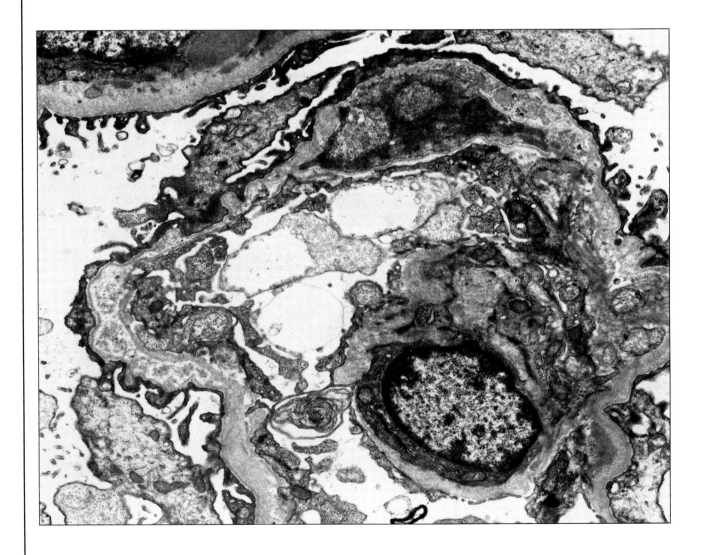

IgM Nephropathy

FIGURE 16.24   Mesangial glomerulonephritis in an adult with nephrotic syndrome, showing mesangial cell proliferation with increased amount of matrix. (H & E × 235)

FIGURE 16.25   Immunofluorescence microscopy from the same case as in Figure 16.24, showing IgM deposits in a mesangial distribution. (× 380)

16.24

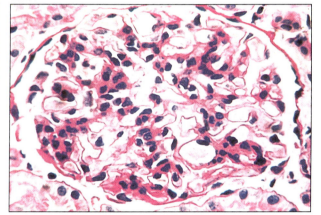

16.25

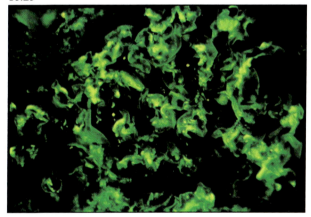

IgM Nephropathy

FIGURE 16.26   Electron micrograph. Same case as in Figure 16.24, showing electron-dense deposits in the mesangium (arrows). The basement membrane over the mesangium varies in thickness. Note prominent endothelial cytofolds in a capillary. (× 7,300)

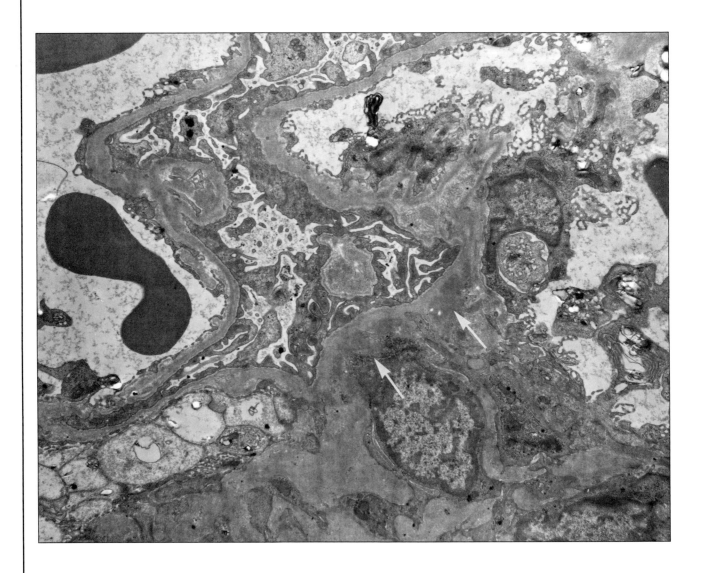

TOXIC NEPHROPATHY

PLANT TOXINS

Death from the consumption of certain plants or plant materials has been known to man since creation, and both ancient and modern writings abound with such reports. The number of poisonous plants is legion; indeed many common garden plants produce toxins with serious effects in man and animals. Wild plants are no exception, and nearly every large family of plants has a proportion capable of producing powerful toxins. The compounding of medicines from plants and their products thus carries a high risk of toxicity, sometimes with damage to the kidneys, more often to the liver.

SEMECARPUS ANACARDIUM

The sap of the marking-nut tree of India is used in dyeing and printing cloth. Although it is best known in India, it is used elsewhere in the tropics and subtropics. The bark and husk contain an extremely irritating, black, caustic juice that causes severe dermatitis and, if taken internally, renal damage with dysuria, hematuria, proteinuria, and acute renal failure.

Renal biopsy shows cytoplasmic necrosis of glomerular cells, extensive damage to the tubules and interstitium, and necrolysis of intertubular arterioles. The basement membrane usually escapes damage.

PITHECOLOBIUM LOBATUM

The djenkol bean belongs to the mimosa family. It resembles the chestnut and emits a strong sulfurous odor, which can be detected on the breath if the bean is eaten. The beans are relished as a food in Indonesia, where they are sold in markets.

Djenkolism and renal damage follow ingestion in a small proportion of people. Two forms are recognized: (1) Mild djenkolism presents with spasmodic loin and suprapubic pain and with proteinuria, hematuria, pyuria, cylindruria, and crystalluria with characteristic needle-shaped crystals. These features resolve in a day or two, and many patients do not seek medical help. (2) Severe djenkolism presents with severe colicky abdominal pain, vomiting, diarrhea, and dysuria. Oliguria progresses to anuria and hypertension. Recovery is the rule, although death has occurred in some cases. Djenkol (sulfurous) factor is detectable in the breath and urine, and diagnosis can be confirmed by demonstration of crystals of djenkolic acid.

MUSHROOMS

Mushroom poisoning is seen the world over but may be more prevalent in Europe. Cases are seen now and again in the tropics, but renal involvement occurs most often in phalloides poisoning due to *Amanita phalloides* (death cap). Mild renal injury may also occur after ingesting *Gallerina venenata*. *A. phalloides* produces two toxins, phallin and amanitin, of which the latter is by far the most important, as phallin is completely hydrolyzed in the stomach. Amanitin is an indole, resistant to hydrolysis by gastric juice.

Pathologic lesions include serous membrane and visceral hemorrhages and damage to the liver, kidneys, heart, and central nervous system. Severe oliguria can progress to total anuria with azotemia. Concomitant jaundice from liver damage aggravates the renal injury, especially in the choleraic forms (*Mycetismus choleriformis*), in which diarrhea and vomiting lead to profound dehydration.

Callilepis Laureola

Callilepis laureola, a member of the family Compositae, is a perennial herb widespread in the grasslands of southern Africa. Chewing and ingesting parts of the plant result in impila poisoning, which is caused by atractyloside, a microcrystalline compound with nephrotoxic and hypoglycemic effects. The plant has a tuberous rootstock that emits a characteristic odor similar to that of peaches. Patients who survive the hypoglycemic renal failure invariably develop centrilobular hepatocellular necrosis. Jaundice occurs, especially in children, and may aggravate renal dysfunction. Hypoglycemia, metabolic acidosis, hyperkalemia, and azotemia are very common. Renal damage occurs in the majority of severe cases.

The kidneys are enlarged and heavy, with a pale, swollen cortex. Tubular necrosis affects both the convoluted tubules and the loops of Henle. Tubules contain casts and may rupture, with extravasation into the interstitium. Edema and intense cellular reaction follow. Tubular cell regeneration may be seen in those who survive the first few days.

Securidaca Longipe Dunculata

A wild bush in the grasslands of eastern and southern Africa is extensively used in traditional infusions and medications for a wide variety of complaints. Its toxin, an amorphous steroid glucoside, gaultherin, causes extensive local tissue destruction. A cupful of the infusion causes death in 12 to 24 hours, with extensive damage to the gut, liver, and kidneys. Acute renal failure may be encountered in severe cases.

Vicis Favus

The broad bean is a very potent trigger of hemolysis in people with hereditary deficiency of the red cell enzyme, glucose-6-phosphate dehydrogenase. Several variants of the deficiency are known, but only two are clinically important: the type caused by a decreased number of enzyme molecules (Caucasian-Mediterranean variety) and the type caused by premature decay (African variety). The enzyme is involved in the smaller pathway (handling 10%) of glucose metabolism in the red cell. *V. favus* contains two active components, divicine and isouramil, which cause hemolysis through iron-catalyzed formation of reactive hydroxyl intermediates. The incidence of deficiency of this enzyme differs in different ethnic groups: 4.5 percent in northern Indians, 22.5 percent in Ghanians, 10 to 15 percent in the Bantu of the eastern African plateau, 0.5 percent in northern Europeans, and 45 to 50 percent among people of Sardinian stock and isolated communities of the Mountains of the Moon (Mt. Ruwenzori in Uganda).

Hemolysis may be triggered by a variety of agents: infections of any kind, drugs and chemicals, diabetic ketoacidosis, uremia, and ingestion or inhalation of foods or plant material.

Reversible acute renal failure occurs occasionally but does not necessarily correlate with severity of hemolysis. Histopathologic studies show degeneration and regeneration of tubular epithelial cells.

Mercury Nephropathy (Chronic Cutaneous Absorption)

Mercurial toxicity to the kidneys presents itself in three ways: (1) Acute intoxication usually by accidental or suicidal ingestion of inorganic mercurial compounds. This presents with acute tubular necrosis and severe gastroenteritis. (2) Subacute intoxication generally by industrial exposure, presenting with chronic tubulointerstitial nephritis. (3) Chronic cutaneous absorption through the application of dermatologic or cosmetic creams. This variety presents with epimembranous glomerulonephritis and nephrotic syndrome. (1) and (2) are described fully in *Classification and Atlas of Tubulointerstitial Diseases*. (3) will be described here.

Mercuric dermatologic creams and ointments have been withdrawn from clinical use. Mercury-containing cosmetics with 5 to 10 percent ammoniated mercuric chloride have, however, been in vogue until very recently, and it is possible that some are still in use today. These creams are used primarily by young women and sometimes by young men of the colored races for skin lightening.

Clinical and Pathologic Manifestations

A small percentage of users develop nephrotic syndrome after continuous use for an average of 13 months, although the period may be much shorter in some cases. Features of systemic mercurialism do not accompany the nephrotic syndrome, and resolution follows withdrawal in many cases. Proteinuria may disappear in 3 to 6 months.

Nephrotic syndrome appears when urine mercury levels reach 90 to 250 mg/L.

Light Microscopic Findings.   Mild cases show some mesangial cell proliferation, but more severe cases show changes of membranous glomerulonephritis. The interstitium and blood vessels show no abnormalities.

Electron Microscopic Findings.   Electron microscopy reveals subepithelial deposits along the glomerular basement membrane.

RAW BILE OF GRASS CARP

Ingestion of raw bile of grass carp (*Clenopharyngodon idellus*) by the Chinese as a traditional method of improving visual acuity is known to cause acute renal failure.

Gastrointestinal symptoms, including abdominal pain, nausea, vomiting, and diarrhea, can occur following ingestion. Fever, chills, headache, tachycardia, vertigo, and hypertension may be observed. There may be mild hepatocellular damage. There is acute renal failure, with oliguria and anuria lasting 3 to 4 weeks.

There is patchy tubular degeneration and necrosis, with distal tubules involved the most. Nephrotoxicity is believed to be due to cyprinol.

MALIGNANCIES IN THE TROPICS

BURKITT'S LYMPHOMA

Burkitt's lymphoma is a malignant lymphoma that was recognized first among children in eastern Africa, where it is relatively common. It is found in a belt of low-lying tropical Africa, where rainfall and temperature are high and malaria is endemic. The tumor is also endemic in Papua New Guinea, but it occurs sporadically in western countries, particularly the United States. The endemic and nonendemic forms have several important differences in clinical characteristics and anatomic distribution. The tumor shows a correlation to infection with the Epstein-Barr virus. The kidney may be infiltrated by the lymphoma.

The geographic distribution of Burkitt's lymphoma in endemic malaria areas suggests the possibility of an arthropod-borne vector as a cause of the neoplasm. Epidemiologic, virologic, immunologic, and biochemical data suggest that Epstein-Barr virus (EBV) is important in Burkitt's lymphoma. The EBV genome can be found in the neoplastic cells of African patients, whereas EBV antibody titers are variable in the serum of American patients, and only a small percentage of tumors in nonendemic countries contain the EBV genome.

Clinical and Pathologic Manifestations

Burkitt's lymphoma usually occurs in children aged 5 to 8 years and is rare before the age of 2 years. Tropical African Burkitt's lymphoma presents most commonly (55%) as a single lesion or as multiple jaw tumors. Other presenting features are abdominal swelling (25%) and ovarian tumors (40%), with much less frequent involvement of lymph nodes and the skeletal system. Nontropical Burkitt's lymphoma usually occurs in adolescent patients and involves abdominal organs and the pelvis rather than the jaw. Diffuse bone marrow involvement is less common in tropical than in nontropical cases, and it indicates a bad prognosis. There is a male predominance (2:1) in both groups of patients. Systemic manifestations usually occur as metabolic complications of therapy and include hyperkalemia, hyperuricemia, and lactic acidosis.

Renal involvement by tumor, although common, seldom produces clinically important symptoms. The most important, perhaps, is renal enlargement, which can be detected radiographically or sonographically. Glomerular and tubular functions are little affected.

The diagnosis of Burkitt's lymphoma is based on the criteria of the World Health Organization, which include infiltration by tightly packed lymphoid cells, 10–25μ in diameter, among which vacuolated histiocytes impart a "starry-sky" pattern. Although often prominent, the histiocytes are not specific to Burkitt's lymphoma or necessary for diagnosis. The histiocytes contain large amounts of neutral fat. The principal tumor cells are uniform and cohesive. They contain narrow rims of vacuolated cytoplasm and slightly indented nuclei. The nuclei contain coarse chromatin and prominent nucleoli. Immunologic studies show the neoplastic cells to be B lymphocytes, perhaps related to the small, noncleaved lymphocytes found in normal germinal centers.

Macroscopic Findings. Renal involvement in Burkitt's lymphoma usually occurs in association with disease in other infradiaphragmatic sites or as a complication of disseminated malignancy. Burkitt's lymphoma may involve the kidney as a solitary lesion or multiple circumscribed gray-white nodules, or as a diffuse mass that obliterates the corticomedullary junction.

Light Microscopic Findings. There is usually diffuse infiltration of the interstitium of the renal cortex and medulla by neoplastic cells that surround tubules, displace collecting ducts, and extend beneath the urothelium of the pelvis.

Lymphomatous infiltrates of the kidney may respond dramatically to chemotherapy with maintenance of normal renal function.

SCHISTOSOMIASIS AND CARCINOMA OF THE URINARY BLADDER

Infection by *Schistosoma haematobium* causes chronic inflammation of the urinary bladder with epithelial hyperplasia, cystitis glandularis, cystitis cystica, and metaplasia of the urothelium to squamous epithelium and columnar mucin-secreting cells. There is a high incidence of bladder cancer associated with chronic *S. haematobium* infection. It has been widely quoted that over 90% of bladder cancers in Egypt are due to schistosomiasis (bilharziasis). The age incidence is 20 years lower than in other bladder cancers. This cancer is sit-

uated outside the trigone, whereas the cancers in other countries develop largely in the trigone.

Clinical and Pathologic Manifestations

Most patients with chronic schistosomiasis are asymptomatic, and others complain with symptoms of cystitis. The development of bladder cancer presents with frank hematuria or symptoms of obstruction.

Macroscopic Findings. In the early stages, red and fleshy polypoid lesions are seen in the bladder and ureteric mucosa. These lesions involute and become yellow-brown fibrotic patches. Thin bands of submucosal calcifications may be found in the bladder and ureter. When cancer develops, the tumor appears as a bulky, ulcerated mass usually situated outside the trigone of the bladder. There may be areas of tumor necrosis and associated cystitis, with submucosal bladder fibrosis.

Microscopic Findings. The histologic patterns in schistosomiasis-associated bladder cancers are squamous cell carcinoma (50%), adenocarcinoma (10%), and transitional cell carcinoma (40%).

Squamous cell carcinoma may show varying degrees of differentiation and can be graded I to III. These tumors are derived from metaplastic epithelium, and there is always evidence of an associated chronic cystitis with granulomatous inflammation around the eggs of *S. haematobium*. Frequently, submucosal fibrosis and scar formation are seen around calcified eggs.

The adenocarcinomas are usually mucin-producing cancers, and they are invariably associated with cystitis cystica and glandularis. The third type of cancer, transitional cell carcinoma, shows varying degrees of differentiation.

Burkitt's Lymphoma of the Kidney

FIGURE 18.1   Burkitt's lymphoma involving the kidney. Patient had disseminated malignancy. The kidney is enlarged and diffusely gray-white.

FIGURE 18.2   Another cases of Burkitt's lymphoma with kidney involvement. There is a large white tumor extending into the renal parenchyma from the hilus and extensive involvement of the perinephric tissues.

18.1

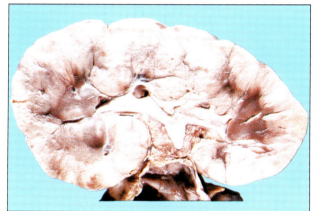

18.2

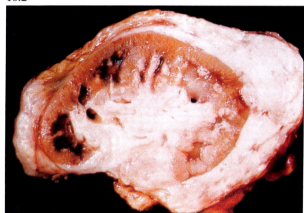

Burkitt's Lymphoma of the Kidney

FIGURE 18.3 The renal interstitium contains a dense infiltrate of large lymphoid cells. Vacuolated histiocytes give the infiltrate a "starry-sky" pattern. Tumor cells are also present in the glomerulus in Bowman's space. (H & E × 140)

FIGURE 18.4 The perinephric tissue shows dense infiltrate of large lymphoid cells, without involvement of the renal parenchyma. (H & E × 50)

FIGURE 18.5 Higher magnification of Figure 18.4. The infiltrate consists of large, relatively uniform lymphocytes with scanty cytoplasm. (H & E × 280)

18.3
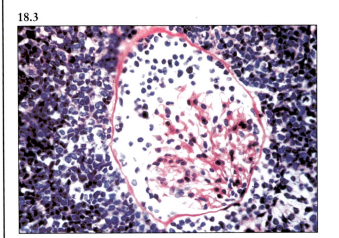

18.4
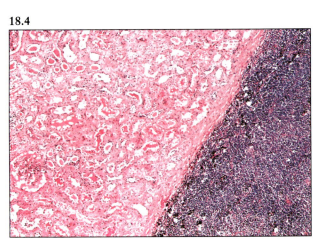

18.5
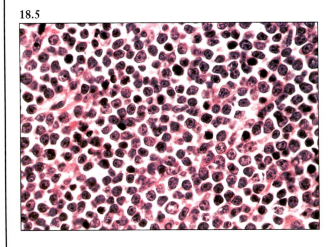

CARCINOMA OF URINARY BLADDER

FIGURE 18.6   Geographic distribution of *Schistosoma haematobium*. (Adapted from multiple sources.)

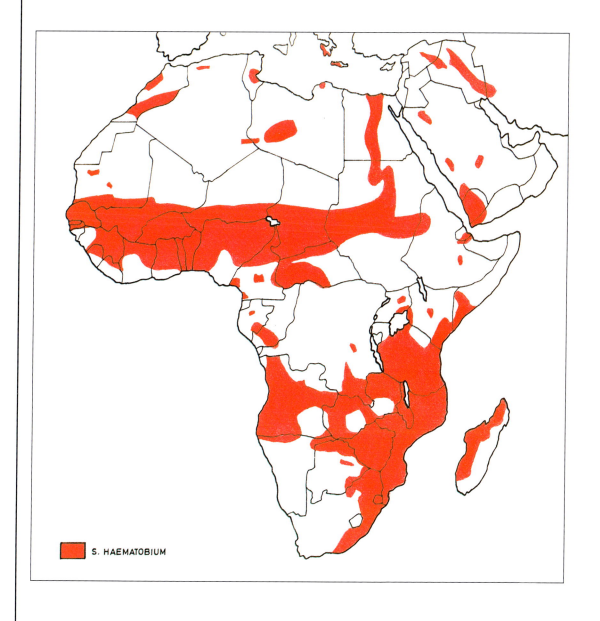

S. HAEMATOBIUM

Carcinoma of Urinary Bladder

FIGURE 18.7   Macroscopic picture. Ulcerating squamous cell carcinoma of urinary bladder in a case of urinary schistosomiasis (*S. haematobium*).

FIGURE 18.8   Macroscopic picture. Fungating carcinoma of urinary bladder in a case of urinary schistosomiasis. Patient was a pregnant woman.

FIGURE 18.9   Light microscopy of carcinoma of bladder associated with urinary schistosomiasis; calcified eggs of *Schistosoma haematobium* are seen in the tissue. (H & E × 140)

18.7

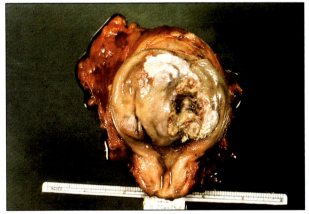

18.8

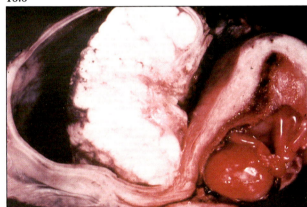

18.9

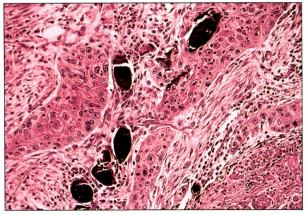

MISCELLANEOUS CONDITIONS

LABREA HEPATITIS

Labrea hepatitis or Labrea black fever is an acute, highly fatal liver disease of unknown etiology apparently confined to the Amazon region. Labrea is the name of a small Brazilian village located deep in the Amazon jungle, where several cases have been observed.

Clinical and Pathologic Manifestations

After a prodromal flu-like illness of 5 to 10 days, the patient shows signs of central nervous system involvement, with convulsions, and soon lapses into coma; death occurs after a few days.

Microscopic Findings.
The liver shows severe diffuse lytic necrosis of hepatocytes as well as acute fatty change and mononuclear cell infiltration.

The kidneys show marked fatty change of the tubular epithelium, with interstitial edema and bile pigment deposits and casts. No glomerular or vascular lesions are seen.

No ultrastructural and immunofluorescent studies have been done to date.

KAWASAKI DISEASE

A systemic febrile disease with lymphadenopathy, rash, oral mucosal inflammation, and coronary arteritis is known as Kawasaki disease (also called mucotaneous lymph node syndrome or infantile polyarteritis nodosa). It also affects the kidney. The cause of Kawasaki disease is unknown, and both infectious and noninfectious etiologies have been considered.

Clinical and Pathologic Manifestations

An exanthem without vesicles is usually present over the trunk; and the palms and soles become erythematous, with brawny edema. The mucous membranes of the mouth and pharynx are inflamed, and there may be conjunctivitis. Dry, fissured lips and a strawberry tongue are characteristically present. The cervical lymph nodes are typically swollen. The fever lasts several weeks and may be accompanied by arthralgia, abdominal pain, diarrhea, and jaundice. Cardiac involvement in the form of myocarditis and coronary arteritis is common. The latter leads to coronary aneurysms and thrombosis, with myocardial infarction as a serious complication. Arteritis develops less often and less consistently in other organs. The disease may be the same as infantile polyarteritis nodosa, although some clinical differences have been described.

Renal involvement occurs in some cases, perhaps one third. Urinary abnormalities include oliguria with moderate proteinuria, hematuria, and mild pyuria. Moderately severe elevations of serum creatinine concentrations are related to diminishing urinary output, followed by subsequent recovery of renal function. Renal enlargement may be a consistent sonographic and radiographic finding. Hemolytic-uremic syndrome, with recovery, has also been described.

Macroscopic Findings. Gross descriptions of the kidney are lacking, but radiographic and sonographic evidence of renal enlargement suggests that kidneys would be grossly swollen, with localized areas of hemorrhage or necrosis in relation to arteritis. Arteritis of the larger branches of the renal artery has been described and may occur in 30 to 40 percent of cases. The affected vessels contain infiltrates of neutrophils in association with fibrinoid necrosis of the vessel wall. Localized vascular necrosis might predispose to subsequent aneurysm formation, but renal arterial aneurysms have not been described as a clinical problem. Recurrent thrombosis of affected vessels in the heart may be an important factor in the development of coronary artery aneurysms, an observation underlying the rationale for anticoagulant therapy. The reparative process leads to intimal fibrosis and medial scarring.

Microscopic Findings. Microscopic studies of the kidneys show perivasculaar edema, in association with perivascular inflammatory cell infiltrates, and localized areas of ischemic necrosis. Arteritic lesions are frequently, but not invariably, associated with renal infarcts. The possibility of glomerular microangiopathic changes requires further investigation. Proliferative glomerulonephritis has been described in polyarteritis nodosa in children, but those cases were thought to be related to prior infection with group A streptococcus.

HEMOLYTIC-UREMIC SYNDROME IN INFECTIONS

Hemolytic-uremic syndrome (HUS) is characterized by a special form of hemolytic anemia (microangiopathic), thrombocytopenia, and vascular damage in the kidneys, often accompanied by thrombosis.

HUS most often follows an infection, but it also occurs as a complication of a variety of noninfectious processes. The infection is usually that of the gastrointestinal or upper respiratory tract and is caused by bacteria (pathogenic *Escherichia coli*, *Salmonella typhi*, *Shigella dysenteriae*, *Pseudomonas*, *Pneumococcus*); spirochetes (*Leptospira*); viruses (*coxsackie*, *influenza*, *echo*, *mumps*, *myxovirus*); or rickettsiae. However, in many cases no specific microorganism can be demonstrated. Noninfectious cases, which occur almost ex-

clusively in adults, include collagen diseases, radiation nephritis, renal transplantation, metastatic carcinomatosis, antineoplastic drugs, malignant hypertension, pregnancy and puerperium and the use of oral contraceptive medication.

Clinical and Pathologic Manifestations

When HUS follows an infection, it usually appears after a symptom-free interval of a few days to 1 or 2 weeks (biphasic course). The onset is abrupt, with weakness, pallor, purpura, oliguria, vomiting, and diarrhea, which is often bloody. Hypertension and volume overload occur in about half the patients. Uremia develops quickly. Urinalysis shows hematuria and proteinuria, and blood studies demonstrate severe hemolytic anemia of a non-immune (Coombs negative) type, with fragmentation of erythrocytes and appearance of "burr," "helmet," "arrowhead," and other abnormal forms. Reticulocytes increase in number. Platelets are decreased, often severely, and fibrinogen levels may be abnormal; but other coagulation factors are generally unchanged.

With proper supportive treatment, mortality in children has been reduced to about 5 percent. Prolonged oliguria or anuria (over 3 weeks) and persistent hypertension are poor prognostic factors. Prognosis is much worse in adults. Improvement has been reported after various forms of therapy, such as heparin, fibrinolytic and antiplatelet agents, steroids, plasma infusion and plasmapharesis, but further evaluation of their efficacy is needed.

Light and Electron Microscopic Findings. Characteristic changes are found in the glomeruli and in the arterial tree. Milder cases involve only glomeruli, showing thickening of the capillary walls with detachment of the endothelium and accumulation of pale fluffy material, containing fibrinogen derivatives, in the subendothelial space. The mesangium is often expanded because of a degree of mesangiolysis. Fragmented erythrocytes may be noted in some glomeruli. Capillary thrombosis is a more serious manifestation. Changes in the arterioles and small arteries generally denote a more severe disease. These changes are similar to those in the glomeruli and consist of endothelial detachment, subendothelial accumulation of fluffy or fibrillar material, and luminal thrombosis; but they may be accompanied by focal or more diffuse tissue infarction and often lead to malignant hypertension and to irreversible renal failure.

CHYLURIA

Chyluria is the passing of milky lymphatic fluid in the urine. It is associated with a variety of diseases, but in the tropics and subtropics is almost invariably caused by filarial infection, commonly with *Wuchereria bancrofti*. Other parasites are *Eustrongylus gigas, Taenia ecchinococcus, Taenia nana*, as well as malaria, ascariasis, and bilharziasis pathogens. Other causes not confined to the tropics and subtropics are retroperitoneal tumors, chronic inflammations such as tuberculosis and abscesses, and aneurysms.

The larvae of *W. bancrofti* multiply at sites of bites in the skin, then migrate to the lympatic vessels and lymph nodes. They mature to worms, which cause lymphadenitis and lymphangitis. When the parasite dies, it produces granulomatous inflammation, resulting in fibrosis and blockage of lymphatic channels and lymph nodes. The obstruction occurs at the level of para-aortic lymph nodes, which drain lymph from both the intestines and the kidneys. The obstruction at this site leads to retrograde flow of chyle into renal pelvic lymphatics, which dilate and subsequently rupture, resulting in chyluria.

The left kidney is involved more often than the right, and, when both are involved, the left more severely than the right.

Clinical and Pathologic Manifestations

The onset of chyluria is sudden and often associated with trauma or straining. There may be back pain, lassitude, renal colic, and the passage of blood clots with the chyluria. Hematuria is common. The attacks last 7 to 14 days, and recurrences are frequent.

Urinalysis shows lymphocytes and fat globules, demonstrated by Sudan Red or Sudan III, in the urine. The urine is milky and on standing shows fat at the top; clear urine in the middle; and red cells, white cells, and debris in the bottom. Microfilariae may be found in the urine. There may be anemia, blood eosinophilia, and lymphocytopenia.

Radiologic Findings. The intravenous pyelogram is usually normal, but reflux and pyelolymphatic backflow may be demonstrated by retrograde pyelography. The lymphangiogram is the most important diagnostic tool in chyluria. It shows dilated and tortuous lymphatics, which have a serpiginous appearance, in the pelvic region; collateral channels in the bladder and scrotum are visible in over one third of cases. Saccular dilatations may be located in the para-aortic region and renal pedicle, and a halo of dilated lymphatic vessels surrounds the minor calices.

The lymph nodes, especially in the para-aortic region, are poorly seen due to fibrosis and obliteration of the lymphatic channels. Usually, there is no thoracic duct obstruction.

PENTASTOMIASIS

Pentastomiasis is an infection caused by Pentastomida, a bloodsucking endoparasite of reptiles, birds, and mammals. Infection in man may be asymptomatic, or there may be pharyngeal involvement or larval stages in tissues. Colon infection is not common, and only rarely obstruction by masses of larvae may occur. Pneumonitis, peritonitis, meningitis, and obstructive jaundice are well recognized complications; there are occasional passing references to renal involvement, but no definite evidence has been presented to date.

LABREA HEPATITIS

FIGURE 19.1   Renal tubules showing small vesicles in the basal portions of the epithelium. (PAS × 470)

FIGURE 19.2   Marked fatty changes in the tubular epithelium accompanied by interstitial edema. (Sudan III × 350)

19.1

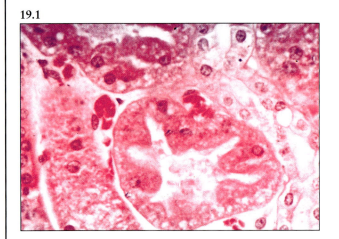

19.2

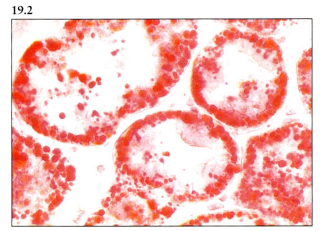

KAWASAKI DISEASE

FIGURE 19.3 Arteritis in Kawasaki disease. Segmental inflammation and destruction of wall of a medium-sized artery in the kidney. (H & E × 60)

FIGURE 19.4 Similar artery under a slightly higher magnification. Destruction of the wall and transmural inflammation are evident. (H & E × 95)

HEMOLYTIC-UREMIC SYNDROME IN INFECTIONS

FIGURE 19.5 Hemolytic-uremic syndrome. Glomerulus shows thickened capillary walls with prominent double outlines. (PAS stain × 380)

19.3

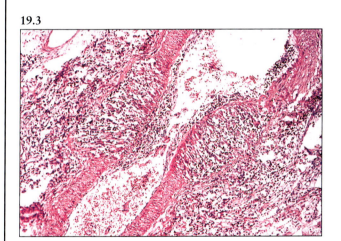

19.4

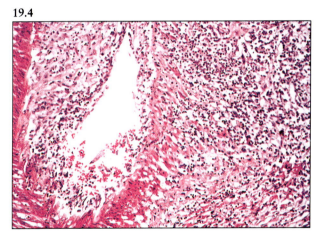

19.5

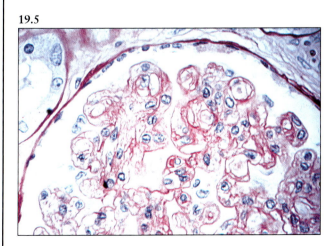

HEMOLYTIC-UREMIC SYNDROME IN INFECTIONS

FIGURE 19.6   Electron micrograph. Hemolytic-uremic syndrome. The epithelial foot processes (top) are partly effaced. The endothelium (lower left) is separated from the basement membrane, and the resulting space is filled with loose fibrilar and granular material and small remnants of cytoplasm. A thin, irregular basement membrane lies adjacent to the endothelium and is presumably responsible for the double outline. ($\times$ 24,100)

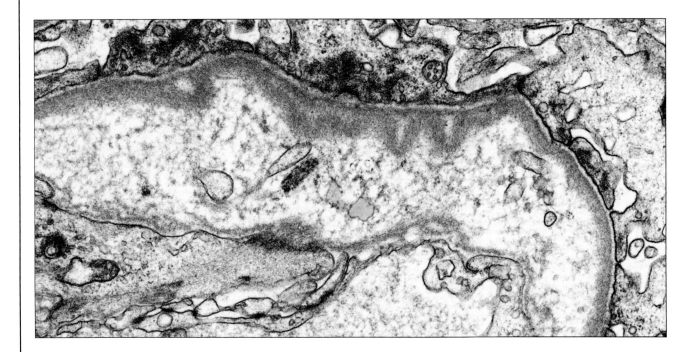

Chyluria

FIGURE 19.7 Lymphatics of the urinary tract. (*1*) Lymphatics of the kidney. (*2*) Lymphatics of the ureter. (*3*) Lymphatics of the ureter. (*4*) Lymphatics of the urinary bladder.

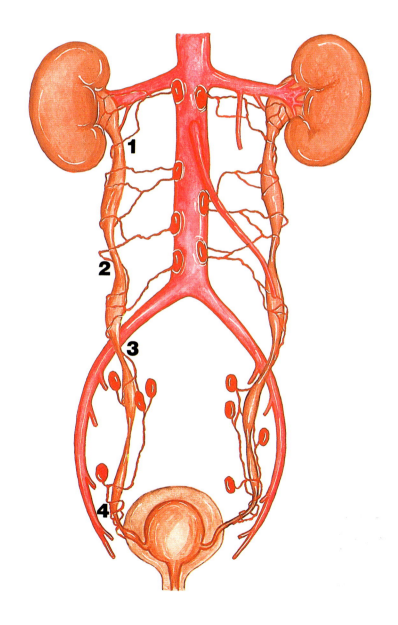

CHYLURIA

FIGURE 19.8   Chyluria. Milky lymphatic fluid in the urine.

FIGURE 19.9   Section of lymph node. Microfilariae of *Brugia malayi* within dilated lymphatics, with surrounding inflammation and fibrosis. (H & E × 120)

FIGURE 19.10   Patient with filariasis and chyluria. Immunofluorescence microscopy shows IgM deposits predominantly in the glomerular mesangium. (× 235)

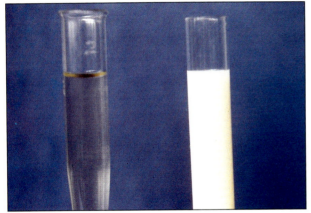

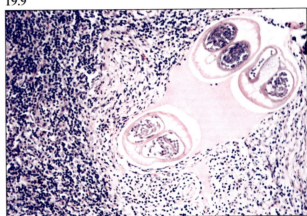

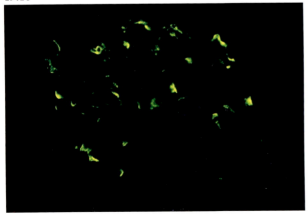

CHYLURIA

FIGURE 19.11   Japanese patient with lymphangioadenopathy of filariasis and chyluria. Lymphangiogram shows cystic type of lymphaticopelvic fistula in the kidney and the para-aortic region.

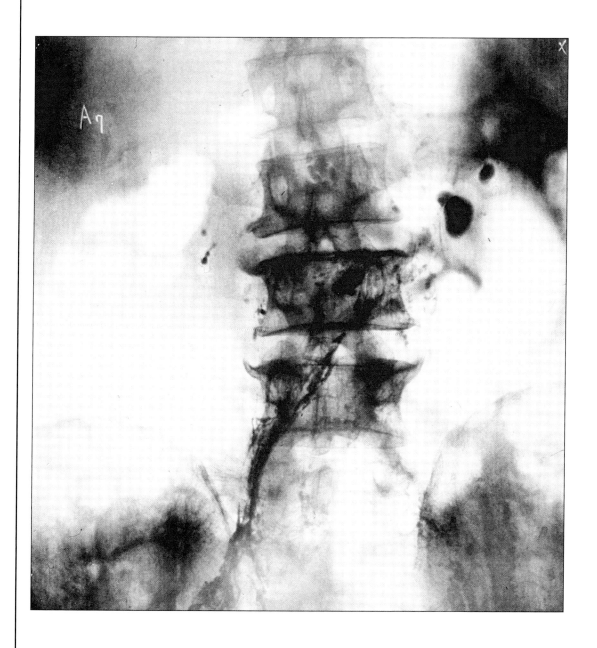

CHYLURIA

FIGURE 19.12   Another Japanese patient with chyluria associated with lymphangioadenopathy of filariasis. Lymphangiogram shows the circular type of lymphaticopelvic fistulization in the kidney and the para-aortic lymphatics.

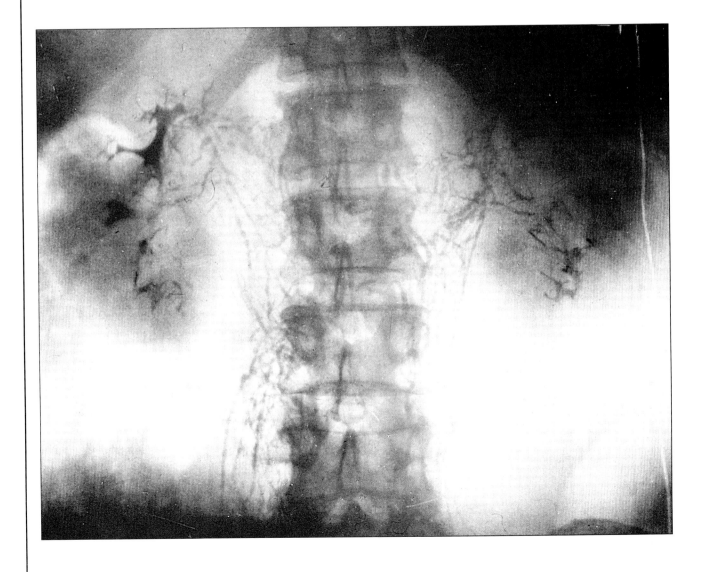

REFERENCES

GENERAL TEXTBOOKS AND MONOGRAPHS

Ash LR, Orihel CC: *Atlas of Human Parasitology*, ed 2. Chicago, ASCP Press, 1984.

Beaver PC, Jung RC, Cupp EW: *Clinical Parasitology*, ed 9. Philadelphia, Lea & Febiger, 1984.

Binford CH, Connor DH (eds): *Pathology of Tropical and Extraordinary Diseases*. Washington, DC, Armed Forces Institute of Pathology, 1976.

Chandler FW, Watts JC: *Pathologic Diagnosis of Fungal Infections*. Chicago, ASCP Press, 1987.

Churg J, Sobin LH: *Renal Disease: Classification and Atlas of Glomerular Diseases*. New York, Igaku-Shoin, 1982.

Churg J, Cotran RS, Sinniah R, et al: *Renal Disease: Classification and Atlas of Tubulo-Interstitial Diseases*. New York, Igaku-Shoin, 1984.

Emmons CW, Binford CH, Utz JP, Kwon-chung KJ: *Medical Mycology*, ed 3. Philadelphia, Lea & Febiger, 1977.

Feigin RD, Cherry JD (eds): *Textbook of Pediatric Infectious Diseases*, ed 2. Philadelphia, WB Saunders & Co, 1987.

Germuth FG, Rodriguez E: *Immunopathology of the Renal Glomerulus: Immune Complex Deposit and Anti-Basement Membrane Disease*. Boston, Little Brown & Co, 1973.

Heptinstall RH: *Pathology of the Kidney*, ed 3. Boston, Little Brown & Co, 1983.

Hoeprich PD (ed): *Infectious Diseases: A Modern Treatise of Infectious Processes*, ed 3. Philadelphia, Harper & Row, 1983.

Kibukamusoke JW: *Nephrotic Syndrome of Quartan Malaria*. London, Edward Arnold, Ltd, 1973.

Kibukamusoke JW (ed): *Tropical Nephrology*. Canberra, Citforge Printery, 1984.

Maegraith B: *Pathological Processes in Malaria and Blackwater Fever*. Oxford, Blackwell Scientific Publications, 1948.

Mandell GL, Douglas RG Jr, Benett JE (eds): *Principles and Practice of Infectious Diseases*, ed 2. New York, John Wiley & Sons, 1985.

Manson-Bahr PEC, Apted FIC: *Manson's Tropical Diseases*, ed 18. London, Bailliere Tindall, 1982.

Marcial-Rojas RA: *Pathology of Protozoal and Helminthic Diseases*. Baltimore, Williams & Wilkins, 1971.

Warren K, Mahmoud A: *Tropical and Geographical Medicine*. New York, McGraw-Hill Book Co, 1984.

Zaman V: *Atlas of Medical Parasitology*, ed 2. Singapore, P.G. Publishers, 1984.

Chapter 1: General Immunologic and Inflammatory Mechanisms

Immunologic Mechanisms

Andres GA, Accinni L, Hsu KC, Zabriskie JB: Electron-microscopic studies of human glomerulonephritis with ferritin-conjugated antibody. *J Exp Med* 123:399, 1966.

Barnes JL, Venkatachalam MA: Enhancement of glomerular immune complex deposition by a circulating polycation. *J Exp Med* 160:286, 1984.

Biesecker G, Noble B, Andres GA, Koffler D: Immunopathogenesis of Heymann's nephritis. *Clin Immunol Immunopathol* 33:333, 1984.

Borges HF, Goldstein C, Kim M, Michael AF: The glomerular mesangium: Kinetics using radiolabelled ferritin and the effects of aggregated IgG. *Clin Immunol Immunopathol* 33:80, 1984.

Churg J, Sobin LH: *Renal Disease: Classification and Atlas of Glomerular Diseases.* New York, Igaku-Shoin, 1982.

Devey ME, Bleasdale K, Stanley C, Steward MW: Failure of affinity maturation leads to increased susceptibility to immune complex glomerulonephritis. *Immunology* 52:377, 1984.

Dixon FJ: Glomerulonephritis and immunopathology. *Hosp Pract* 2:35, 1967.

Dixon FJ: The role of antigen-antibody complexes in disease. *Harvey Lect* 58:21, 1963.

Dixon FJ, Feldman JD, Vasquez JJ: Experimental glomerulonephritis: The pathogenesis of a laboratory model resembling the spectrum of human glomerulonephritis. *J Exp Med* 113:899, 1961.

Doi T, Mayumi M, Kanatsu K, Suehiro F, Hamashima Y: Distribution of IgG subclasses in membranous nephropathy. *Clin Exp Immunol* 58:57, 1984.

Ford PM, Kosatka I: The effect of in-situ formation of antigen-antibody complexes in the glomerulus on subsequent glomerular localization of passively administered immune complexes. *Immunology* 39:337, 1980.

Ford PM, Kosatka I: In-situ formation of antigen-antibody complexes in the mouse glomerulus. *Immunology* 38:473, 1979.

Ford PM, Kosatka I: A mechanism of enhancement of immune complex deposition following in-situ immune complex formation in the mouse glomerulus. *Immunology* 43:433, 1981.

Gauthier VJ, Mannik M, Striker GE: Effect of cationized antibodies in preformed immune complexes on deposition and persistence in renal glomeruli. *J Exp Med* 156:766, 1982.

Gerber MA, Paronetto F: IgE in glomeruli of patients with nephrotic syndrome. *Lancet* 1:1097, 1971.

Germuth FG Jr: A comparative histologic and immunologic study in rabbits of induced hypersensitivity of the serum sickness type. *J Exp Med* 97:257, 1953.

Germuth FG, Rodriguez ER: Effect of human IgM rheumatoid factor on the glomerular site of localization of passively administered immune complexes in mice. *Immunology* 53:395, 1984.

Germuth FG, Rodriguez E: *Immunopathology of the Renal Glomerulus: Immune Complex Deposit and Anti-Basement Membrane Disease.* Boston, Little Brown & Co, 1973.

Henson PM, Cochrane CG: Acute immune complex disease in rabbits: The role of complement and of a leukocyte-dependent release of vasoactive amines from platelets. *J Exp Med* 133:554, 1971.

Houba V: Immunologic aspects of renal lesions associated with malaria. *Kidney Int* 16:3, 1979.

Houba V, Lambert PH: Immunological studies on tropical nephropathies. *Adv Biosci* 12:617, 1974.

Houba V, Lambert PH, Voller A, Soyanwo MAO: Clinical and experimental investigation of immune complexes in malaria. *Clin Immunol Immunopathol* 6:1, 1976.

Houba V, Sturrock RF, Butterworth AE: Kidney lesions in baboons infected with *Schistosoma mansoni. Clin Exp Immunol* 30:439, 1977.

Hyman LR, Jenis EH, Hill GS, et al: Alternate C_3 pathway activation in pneumococcal glomerulonephritis. *Am J Med* 58:810, 1975.

Isaacs KL, Miller F: Antigen size and charge in immune complex glomerulonephritis. II. Passive induction of immune deposits with dextran-antidextran immune complexes. *Am J Pathol* 111:298, 1983.

Izui S, Lambert PH, Miescher PA: In-vitro demonstration of a particular affinity of glomerular basement membrane and collagen for DNA: A possible basis for a local formation of DNA–anti–DNA complexes in systemic lupus erythematosus. *J Exp Med* 144:428, 1976.

Jeraj K, Fish AJ, Yoshioka K, Michael AF: Development and heterogeneity of antigens in the immature nephron. *Am J Pathol* 117:180, 1984a.

Jeraj K, Vernier RL, Sisson SP, Michael AF: A new glomerular antigen in passive Heymann's nephritis. *Br J Exp Pathol* 65:485, 1984b.

Lambert PH, Houba V: Immune complexes in parasitic diseases, in Brent L, Holborow J (eds): *Progress in Immunology*, II. Amsterdam, North Holland Publishing Co, 1974, vol 5, pp 57–67.

Lambert PH, Bricteux N, Salmon J, Miescher PA: Dynamics of immune complex nephritis during antibody excess. *Int Arch Allergy* 45:185, 1973.

Lawley TJ, Bielory L, Gascon P, et al: A prospective clinical and immunologic analysis of patients with serum sickness. *N Engl J Med* 311:1407, 1984.

Lehman DH, Marquardt H, Wilson CB, Dixon FJ: Specificity of autoantibodies to tubular and glomerular basement membranes induced in guinea pigs. *J Immunol* 112:241, 1974.

Lew AM, Steward MW: Glomerulonephritis: The use of grafted hybridomas to investigate the role of epitope density, antibody affinity and antibody isotype in active serum sickness. *Immunology* 52:367, 1984.

Lew AM, Staines NA, Steward MW: Glomerulonephritis induced by pre-formed immune complex containing monoclonal antibodies of defined affinity and isotype. *Clin Exp Immunol* 57:413, 1984.

McCluskey RT, Bhan AK: Cell-mediated immunity in renal disease. *Hum Pathol* 17:146, 1986.

Michael AF Jr, Drummond KM, Good RA, Vernier R: Acute poststreptococcal glomerulonephritis: Immune deposit disease. *J Clin Invest* 45:237, 1966.

Murphy-Ullrich JE, Oberley TD, Mosher DF: Detection of autoantibodies and glomerular injury in rabbits immunized with denatured human fibronectin monomer. *Am J Pathol* 117:1, 1984.

Parra G, Platt JL, Falk RJ, et al: Cell populations and membrane attack complex in glomeruli of patients with poststreptococcal glomerulonephritis: Identification using monoclonal antibodies by indirect immunofluorescence. *Clin Immunol Immunopathol* 33:324, 1984.

Pertschuk LP, Bruce A, Vuletin JC, et al: Glomerulonephritis due to *Staphylococcus aureus* antigen. *Am J Clin Pathol* 65:301, 1976.

Rose LM, Lambert PH: The natural occurrence of circulating idiotype–anti–idiotype complexes during a secondary immune response to phosphorylcholine. *Clin Immunol Immunopathol* 15:481, 1980.

Stachura I, Whiteside TL, Kelly RH: Circulating and deposited immune complexes in patients with glomerular disease. *Am J Pathol* 103:21, 1981.

Steward MW: The biological significance of antibody affinity. *Immunology Today* 2:134, 1981.

Steward MW: Chronic immune complex disease in mice: The role of antibody affinity. *Clin Exp Immunol* 38:414, 1979.

Theofilopoulos AN, Dixon FJ: The biology and detection of immune complexes. *Adv Immunol* 28:89, 1979.

Tresser G, Semar M, McVicar M, et al: Antigenic streptococcal components in acute glomerulonephritis. *Science* 163:676, 1969.

Unanue ER, Dixon FJ: Experimental glomerulonephritis. V. Studies on the interaction of nephrotoxic antibodies with tissues of the rat. *J Exp Med* 121:697, 1965.

Unanue ER, Dixon FJ: Experimental glomerulonephritis: Immunological events and pathogenetic mechanisms. *Adv Immunol* 6:1, 1967.

WHO: The role of immune complexes in disease. Technical Report Series, 606. Geneva, World Health Organization, 1977.

Wiggins RG, Cochrane CG: Current concepts in immunology: Immune complex mediated biological effects. *N Engl J Med* 304:518, 1981.

Williams DG, Bartlett A, Dufus P: Identification of nephritic factor as an immunoglobulin. *Clin Exp Immunol* 33:425, 1978.

Wilson CB: Nephritogenic antibody mechanisms involving antigens within the glomerulus. *Immunol Rev* 55:257, 1981.

Wu, MJ, Moorthy AV: Suppressor cell function in patients with primary glomerular disease. *Clin Immunol Immunopathol* 22:442, 1982.

Yamamoto T, Kihara I, Morita T, Oite T: Attachment

of polymorphonuclear leukocytes to glomeruli with immune deposits. *J Immunol Meth* 26:315, 1979.

Yoshizawa N, Tresser G, Sagel I: Demonstration of antigenic sites in glomeruli of patients with acute post-streptococcal glomerulonephritis by immunofluorescein and immunoferritin techniques. *Am J Pathol* 70:131, 1973.

Inflammatory Reactions

Couser WG: Mechanisms of glomerular injury in immune-complex disease. *Kidney Int* 28:569, 1985.

Fantone JC, Ward PA: Role of oxygen derived free radicals and metabolites in leukocyte dependent inflammatory reactions. *Am J Pathol* 107:395, 1982.

Johnson KJ, Ward PA: Biology of disease: Newer concepts in the pathogenesis of immune complex–induced tissue injury. *Lab Invest* 47:218, 1982.

Klebanoff SJ: Oxygen metabolism and the toxic properties of phagocytes. *Ann Intern Med* 93:480, 1980.

Rehan A, Johnson KJ, Wiggins RC, et al: Evidence for the role of oxygen radicals in acute nephrotoxic nephritis. *Lab Invest* 51:396, 1984.

CHAPTER 2: PROTOZOAL INFECTIONS

Malaria

Aikawa M, Suzuki M, Gutierrez Y: Pathology of malaria, in Kreier JP (ed): *Malaria*. New York, Academic Press, 1980, pp 47–102.

Berger M, Birch LM, Conte NF: The nephrotic syndrome secondary to acute glomerulonephritis during falciparum malaria. *Ann Intern Med* 67:1167, 1967.

Bhamarapravati N, Boonpucknavig S, Boonpucknavig V, Yaemboonruang C: Glomerular changes in acute *Plasmodium falciparum* infection: An immunologic study. *Arch Pathol* 96:289, 1973.

Boonpucknavig V, Sitprija V: Renal disease in acute *Plasmodium falciparum* infection in man. *Kidney Int* 16:44, 1979.

Boonpucknavig V, Srichaikul T, Punyagupta S: Clinical pathology of malaria, in Peters W, Richards WHG (eds): *Antimalarial Drugs: Biological Background, Experimental Methods and Drug Resistance*. Berlin, Springer-Verlag, 1984, pp 127–176.

Futrakul P, Boonpucknavig V, Boonpucknavig S, et al:

Acute glomerulonephritis complicating *Plasmodium falciparum* infection. *Clin Pediatr* 13:281, 1974.

Hendrickse RG, Adeniyi A: Quartan malarial nephrotic syndrome in children. *Kidney Int* 16:64, 1979.

Hendrickse RG, Andeniyi A, Edington GM, et al: Quartan malarial nephrotic syndrome. Collaborative clinico-pathological study in Nigerian children. *Lancet* 1:1143, 1972.

Houba V: Immunologic aspects of renal lesions associated with malaria. *Kidney Int* 16:3, 1979.

Houba V: Immunopathology of nephropathies associated with malaria. *Bull WHO* 52:199, 1975.

Hutt MSR: Pathology, in Kibukamusoke JW (ed): *Nephrotic Syndrome of Quartan Malaria*. London, Edward Arnold Publishers, 1973, pp 61–74.

Miller LH, Makaranond P, Sitprija V, et al: Hyponatremia in malaria. *Ann Trop Med Parasitol* 61:265, 1967.

Rosen S, Hano JE, Inman NM, et al: The kidney in blackwater fever. *Am J Clin Pathol* 49:358, 1968.

Sitprija V: Renal involvement in malaria. *Trans R Soc Trop Med Hyg* 64:695, 1970.

Sitprija V, Vongthongsri M, Poshyachinda V, Arthachinta S: Renal failure in malaria: A pathophysiologic study. *Nephron* 18:277, 1977.

Stone WJ, Hanchett JE, Knepshell JH: Acute renal insufficiency due to falciparum malaria. *Arch Intern Med* 129:620, 1972.

Voller A: Immunopathology of malaria. *Bull WHO* 50:177, 1974.

WHO: Immunopathology of nephritis in Africa. *Bull WHO* 46:387, 1972.

Visceral Leishmaniasis

Andrade ZA, Iabuki K: A nefropatia do calazar. *Rev Inst Med Trop Sao Paulo* 14:51, 1972.

Brito T, Hoshino-Shimizu S, Amato-Neto V, et al: Glomerular involvement in human Kala-azar: A light, immunofluorescent and electron microscopic study based on kidney biopsies. *Am J Trop Med Hyg* 24:9, 1975.

Duarte MIS, Silva MRR, Goto H, et al: Interstitial nephritis in human Kala-azar. *Trans R Soc Trop Med Hyg* 77:531, 1983.

Dutra M, Martinelli R, de Carvalho EM, et al: Renal

involvement in visceral leishmaniasis. *Am J Kidney Dis* 6:22, 1985.

Galvao Castro B, Ferreira YAS, Marzochi KF, et al: Polyclonal B-cell activation circulating immune complexes and autoimmunity in human American visceral leishmaniasis. *Clin Exp Immunol* 56:58, 1984.

Oliveira AV, Roque-Barreira MC, Sartori A, et al: Mesangial proliferative glomerulonephritis associated with progressive amyloid deposition in hamsters experimentally infected with *Leishmania donovani*. *Am J Pathol* 120:256, 1985.

American Trypanosomiasis (Chagas' Disease)

Andrade ZA, Andrade SG: Chagas' disease (American trypanosomiasis), in Marcial-Rojas RA (ed): *Pathology of Protozoal and Helminthic Disease*. Baltimore, Williams & Wilkins, 1971, chap 2.

Toxoplasmosis

Frankel JK: Toxoplasmosis: Mechanisms of infection, laboratory diagnosis and management. *Curr Top Pathol* 54:28, 1971.

Amebiasis

Brandt H, Pérez Tamayo: Pathology of human amebiasis. *Hum Pathol* 1:351, 1970.

Connor DH, Neafie RC, Meyers WH: Amebiasis, in Binford CH, Connor DH (eds): *Pathology of Tropical and Extraordinary Diseases*. Washington, DC, Armed Forces Institute of Pathology, 1976, pp 308–316.

Craig CF: The complications and sequelae of amebiasis, in *The Etiology, Diagnosis and Treatment of Amebiasis*. Baltimore, Williams & Wilkins, 1944, pp 150–180.

Ross JA: Amebic perinephric abscess. *Br J Radiol* 17:289, 1944.

Sinniah R: Renal involvement in amebiasis (unpublished results, Department of Pathology, National University of Singapore).

Watson JM: Urinary amebiasis: A critical review. *Trop Dis Bull* 42:947, 1945.

Wilmot AJ: Other complications of amoebiasis and some associated conditions. In *Clinical Amoebiasis*. Oxford, Blackwell Scientific Publications, 1962, pp 118–124.

CHAPTER 3: FILARIAL NEMATODE INFECTIONS

Bariety J, Bárbier M, Laigre MC, et al: Proteinurie et loase: Etude histologique optique et electronique d'un cas. *Bull Soc Med* 118:1015, 1967.

Chugh KS, Singhal PC, Tewari SC, et al: Acute glomerulonephritis associated with filariasis. *Am J Trop Med Hyg* 27:630, 1978.

Meyers WH, Neafie RC, Connor DH: Bancroftian and Malayan filariasis, in Binford CM, Connor DH (eds): *Pathology of Tropical and Extraordinary Diseases*. Washington, DC, Armed Forces Institute of Pathology, 1976, pp 340–355.

Meyers WM, Neafie RC, Connor DH: Onchocerciasis: Invasion of deep organs by *Onchocerca volvulus*. *Am J Trop Med Hyg* 26:650, 1977.

Ngu JL, Chatelanat F, Leke R, et al: Nephropathy in Cameroon: Evidence for filarial derived immune-complex pathogenesis in some cases. *Clin Nephrol* 24:128, 1985.

CHAPTER 4: NEMATODE INFECTIONS

Trichinosis

Guattery JM, Milne J, House RK: Observations on hepatic and renal dysfunction in trichinosis. *Am J Med* 21:576, 1956.

Mikhail EG, Milad M, Sabet S, Abdallah A: Experimental trichinosis. I. A pathological study of hepatic, renal and gonadal involvement. *J Egypt Public Health Assoc* 53:327, 1978.

Schoenfeld MR, Edis GT: Trichinosis and glomerulonephritis. *Arch Pathol* 84:625, 1967.

Sitprija V, Keoplug M, Boonpucknavig V, Boonpucknavig S: Renal involvement in human trichinosis. *Arch Intern Med* 140:544, 1980.

Trandafirescu V, Georgescu L, Schwarzkopf A, et al: Trichinous nephropathy. *Morphol Embryol* 25:133, 1979.

Dioctophymiasis

Fernando SSE: The giant kidney worm (*Dioctophyma renale*), infection in man in Australia. *Am J Surg Pathol* 7:281, 1983.

Hanjani AA, Sadinghian A, Nikakhtar B, Arfaa F: The first report of human infection with *Dioctophyma* renale in Iran. *Trans R Soc Trop Med Hyg* 62:647, 1968.

Karmanova EM: The life cycle of the *Dioctophyma renale* (Goeze, 1782): A parasite in the kidneys of carnivora and of man. *Doklady Biol Sci Sec* 132:456, 1960.

Tuur SM, Nelson AM, Gibson DW, et al: Liesegang rings in tissue: How to distinguish Liesegang rings from the giant kidney worm, *Dioctophyma renale*. *Am J Surg Pathol* 11:598–605, 1987.

CHAPTER 5: TREMATODE INFECTIONS

Schistosomiasis

Andrade ZA, Rocha H: Schistosomal glomerulopathy. *Kidney Int* 16:23, 1979.

Andrade ZA, Andrade SG, Susin M: Pathological changes due to massive schistosomal infection in man. *Rev Inst Med Trop Sao Paulo* 16:171, 1974.

Falcao H, Gould DB: Immune complex nephropathy in schistosomiasis. *Ann Intern Med* 83:148, 1975.

Hoshino-Shimizu S, Brito T, Kanamura HY, et al: Human schistosomiasis: *Schistosoma mansoni* antigen detection in renal glomeruli. *Trans R Soc Trop Med Hyg* 70:492, 1976.

Moriearty PL, Brito E: Elution of renal antischistosome antibodies in human schistosomiasis mansoni. *Am J Trop Med Hyg* 26:717, 1977.

Robinson A, Lewert RM, Spargo BH: Immune complex glomerulonephritis and amyloidosis in *Schistosoma japonicum* infected rabbits. *Trans R Soc Trop Med Hyg* 76:214, 1982.

Sinniah R: Heterogeneous IgA glomerulonephropathy in liver cirrhosis. *Histopathology* 8:947, 1984.

Tada T, Kondo YM, Okumura K, et al: Schistosoma japonicum: Immunopathology of nephritis in Macaca fascicularis. *Exp Parasitol* 38:291, 1975.

Van Marck E: Presence of the circulating polysaccharide antigen in the liver of mice infected with *Schistosoma mansoni*. *Ann Soc Belg Med Trop* 55:373, 1975.

CHAPTER 6: CESTODE INFECTIONS

Echinococcosis

Kung'u A: Glomerulonephritis following chemotherapy of hydatid disease with mebendazole. *East Afr Med J* 59:404, 1982.

Poole JB, Marchial-Rojas RA: Echinococcosis, in Marcial-Rojas RA (ed): *Pathology of Protozoal and Helminthic Diseases*. Baltimore, Williams & Wilkins, 1971.

Cysticercosis

Marquez-Monter H: Cysticercosis, in Marcial-Rojas RA (ed): *Pathology of Protozoal and Helminthic Diseases*. Baltimore, Williams & Wilkins, 1971.

CHAPTER 7: VIRAL INFECTIONS

Hantavirus (Bunyaviridae)

Collan Y, Lähdevirta J, Jokinen EJ: Electron microscopy of nephropathia epidemica: Glomerular changes. *Virchows Arch [A]* 377:129, 1978.

Desmyter J, Johnson KM, Deckers C, et al: Laboratory rat associated outbreak of hemorrhagic fever with renal syndrome due to Hantaan-like virus in Belgium. *Lancet* 2:1445, 1983.

Hurault de Ligny B, Prieur JP, Schmitt JL, et al: Ten new cases of HFRS in north-eastern France. *Lancet* 2:864, 1984.

Lahdevirta J: Nephropathia epidemica in Finland. *Ann Clin Res* 3:12, 1971.

Lee HW: Korean hemorrhagic fever. *Prog Med Virol* 28:96, 1982.

Lukes RJ: The pathology of thirty-nine fatal cases of epidemic hemorrhagic fever. *Am J Med* 16:639, 1954.

Van Ypersele de Strihou C, Van der Groen G, Desmyter J: Hantavirus nephropathy in western Europe: Ubiquity of hemorrhagic fevers with renal syndrome, in Grünfeld JP, Bach JF, Crosnier J, et al (eds): *Advances in Nephrology*. Chicago, Year Book Medical Publishers, 1986, vol 15, pp 143–172.

Arenaviridae

Casals J: Serological studies on Junin and Tacaribe viruses. *Am J Trop Med Hyg* 14:794, 1965.

Child P, Mackenzie RB, Valverde LRC, Johnson KM: Bolivian hemorrhagic fever: A pathologic description. *Arch Pathol* 83:434, 1967.

Cossio P, Laguens R, Arana R, et al: Ultrastructural and immunohistochemical study of the human kidney in Argentine hemorrhagic fever. *Virchows Arch [A]* 368:1, 1975.

Elsner B, Schwarz E, Mando OG, et al: Pathology of 12 fatal cases of Argentine hemorrhagic fever. *Am J Trop Med Hyg* 22:229, 1973.

Johnson KM, Wiebenga NH, Mackenzie RB, et al: Virus isolations from human cases of hemorrhagic fever in Bolivia. *Proc Soc Exp Biol Med* 118:113, 1965.

Johnson KM, Halstead SB, Cohen SN: Hemorrhagic fevers of Southeast Asia and South America: A comparative appraisal. *Prog Med Virol* 9:105, 1967.

Maiztegui JI, Laguens RP, Cossio P, et al: Ultrastructural and immunohistochemical studies in five cases of Argentine hemorrhagic fever. *J Infect Dis* 132:35, 1975.

Mettler N, Casals J, Shope RE: Study of the antigenic relationships between Junin virus, the etiological agent of Argentinian hemorrhagic fever and other arthropod-borne viruses. *Am J Trop Med Hyg* 12:647, 1963.

Pinheiro FP, Shope RE, Andrade AHP, et al: Amapari, a new virus of the Tacaribe group from rodents and mites of Amapa Territory, Brazil. *Proc Soc Exp Biol Med* 122:531, 1966.

Togaviridae (Alphavirus and Flavivirus)

Boonpucknavig V, Bhamarapravati N, Boonpucknavig S, et al: Glomerular changes in dengue hemorrhagic fever. *Arch Pathol Lab Med* 100:206, 1976.

Francis TI, Moore DL: A clinicopathological study of human yellow fever. *Bull WHO* 46:659, 1972.

Nimmannitya S, Halstead SB, Cohen SN, et al: Dengue and chikungunya virus infection in man in Thailand, 1962–1964. I. Observation on hospitalized patients with hemorrhagic fever. *Am J Trop Med Hyg* 18:957, 1969.

Ruangjirachuporn W, Boonpucknavig S, Nimmannitya S: Circulating immune complexes in serum from patients with dengue hemorrhagic fever. *Clin Exp Immunol* 36:46, 1979.

Sinniah R: Pathology of dengue hemorrhagic fever: An autopsy study (unpublished results, Department of Pathology, National University of Singapore).

Viral Hepatitis

Amemiya S, Ito H, Kato H, et al: A case of membranous proliferative glomerulonephritis type III (Burkholder) with the deposition of both HBeAg and HBsAg. *Int J Pediatr Nephrol* 4:267, 1983.

Drueke T, Barbanel C, Jungers P, et al: Hepatitis B antigen–associated periarteritis nodosa in patients undergoing long-term hemodialysis. *Am J Med* 68:86, 1980.

Hirose H, Udo K, Kojima M, et al: Deposition of hepatitis B e antigen in membranous glomerulonephritis: Identification by F(ab′)$_2$ fragments of monoclonal antibody. *Kidney Int* 26:338, 1984.

Hsu HC, Lin GH, Chang MH, Chen CH: Association of hepatitis B surface (HBs) antigenemia and membranous glomerulonephropathy in children in Taiwan. *Clin Nephrol* 20:121, 1983.

Nagy J, Bajtai G, Brasch H, et al: The role of hepatitis B surface antigen in the pathogenesis of glomerulonephritis. *Clin Nephrol* 12:109, 1979.

Ronco P, Verroust P, Mignon F, et al: Immunopathological studies of polyarteritis nodosa and Wegener's granulomatosis: A report of 43 patients with 51 renal biopsies. *Q J Med* 52:212, 1983.

Tarantino A, de Vecchi A, Montagnino G, et al: Renal disease in essential mixed cryoglobulinemia. *Q J Med* 50:1, 1981.

Wiggelinkhuizen J, Sinclair-Smith C, Stannard LM, Smuts H: Hepatitis b virus associated membranous glomerulonephritis. *Arch Dis Child* 58:488, 1983.

Yoshikawa N, Ito H, Yamada Y, et al: Membranous glomerulonephritis associated with hepatitis B antigen in children: A comparison with idiopathic membranous glomerulonephritis. *Clin Nephrol* 23:28, 1985.

AIDS Virus
(HIV: Human Immunodeficiency Virus)

Gardenswartz MH, Lerner CW, Seligson GR, et al: Renal disease in patients with AIDS: A clinicopathologic study. *Clin Nephrol* 21:197, 1984.

Pardo V, Aldana M, Colton RM, et al: Glomerular lesions in the acquired immunodeficiency syndrome. *Ann Intern Med* 101:429, 1984.

Rao TKS, Filippone EJ, Nicastri AD, et al: Associated focal and segmental glomerulosclerosis in the acquired immunodeficiency syndrome. *N Engl J Med* 310:669, 1984.

Welch K, Finkbeiner W, Alpers CE, et al: Autopsy findings in the acquired immune deficiency syndrome. *JAMA* 252:1152, 1984.

Other Viral Infections of the Kidney

Behan PO, Lowenstein LM, Stilmant M, Sax DS: Landry-Guillain-Barré-Strohl syndrome and immune complex nephritis. *Lancet* 1:850, 1973.

Brun C, Madsen S, Olsen S: Infectious mononucleosis with hepatic and renal involvement. *Scand J Gastroenterol* (suppl) 7:89, 1970.

Burch G, Harb J, Hiramoto Y: Coxsackie B4 viral infection of the human kidney. *J Urol* 112:714, 1974.

Donnellan WL, Chantra-Umporn S, Kidd JM: The cytomegalic inclusion cell. *Arch Pathol* 82:336, 1966.

Herrera GA, Alexander RW, Cooley CF, et al: Cytomegalovirus glomerulopathy: A controversial lesion. *Kidney Int* 29:725, 1986.

Jensen MM: Viruses and kidney disease: Review. *Am J Med* 43:897, 1967.

Krebs RA, Burvant MU: Nephrotic syndrome in association with varicella. *JAMA* 222:325, 1972.

Lin CY, Hsu HC: Measles and acute glomerulonephritis. *Pediatrics* 71:398, 1983.

Lin CY, Hsu HC, Hung YY: Nephrotic syndrome associated with varicella infection. *Pediatrics* 75:1127, 1985.

Minkowitz S, Wenk R, Friedman E, et al: Acute glomerulonephritis associated with varicella infection. *Am J Med* 44:489, 1968.

Rodriguez-Iturbe B, Garcia R, Rubio L, et al: Acute glomerulonephritis in the Guillain-Barré-Strohl syndrome: Report of nine cases. *Ann Intern Med* 78:391, 1973.

Shields AF, Hackman RD, Fife KH, et al: Adenovirus infections in patients undergoing bone-marrow transplantation. *N Engl J Med* 312:529, 1985.

Smith RD, Aquino J: Viruses and the kidney. *Med Clin North Am* 55:89, 1971.

Woodroffe AJ, Row PG, Meadows R, Lawrence JR: Nephritis in infectious mononucleosis. *Q J Med* 171:451, 1974.

Yuceoglu AM, Berkovich S, Minkowitz S: Acute glo-

merulonephritis associated with ECHO virus type 9 infection. *J Pediatr* 69:603, 1966.

CHAPTER 8: RICKETTSIAL INFECTIONS

Allen AC, Spitz S: A comparative study of the pathology of scrub typhus (tsutsugamushi disease) and other rickettsial diseases. *Am J Pathol* 21:603, 1945.

Bradford WD, Croker BP, Tisher CC: Kidney lesions in Rocky Mountain spotted fever: A light, immunofluorescent-, and electron-microscopic study. *Am J Pathol* 97:381, 1979.

Pinkerton H, Strano AJ: Rickettsial diseases, in Binford CH, Connor DH (eds): *Pathology of Tropical and Extraordinary Diseases*. Washington, DC, Armed Forces Institute of Pathology, 1976, pp 87–100.

Wear DJ, Connor DH: Rocky Mountain spotted fever: Demonstration of Rickettsia rickettsii in endothelial cells, using the Brown-Hopps tissue Gram stain (unpublished results, Department of Infectious and Parasitic Disease Pathology, Armed Forces Institute of Pathology).

CHAPTER 9: SPIROCHETE INFECTIONS

Leptospirosis

Davila de Arriga AJ, Rocha AS, Yasuda PH, de Brito T: Morphofunctional patterns of kidney injury in the experimental leptospirosis of the guinea pig (*L. icterohaemorrhagiae*). *J Pathol* 138:145, 1982.

De Brito T, Bohm GM, Yasuda PH: Vascular damage in acute experimental leptospirosis of the guinea pig. *J Pathol* 128:177, 1979.

Lai KN, Aarons I, Woodroffe AJ, Clarkson AR: Renal lesions in leptospirosis. *Aust NZ J Med* 12:276, 1982.

Sitprija V: Renal involvement in leptospirosis, in Robinson RR (ed): *Nephrology*. Proceedings of the ninth International Congress of Nephrology. New York, Springer-Verlag, 1984, pp 1041–1052.

Sitprija V, Evans H: The kidney in human leptospirosis. *Am J Med* 49:780, 1970.

Sitprija V, Pipatanagul V, Mertowidjojo K, et al: Pathogenesis of renal disease in leptospirosis: Clinical and experimental studies. *Kidney Int* 17:827, 1980.

Relapsing Fever

Anderson TR, Zimmerman LE: Relapsing fever in Korea: A clinicopathologic study of eleven fatal cases with special attention to association with salmonella infections. *Am J Pathol* 31:1083, 1955.

Bryceson ADM, Parry EHO, Perine PL, et al: Louse-borne relapsing fever: A clinical and laboratory study of 62 cases in Ethiopia and a reconsideration of the literature. *Q J Med* 39:129, 1970.

Judge DM, Samuel I, Perine PL, Vukotic D: Louse-borne relapsing fever in man. *Arch Pathol* 97:136, 1974.

Treponematoses

Losito A, Bucciarelli E, Massi-Benedetti F, Lato M: Membranous glomerulonephritis in congenital syphilis. *Clin Nephrol* 12:32, 1979.

Walker PD, Deeves EC, Sahba G, et al: Rapidly progressive glomerulonephritis in a patient with syphilis: Identification of antitreponemal antibody and treponemal antigen in renal tissue. *Am J Med* 76:1106, 1984.

CHAPTER 10: BACTERIAL INFECTIONS

Renal Involvement in Enteric Infections

Amerio A, Pastore G, Campese V, et al: Complicanze renali nel colera asiatico. *Ann Sclavo* 17:419, 1975.

Baker NM, Mills AE, Rachman I, Thomas JEP: Haemolytic uraemic syndrome in typhoid fever. *Br Med J* 2:84, 1974.

Benyajati C, Keoplung M, Beisel WR, et al: Acute renal failure in Asiatic cholera: Clinicopathologic correlation with acute tubular necrosis and hypokalemic nephropathy. *Ann Intern Med* 52:960, 1960.

De SN, Sengupta KP, Chanda NN: Renal changes including total cortical necrosis in cholera. *Arch Pathol* 57:505, 1954.

Faierman D, Ross FA, Seckler SG: Typhoid fever complicated by hepatitis, nephritis, and thrombocytopenia. *JAMA* 221:60, 1972.

Indraprasit S, Boonpucknavig V, Boonpucknavig S: IgA nephropathy associated with enteric fever. *Nephron* (in press).

Koster FT, Boonpucknavig V, Sujaho S, et al: Renal

histopathology in the hemolytic-uremic syndrome following shigellosis. *Clin Nephrol* 21:126, 1984.

Koster F, Levin J, Walker L, et al: Hemolytic-uremic syndrome after shigellosis: Relation to endotoxemia and circulating immune complexes. *N Engl J Med* 298:927, 1978.

Lwanga D, Wing AJ: Renal complications associated with typhoid fever. *E Afr Med J* 47:146, 1970.

Musa AM, Saleh SY, Abu Asha H: Transient nephritis during typhoid fever in five Sudanese patients. *Ann Trop Med Hyg* 75:181, 1981.

Rheingold OJ, Greenwald RA, Hayes PJ, et al: Myoglobinuria and renal failure associated with typhoid fever. *JAMA* 238:341, 1977.

Sitprija V, Pipatanagul V, Boonpucknavig V, Boonpucknavig S: Glomerulitis in typhoid fever. *Ann Intern Med* 81:210, 1974.

Brucella Infection

Doregatti C, Volpi A, Tarelli LT, et al: Acute glomerulonephritis in human brucellosis. *Nephron* 41:365, 1985.

Dunea G, Kark RM, Lannigan R, et al: Brucella nephritis. *Ann Intern Med* 70:783, 1969.

Kelalis PP, Greene LF, Weed LA: Brucellosis of the urogenital tract: A mimic of tuberculosis. *J Urol* 88:347, 1962.

Wasserheit JN, Dugdale DC, Agosti JM: Rhabdomyolysis and acute renal failure: A new presentation of acute brucellosis. *J Infect Dis* 150:782, 1984.

Legionella Infection

Dorman SA, Hardin NJ, Winn WC Jr: Pyelonephritis associated with legionella pneumophila, serogroup 4. *Ann Intern Med* 93:835, 1980.

Fenves AZ: Legionnaires' disease associated with acute renal failure: A report of two cases and review of the literature. *Clin Nephrol* 23:96, 1985.

Botryomycosis

Auger C: Human actinobacillary and staphylococcic actinophytosis. *Am J Clin Pathol* 18:645, 1948.

Brunken RC, Lichon-Chao N, van den Broeck H: Immunologic abnormalities in botryomycosis. *J Am Acad Dermatol* 9:428, 1983.

Winslow DJ: Botryomycosis. *Am J Pathol* 35:153, 1959.

Winslow DJ, Chamblin SA: Disseminated visceral botryomycosis: Report of a fatal case probably caused by *Pseudomonas aeruginosa*. *Am J Clin Pathol* 33:43, 1960.

Malacoplakia

Cadnapaphornchai P, Rosenberg BF, Taher S, et al: Renal parenchymal malakoplakia: An unusual cause of renal failure. *N Engl J Med* 299:1110, 1978.

Damjanov I, Katz SM: Malakoplakia. *Pathol Annu* 16(2):103, 1981.

McClure J: Malakoplakia. *J Pathol* 140:275, 1983.

McClurg FV, D'Agostino AN, Martin JH, Race GJ: Ultrastructural demonstration of intracellular bacteria in three cases of malakoplakia of the bladder. *Am J Clin Pathol* 60:780, 1973.

Voigt J: Malacoplakia of the urinary tract. *Acta Pathol Microbiol Scand* 44:377, 1958.

Xanthogranulomatous Pyelonephritis

Goldman SM, Hartman DS, Fishman EK, et al: CT of xanthogranulomatous pyelonephritis: Radiologic-pathologic correlation. *AJR* 141:963, 1984.

Goodman M, Curry T, Russel T: Xanthogranulomatous pyelonephritis (XGP): A local disease with systemic manifestations. Report of 23 patients and review of the literature. *Medicine* 58:171, 1979.

Hartman DS, Davis CJ Jr, Goldman SM, et al: Xanthogranulomatous pyelonephritis: Sonographic-pathologic correlation of 16 cases. *J Ultrasound Med* 3:481, 1984.

Khalyl-Mawad, J, Greco MA, Schinella RA: Ultrastructural demonstration of intracellular bacteria in xanthogranulomatous pyelonephritis. *Hum Pathol* 13:41, 1982.

Parsons MA, Harris SC, Longstaff AJ, Grainger RG: Xanthogranulomatous pyelonephritis: A pathological, clinical and aetiological analysis of 87 cases. *Diagn Histopathol* 6:203, 1983.

Glomerulonephritis in Chronic Sepsis

Beaufils M: Glomerular disease complicating abdominal sepsis [clinical conference]. *Kidney Int* 19:609, 1981.

Beaufils M, Morel-Maroger L, Sraer JD, et al: Acute renal failure of glomerular origin during visceral abscesses. *N Engl J Med* 295:185, 1976.

Dormont J, Delfraissy JF: The kidney in infectious diseases, in Hamburger J, Grunfeld JP (eds): *Nephrology*. New York, John Wiley & Sons, 1979, pp 767–790.

Forrest JW Jr, John F, Mills LR, et al: Immune complex glomerulonephritis associated with *Klebsiella pneumoniae* infection. *Clin Nephrol* 7:76, 1977.

Levy RL, Hong R: The immune nature of subacute bacterial endocarditis (SBE) nephritis. *Am J Med* 54:645, 1973.

Schena FP: Renal manifestations in bacterial infections. *Contr Nephrol* 48:125, 1985.

Williams RC Jr, Kunkel HG: Rheumatoid factor, complement and conglutinin aberrations in patients with subacute bacterial endocarditis. *J Clin Invest* 41:666, 1962.

CHAPTER 11: MYCOBACTERIAL INFECTIONS

Leprosy

Bjorvatn B, Barnetson RS, Kronvall G, et al: Immune complexes and complement hypercatabolism in patients with leprosy. *J Clin Exp Immunol* 26:388, 1976.

Date A, Thomas A, Mathal R, Johny KV: Glomerular pathology in leprosy: An electron microscopic study. *Am J Trop Med Hyg* 26:266, 1977.

Drutz DJ, Gutman RA: Renal manifestations of leprosy: Glomerulonephritis, a complication of erythema nodosum leprosum. *Am J Trop Med Hyg* 22:496, 1973.

Editorial: Amyloidosis and leprosy. *Lancet* 2:589, 1975.

Johny KV, Karat ABA, Rao PSS, Date A: Glomerulonephritis in leprosy: A percutaneous renal biopsy study. *Leprosy Rev* 46:29, 1975.

Tin Shwe: Immune complexes in glomeruli of patients with leprosy. *Leprosy Rev* 42:282, 1972.

Tuberculosis

Bhat HS: Observations on urogenital tuberculosis in India. *Ann Ind Acad Med Sci* 12:65, 1976.

Christensen WI: Genito-urinary tuberculosis: Review of 102 cases. *Medicine* 53:377, 1974.

Gow JG: Genito-urinary tuberculosis. *Br J Urol* 51:239, 1979.

Kollins SA, Hartman GW, Carr DT, et al: Roentgenographic findings in urinary tract tuberculosis. *Am J Roentgenol Rad Ther Nucl Med* 121:487, 1974.

Sharma SK, Chugh KS: Genito-urinary tuberculosis in India. *J Assoc Phys Ind* 25:813, 1977.

Chapter 12: Fungal and Actinomycetal Infections

Cohen J: Antifungal chemotherapy. *Lancet* 2:532, 1982.

Grocott RG: A stain for fungi in tissue sections and smears using Gomori's methenamine-silver nitrate technic. *Am J Clin Pathol* 25:975, 1955.

Kaplan W, Kraft DE: Demonstration of pathogenic fungi in formalin-fixed tissues by immunofluorescence. *Am J Clin Pathol* 52:420, 1969.

Michigan S: Genitourinary fungal infections. *J Urol* 116:390, 1976.

Orr WA, Mulholland SG, Walzak MP: Genitourinary tract involvement with systemic mycoses. *J Urol* 107:1047, 1972.

Candidiasis

Eckstein CW, Kass EJ: Anuria in a newborn secondary to bilateral ureteropelvic fungus balls. *J Urol* 127:109, 1982.

Gerle RD: Roentgenographic features of primary renal candidiasis: Fungus ball of the renal pelvis and ureter. *Am J Roentgenol* 119:731, 1973.

Heel RC: Systemic candidosis and candiduria, in Levine HB (ed): *Ketoconazole in the Management of Fungal Disease.* New York, ADIS Press, 1982, pp 116–118.

Hughes WT: Systemic candidiasis: A study of 109 fatal cases. *Pediatr Infect Dis* 1:11, 1982.

Lehner T: Systemic candidiasis and renal involvement. *Lancet* 1:1414, 1964.

Myerowitz RL, Pazin GJ, Allen CM: Disseminated candidiasis: Changes in incidence, underlying diseases and pathology. *Am J Clin Pathol* 68:29, 1977.

Odds FC: Candidosis of the urinary tract, in *Candida and Candidosis.* Baltimore, University Park Press, 1979, pp 147–153.

Tomashefski JF, Abramowsky CR: Candida-associated renal papillary necrosis. *Am J Clin Pathol* 75:190, 1981.

Torulopsosis

Berkowitz ID, Robboy SJ, Karchmer AW, Kunz LJ: Torulopsis glabrata fungemia: A Clinical pathological study. *Medicine* 58:430, 1979.

Grimley PM, Wright LD, Jennings AE: Torulopsis glabrata infection in man. *Am J Clin Pathol* 43:216, 1965.

Kauffman CA, Tan JS: Torulopsis glabrata renal infection. *Am J Med* 57:217, 1974.

Khauli RB, Kalash S, Young JD Jr: Torulopsis glabrata perinephric abscess. *J Urol* 130:968, 1983.

Takeuchi H, Tomoyoshi T: Torulopsis infection extensively involving urinary tract. *Urology* 22:173, 1983.

Vordermark JS II, Modarelli RO, Buck AS: Torulopsis pyelonephritis associated with papillary necrosis: A case report. *J Urol* 123:96, 1980.

Cryptococcosis

Hellman RN, Hinrichs J, Sicard G, et al: Cryptococcal pyelonephritis and disseminated cryptococcosis in a renal transplant patient. *Arch Intern Med* 141:128, 1981.

Kaplan MH, Rosen PP, Armstrong D: Cryptococcosis in a cancer hospital. *Cancer* 39:2265, 1977.

Randall RE, Stacy WK, Toone EC, et al: Cryptococcal pyelonephritis. *N Engl J Med* 279:60, 1968.

Sayler WR, Salyer DC: Involvement of the kidney and prostate in cryptococcosis. *J Urol* 109:695, 1973.

Blastomycosis

Busey JF: Blastomycosis. I. A review of 198 collected cases in the Veterans Administration hospitals. *Am Rev Respir Dis* 89:659, 1964.

Eickenberg HU, Amin M, Lich R Jr: Blastomycosis of the genitourinary tract. *J Urol* 112:650, 1975.

Rolnick D, Baumrucker GO: Genitourinary blastomycosis: Case report and review of literature. *J Urol* 79:315, 1958.

Sarosi GA, Davies SF: Blastomycosis. *Am Rev Respir Dis* 120:911, 1979.

Schwarz J, Salfelder K: Blastomycosis: A review of 152 cases, in Grudmann E, Kirsten WH (eds): *Current Topics in Pathology.* Berlin, Springer-Verlag, 1977, vol 65, pp 165–200.

Tenenbaum MJ, Greenspan J, Kerkering TM: Blastomycosis. *CRC Crit Rev Microbiol* 9:139, 1982.

Histoplasmosis

Baker RD: Histoplasmosis in routine autopsies. *Am J Clin Pathol* 41:457, 1964.

Goodwin RA Jr, Des Prez RM: Histoplasmosis. *Am Rev Respir Dis* 117:929, 1978.

Goodwin RA Jr, Shapiro JL, Thurman GH, et al: Disseminated histoplasmosis: Clinical and pathological correlations. *Medicine* 59:1, 1980.

Sathapatayavongs B, Batteiger BE, Wheat J, et al: Clinical and laboratory features of disseminated histoplasmosis during two large urban outbreaks. *Medicine* 62:263, 1983.

Schwarz J: African histoplasmosis (part 2), in Baker RD (ed): *The Pathologic Anatomy of Mycoses: Human Infection with Fungi, Actinomycetes and Algae*. Berlin, Springer-Verlag, 1971, pp 139–146.

Straus SE, Jacobson ES: The spectrum of histoplasmosis in a general hospital: A review of 55 cases diagnosed at Barnes Hospital between 1966 and 1977. *Am J Med Sci* 279:147, 1980.

Williams AO, Lawson EA, Lucas AO: African histoplasmosis due to *Histoplasma duboisii*. *Arch Pathol* 92:306, 1971.

Paracoccidioidomycosis (South American Blastomycosis)

Angulo-Ortega A, Pollak L: Paracoccidioidomycosis, in Baker RD (ed): *The Pathologic Anatomy of Mycoses: Human Infection with Fungi, Actinomycetes and Algae*. Berlin, Springer-Verlag, 1971, pp 507–576.

Restrepo A, Robledo M, Gutierrez F, et al: Paracoccidioidomycosis (South American blastomycosis): A study of 39 cases observed in Medellin, Colombia. *Am J Trop Med Hyg* 19:68, 1970.

Salfelder K, Doehnert G, Doehnert HR: Paracoccidioidomycosis: Anatomic study with complete autopsies. *Virchows Arch [A]* 348:51, 1969.

Coccidioidomycosis

Conner WT, Drach GW, Bucher WC: Genitourinary aspects of disseminated coccidioidomycosis. *J Urol* 113:82, 1975.

Drutz DJ, Catanzaro A: Coccidioidomycosis, parts I and II. *Am Rev Respir Dis* 117:559 and 727, 1978.

Huntington RW, Waldmann WJ, Sargent JA, et al: Pathologic and clinical observations on 142 cases of fatal coccidioidomycosis with necropsy, in Ajello L (ed): *Coccidioidomycosis*. Second Symposium on Coccidioidomycosis. Tucson, University of Arizona Press, 1967, pp 143–167.

Petersen EA, Friedman BA, Crowder ED, Rifkind D: Coccidioiduria: Clinical significance. *Ann Intern Med* 85:34, 1976.

Rohn JG, Davila JC, Gibson TE: Urogenital aspects of coccidioidomycosis: Review of the literature and report of two cases. *J Urol* 65:660, 1951.

Winn WR, Finegold SM, Huntington RW: Coccidioidomycosis with fungemia, in Ajello L (ed): *Coccidioidomycosis*. Second Symposium on Coccidioidomycosis. Tucson, University of Arizona Press, 1967, pp 93–109.

Aspergillosis

Flechner SM, McAninch JW: Aspergillosis of the urinary tract: Ascending route of infection and evolving patterns of disease. *J Urol* 125:598, 1981.

Meyer RD, Young LS, Armstrong D, Yu B: Aspergillosis complicating neoplastic disease. *Am J Med* 54:6, 1973.

Torrington KG, Old CW, Urban ES, Carpenter JL: Transurethral passage of aspergillus fungus balls in acute myelocytic leukemia. *South Med J* 72:361, 1979.

Warshawsky AB, Keiller D, Gittes RF: Bilateral renal aspergillosis. *J Urol* 113:8, 1975.

Young RC, Bennett JE, Vogel CL, et al: Aspergillosis: The spectrum of the disease in 98 patients. *Medicine* 49:147, 1970.

Mucormycosis (Zygomycosis)

Baker RD: Mucormycosis, in Baker RD (ed): *The Pathologic Anatomy of Mycoses: Human Infection with Fungi, Actinomycetes and Algae*. Berlin, Springer-Verlag, 1971, pp 832–918.

Dansky AS, Lynne CM, Politano VA: Disseminated mucormycosis with renal involvement. *J Urol* 119:275, 1978.

Langston C, Roberts DA, Porter GA, Bennett WM: Renal phycomycosis. *J Urol* 109:941, 1973.

Low AI, Tulloch AGS, England EJ: Phycomycosis of the kidney associated with a transient immune defect and treated with clotrimazole. *J Urol* 111:732, 1974.

Meyer RD, Rosen P, Armstrong D: Phycomycosis complicating leukemia and lymphoma. *Ann Intern Med* 77:871, 1972.

Prout GR, Goddard AR: Renal mucormycosis: Survival after nephrectomy and amphotericin B therapy. *N Engl J Med* 263:1246, 1960.

Actinomycosis

Brown JR: Human actinomycosis: A study of 181 subjects. *Hum Pathol* 4:319, 1973.

Burkman R, Schlesselman S, McCaffrey L, et al: The relationship of genital tract actinomycetes and the development of pelvic inflammatory disease. *Am J Obstet Gynecol* 143:585, 1982.

Causey WA: Actinomycosis, in Vinken PJ, Bruyn GW (eds): *Handbook of Clinical Neurology: Infections of the Nervous System*, Part III. Amsterdam, North Holland Publishing Co, 1978, pp 383–394.

Wajszczuk CP, Logan TF, Pasculle AW, Ho M: Intra-abdominal actinomycosis presenting with sulfur granules in the urine. *Am J Med* 77:1126, 1984.

Weese WC, Smith IM: A study of 57 cases of actinomycosis over a 36-year period. *Arch Intern Med* 135:1562, 1975.

Nocardiosis

Causey WA, Lee R: Nocardiosis, in Vinken PJ, Bruyn GW (eds): *Handbook of Clinical Neurology: Infections of the Nervous System*, Part III. Amsterdam, North Holland Publishing Co, 1978, pp 517–530.

Frazier AR, Rosenow EC, Roberts GD: Nocardiosis: A review of 25 cases occurring during 24 months. *Mayo Clin Proc* 50:657, 1975.

Mahvi TA: Disseminated nocardiosis caused by *Nocardia brasiliensis*. *Arch Dermatol* 89:426, 1964.

Palmer DL, Harvey RL, Wheeler JK: Diagnostic and therapeutic considerations in *Nocardia asteroides* infection. *Medicine* 53:391, 1974.

CHAPTER 13: ARTHROPOD AND VENOMOUS ANIMAL BITES AND STINGS

Snakebites

Chugh KS, Pal Y, Chakravarty RN, et al: Acute renal failure following poisonous snake bite. *Am J Kidney Dis* 4:30, 1984.

Date A, Shastry JCM: Renal ultrastructure in cortical

necrosis following Russell's viper envenomation. *J Trop Med Hyg* 84:3, 1981.

Date A, Shastry JCM: Renal ultrastructure in acute tubular necrosis following Russell's viper envenomation. *J Pathol* 137:225, 1982.

Minton SA (ed): *Snake Venoms and Envenomation*. New York, Marcel Dekker, 1971.

Reid HA: Myoglobinuria and sea snake bite poisoning. *Br Med J* 1:1284, 1961.

Seedat YK, Reddy J, Edington DA: Acute renal failure due to proliferative nephritis from snake bite poisoning. *Nephron* 13:455, 1974.

Sitprija V, Boonpucknavig V: Snake venoms and nephrotoxicity, in Lee CY (ed): *Snake Venoms*. Berlin, Springer-Verlag, 1979, pp 997–1018.

Arthropod Stings

Bazolet L: Scorpionism in the Old World, in Bucherl W, Buckley E (eds): *Venomous Animals and Their Venoms*. Vol IV. *Venomous Invertebrates*. New York, Academic Press, 1971, p 349.

Bucherl W, Spiders K: In Bucherl W, Buckley E (eds): *Venomous Animals and Their Venoms*. Vol IV.—*Venomous Invertebrates*. New York, Academic Press, 1971, pp 197–277.

Kibukamusoke JW, Chugh KS, Sakhuja V: Other venomous stings, in Kibukamusoke JW (ed): *Tropical Nephrology*. Canberra: Citforge Printery, 1984, pp 188–195.

Shilkin KB, Chen BTM, Khoo OT: Rhabdomyolysis caused by hornet venom. *Br Med J* 1:156, 1972.

CHAPTER 14: CONSEQUENCES OF METABOLIC DERANGEMENTS IN TROPICAL CLIMATES

Acute Rhabdomyolysis and Myoglobinuria

Flamenbaum W, Gehr M, Gross M, et al: Acute renal failure associated with myoglobinuria and hemoglobinuria, in Brenner BM, Lazarus JM (eds): *Acute Renal Failure*. Philadelphia, WB Saunders Co, 1983, chap 12.

Grossman RA, Hamilton RW, Morse BM, et al: Nontraumatic rhabdomyolysis and acute renal failure. *N Engl J Med* 291:807, 1974.

Kagen LJ: Immunofluorescent demonstration of myoglobin in the kidney: Case report and review of 43 cases of myoglobinemia and myoglobinuria identified immunologically. *Am J Med* 48:649, 1970.

Knochel JP: Renal injury in muscle disease, in Suki WN, Eknoyan G (eds): *The Kidney in Systemic Disease*. New York, John Wiley & Sons, 1976, p 129.

Koffler A, Friedler RM, Massry SG: Acute renal failure due to nontraumatic rhabdomyolysis. *Ann Intern Med* 85:23, 1976.

Schrier RW, Henderson HS, Tisher CC, Tannen RL: Nephropathy associated with heat stress and exercise. *Ann Intern Med* 67:356, 1967.

Schrier RW, Hano J, Keller HI, et al: Renal, metabolic, and circulatory responses to heat and exercise: Studies in military recruits during summer training, with implications for acute renal failure. *Ann Intern Med* 73:213, 1970.

Heat Stroke

Chao TC, Sinniah R, Pakiam JE: Acute heat stroke deaths. *Pathology* 13:145, 1981.

Kew MC, Abrahams C, Levin MW, et al: The effects of heat stroke on the function and structure of the kidney. *Q J Med* 36:277, 1967.

Knochel JP, Beisel WR, Herndon EG, et al: The renal, cardiovascular, hematologic and serum electrolyte abnormalities of heat stroke. *Am J Med* 30:299, 1961.

Malamud N, Haymaker W, Custer RP: Heat stroke: A clinicopathological study of 125 fatal cases. *Milit Surg* 99:397, 1946.

Sohal RS, Sun SC, Colcolough HL, et al: Heat stroke: An electron microscopic study of endothelial cell damage and disseminated intravascular coagulation. *Arch Intern Med* 122:43, 1968.

Fluid and Electrolyte Depletion

Adu D, Anim-Addoy, Foli AK, et al: Acute renal failure in tropical Africa. *Br Med J* 1:890, 1976.

Chugh KS, Singhal PC: Pattern of acute renal failure in the developing countries: Influence of socio-economic and environmental factors, in Eliahou HE (ed): *Acute Renal Failure*. London, John Libbey, 1982, pp 156–160.

Chugh KS, Singhal PC, Sharma BK, et al: Acute renal failure due to intravascular hemolysis in north Indian patients. *Am J Med Sci* 274:139, 1977.

CHAPTER 15: BLOOD DYSCRASIAS

Sickle Cell Diseases

Alleyne GAO, Statius Van Eps LW, Addae SK, et al: The kidney in sickle cell anemia. *Kidney Int* 7:371, 1975.

Bernstein J, Whitten CF: A histologic appraisal of the kidney in sickle cell anemia. *Arch Pathol* 70:407, 1960.

Buckalew VM Jr: Sickle cell nephropathy, in Robinson RR (ed): *Nephrology*. Proceedings of the Ninth International Congress of Nephrology. New York, Springer-Verlag, 1984, pp 916–925.

Elfenbein L, Patchefsky A, Schwartz AW, Weinstein AG: Pathology of the glomerulus in sickle cell anemia with and without the nephrotic syndrome. *Am J Pathol* 77:357, 1974.

de Jong PE, Statius Van Eps LW: Sickle cell nephropathy: New insights into its pathophysiology. *Kidney Int* 27:711, 1985.

McCoy RC: Ultrastructural alterations in the kidney with sickle cell disease and the nephrotic syndrome. *Lab Invest* 21:85, 1969.

Martinez-Maldonado M: The kidney in sickle cell disease and multiple myeloma, in Suki WN, Eknoyan G (eds): *The Kidney in Systemic Disease*. New York, John Wiley & Sons, 1976.

Statius Van Eps LW, Penedo-Veels C, de Vries GH, de Koning J: Nature of concentrating defect in sickle cell nephropathy. *Lancet* 1:450, 1970.

Wintrobe MM, Lee GR, Boggs DF, et al: *Clinical Hematology*, ed 8. Philadelphia, Lea & Febiger, 1981.

Thalassemia

Bhamarapravati N, Na-Nakorn S, Wasi P, et al: Pathology of abnormal hemoglobin diseases seen in Thailand. *Am J Clin Pathol* 47:745, 1967.

Dubovsky D, Jacobs P: Acute uric acid nephropathy in thalassemia. *S Afr Med J* 49:243, 1975.

Grossman H, Dische MR, Winchester PH, et al: Renal enlargement in thalassemia major. *Radiology* 100:645, 1971.

Mastrangelo F, Lopez T, Rizzelli S, et al: Function of the kidney in adult patients with Cooley's anemia. *Nephron* 14:229, 1975.

Tanphaichitr P, Banchet P, Petchclai B, et al: The association between thalassemic diseases and traits and post-streptococcal acute glomerulonephritis. *Southeast Asian J Trop Med Public Health* 8:121, 1977.

Wasi P: Streptococcal infection leading to cardiac and renal involvement in thalassemia. *Lancet* 1:949, 1971.

G-6-PD Deficiency and Hemolysis

Kibukamusoke JW: Malaria and acute renal failure, in Kibukamusoke JW (ed): *Tropical Nephrology.* Canberra, Citforge Printery, 1984, pp 76–84.

CHAPTER 16: RENAL DISEASE OF GEOGRAPHIC IMPORTANCE

Tropical Nephropathy and Extramembranous (Membranous) Glomerulonephritis

Coovadia HM, Adhikari M, Morel-Maroger L: Clinical-pathological features of the nephrotic syndrome in South African children. *Q J Med* 48:77, 1979.

Morel-Maroger L, Verroust P, Sloper JC, Saimot G: Extramembranous proliferative glomerulonephritis in West African children, in Giovannetti S, Bonomini V, D'Amico G (eds): Proceedings of the Sixth International Congress of Nephrology. Florence, 1975. Basel, S. Karger, 1976, pp 457–461.

Morel-Maroger L, Saimot AG, Sloper JC, et al: "Tropical nephropathy" and tropical extramembranous glomerulonephritis of unknown aetiology in Senegal. *Br Med J* 1:541, 1975.

Poststreptococcal Glomerulonephritis

Axema P, Freij L, Hadgu P, et al: Streptococcal types in impetigo and acute glomerulonephritis among children in Addis Ababa. *Scand J Inf Dis* 8:161, 1976.

Dillon HC, Reeves MS, Maxted WR: Acute glomerulonephritis following skin infection due to streptococci of M-type 2. *Lancet* 1:543, 1968.

Hersch C: Acute glomerulonephritis due to skin disease with special reference to scabies. *S Afr Med J* 1:29, 1967.

Kaplan EL, Anthony BF, Chapman SS, Wannamaker LW: Epidemic acute glomerulonephritis associated with type 49 streptococcus pyoderma. *Am J Med* 48:9, 1970.

Koshi G, Webb JKG, Myers RM: Association of preceding streptococcal skin infection and acute glomerulonephritis in children in south India. *Ind J Med Res* 56:951, 1968.

Lasch EE, Frankel V, Vardy PA, et al: Epidemic glomerulonephritis in Israel. *J Infect Dis* 124:141, 1971.

McDowall MF, Ramkissoon R, Basset DCJ: Epidemic and endemic pattern of childhood nephritis. *Clin Pediatr* 9:580, 1970.

Poon-King T, Mohammed I, Cox R, et al: Recurrent epidemic nephritis in south Trinidad. *N Engl J Med* 277:728, 1967.

Poon-King T, Potter EV, Svartman M, et al: Acute glomerulonephritis with reappearance of M-Type 55 Streptococci in Trinidad. *Lancet* 1:475, 1973.

Potter EV, Svartman M, Burt EG, et al: Relationship of acute rheumatic fever to acute glomerulonephritis in Trinidad. *J Infect Dis* 125:619, 1972.

Rodriguez-Iturbi B, Garcia R, Rubio L, et al: Epidemic glomerulonephritis in Maracaibo: Evidence for progression to chronicity. *Clin Nephrol* 5:197, 1976.

Smith EV, Claypoole TF: Canine scabies in dogs and in humans. *JAMA* 199:59, 1967.

Stetson CA, Rammelkamp CH Jr, Krause RM, et al: Epidemic acute nephritis. *Medicine* 34:431, 1955.

Svartman M, Potter EV, Finklea J, et al: Epidemic scabies and acute glomerulonephritis in Trinidad. *Lancet* 1:249, 1972.

Symonds BER: Epidemic nephritis in south Trinidad. *J Pediatr* 56:420, 1960.

Mesangial IgA Nephropathy

Berger J: IgA glomerular deposits in renal disease. *Transplant Proc* 1:934, 1969.

Clarkson AR, Seymour AE, Thompson AJ, et al: IgA nephropathy: A syndrome of uniform morphology, diverse clinical features, and uncertain prognosis. *Clin Nephrol* 8:459, 1977.

D'Amico G: Natural history and treatment of idiopathic IgA nephropathy, in Robinson RR, et al (eds): *Nephrology.* Proceedings of the Ninth International Congress of Nephrology. New York, Springer-Verlag, 1984, vol 1, pp 686–701.

Droz D: Natural history of primary glomerulonephritis with mesangial deposits of IgA. *Contr Nephrol* 2:150, 1976.

Kurt Lee SM, Rao VM, Franklin WA, et al: IgA nephropathy: Morphologic predictors of progressive renal disease. *Hum Pathol* 13:314, 1982.

Levy M, Beaufils H, Gubler MC, Habib R: Idiopathic recurrent macroscopic hematuria and mesangial IgA-IgG deposits in children (Berger's disease). *Clin Nephrol* 1:63, 1973.

McCoy RC, Abramowsky CR, Tisher CC: IgA nephropathy. *Am J Pathol* 76:123, 1974.

Shigematsu H, Kobayashi Y, Tateno S, et al: Ultrastructural glomerular loop abnormalities in IgA nephropathy. *Nephron* 30:1, 1982.

Shirai T, Tomino Y, Sato M, et al: IgA nephropathy: Clinicopathology and immunopathology. *Contr Nephrol* 9:88, 1978.

Sinniah R: IgA mesangial nephropathy: Berger's disease. Editorial review. *Am J Nephrol* 5:73, 1985.

Sinniah R, Churg J: Effect of IgA deposits on the glomerular mesangium in Berger's disease. *Ultrastruct Pathol* 4:9, 1983.

Sinniah R, Ku G: Clinicopathologic correlations in IgA nephropathy, in Robinson RR, et al (eds): *Nephrology.* Proceedings of the Ninth International Congress of Nephrology. New York, Springer-Verlag, 1984, vol 1, pp 665–685.

Sinniah R, Javier AR, Ku G: The pathology of mesangial IgA nephritis with clinical correlations. *Histopathology* 5:469, 1981.

Sinniah R, Pwee HS, Lim CH: Glomerular lesions in asymptomatic microscopic hematuria discovered on routine medical examination. *Clin Nephrol* 5:216, 1976.

Ueda Y, Sakai O, Yamagata M, et al: IgA glomerulonephritis in Japan. *Contr Nephrol* 4:36, 1977.

Mesangial IgM Nephropathy

Bhasin HK, Abuelo JG, Nayak R, Esparza AR: Mesangial proliferative glomerulonephritis. *Lab Invest* 39:21, 1978.

Cohen AH, Border WA, Glassock RJ: Nephrotic syndrome with glomerular mesangial IgM deposits. *Lab Invest* 38:610, 1978.

Kobayashi Y, Shigematsu H, Tateno S, Hiki Y: Nephrotic syndrome with diffuse mesangial IgM deposits. *Acta Pathol Jpn* 32:307, 1982.

Sitprija V: The kidney in acute tropical disease, in Ki-

bukamusoke JW (ed): *Tropical Nephrology.* Canberra, Citforge Printery, 1984, pp 148–169.

Waldherr R, Gubler MC, Levy M, et al: The significance of pure diffuse mesangial proliferation in idiopathic nephrotic syndrome. *Clin Nephrol* 10:171, 1978.

Secondary Amyloidosis

Chugh KS, Singhal PC, Sakhuja V, et al: Pattern of renal amyloidosis in Indian patients. *Postgrad Med J* 57:31, 1981.

Cohen AS: Amyloidosis. *N Engl J Med* 277:522, 574 and 628, 1967.

Cooke RA, Champness LT: Amyloidosis in Papua and New Guinea. *Papua New Guinea Med J* 10:43, 1967.

McAdam KPWJ: Endemic amyloidosis and the pathogenesis of secondary amyloidosis, in Zurukzoglu W et al (eds): Proceedings of the Eighth International Congress of Nephrology. Basel, S Karger, 1981, pp 1225–1231.

Sokmen C, Ozdemir AI: The spectrum of renal diseases found by kidney biopsy in Turkey. *Ann Intern Med* 67:603, 1967.

CHAPTER 17: TOXIC NEPHROPATHY

Plant Toxins

Berndt WO: The nephrotoxicity of mycotoxins and botanicals, in Bach PH et al (eds): *Nephrotoxicity: Assessment and Pathogenesis.* Monographs in Applied Toxicology. Chichester, John Wiley & Sons, 1982, vol 1, pp 378–395.

Chugh KS, Singhal PC, Sharma BK, et al: Acute renal failure due to intravascular hemolysis in north Indian patients. *Am J Med Sci* 274:139, 1977.

Kibukamusoke JW, Coovadia HM: Renal hazards from plant products, in Kibukamusoke JW (ed): *Tropical Nephrology.* Canberra, Citforge Printery, 1984, chap 15.

Minerals, Including Mercury and Copper

Becker CG, Becker EL, Maher JF, Schreiner GE: Nephrotic syndrome after contact with mercury. A report of five cases, three after the use of ammoniated mercury ointment. *Arch Intern Med* 110:178, 1962.

Cameron JS, Trounce JR: Membranous glomerulonephritis and the nephrotic syndrome appearing during Mersalyl therapy. *Guy Hosp Rep* 114:101, 1965.

Kazantzis G, Schiller KF, Asscher AW, Drew RG: Albuminuria and the nephrotic syndrome following exposure to mercury and its compounds. *Q J Med* 31:403, 1962.

Kibukamusoke JW, Davies DR, Hutt MSR: Membranous nephropathy due to skin-lightening cream. *Br Med J* 2:646, 1974.

Mandema E, Arends A, Van Zeijst J, et al: Mercury and the kidney. *Lancet* 1:1266, 1963.

Bile of Grass Carp

Chen WY, Yen TD, Cheng JT, et al: Acute renal failure due to raw bile of grass carp (*Clenopharyngodon idellus*). *J Med Assoc Thailand* 61(suppl 1):63, 1978.

CHAPTER 18: MALIGNANCIES IN THE TROPICS

Burkitt's Lymphoma of the Kidney

Banks PM, Arseneau JC, Gralnick HR, et al: American Burkitt's lymphoma: A clinicopathologic study of 30 cases. II. Pathologic correlations. *Am J Med* 58:322, 1975.

Berard C, O'Conor GT, Thomas LB, Torloni H: Histopathological identification of Burkitt's tumor. *Bull WHO* 40:601, 1969.

Burkitt D, O'Conor GT: Malignant lymphoma in African children. I. A clinical syndrome. *Cancer* 14:258, 1961.

O'Conor GT: Malignant lymphoma in African children. *Cancer* 14:270, 1961.

ten Seldam REJ, Cooke R, Atkinson L: Childhood lymphoma in the territories of Papua and New Guinea. *Cancer* 19:437, 1966.

Wright DH: Burkitt's lymphoma: A review of the pathology, immunology and possible etiologic factors. *Pathol Annu* 6:337, 1971.

Schistosomiasis and Carcinoma of the Urinary Bladder

Lehman JS Jr, Farid Z, Smith JH, et al: Urinary schistosomiasis in Egypt: Clinical, radiological, bacteriological and parasitological correlations. *Trans R Soc Trop Med Hyg* 67:384, 1973.

Mostofi FK (ed): Bilharziasis. International Academy of Pathology special monograph. New York, Springer-Verlag, 1967.

von Lichtenberg F, Edington GM, Nwabuebo L, et al: Pathologic effects of schistosomaisis in Ibadan, western state of Nigeria. II. Pathogenesis of lesions of the bladder and ureters. *Am J Trop Med Hyg* 20:244, 1971.

CHAPTER 19: MISCELLANEOUS CONDITIONS

Labrea Hepatitis

Andrade ZA, Santos JB, Prata A, Dourado H: Histopatologia da hepatite de Labrea. *Rev Soc Bras Med Trop* 16:31, 1983.

De Paola D, Strano AJ, Hopps HC: Labrea hepatitis (black fever): A problem in geographic pathology. *Bull Int Acad Pathol* 9:43, 1968.

Kawasaki Disease

Kawasaki T: MCLS showing particular skin desquamation from the finger and toe in infants. (In Japanese.) *Allergy* 16:178, 1967.

Tanaka N, Sekimoto K, Naoe S: Kawasaki disease: Relationship with infantile periarteritis nodosa. *Arch Pathol Lab Med* 100:81, 1976.

Hemolytic-Uremic Syndrome in Infections

Baker NM, Mills AE, Rachman I, Thomas JEP: Hemolytic uremic syndrome in typhoid fever. *Br Med J* 2:84, 1974.

Churg J, Strauss L: Renal involvement in thrombotic microangiopathies, in *Seminars in Nephrology*. New York, Grune & Stratton, 1985, vol 5, pp 46–56.

Koster FT, Boonpucknavig V, Sujaho S, et al: Renal histopathology in the hemolytic-uremic syndrome following shigellosis. *Clin Nephrol* 21:126, 1984.

Rapaport SI, Tatter D, Coeur-Barron N, et al: Pseudomonas septicemia with intravascular clotting leading to the generalized Shwartzman reaction. *N Engl J Med* 271:80, 1964.

Chyluria

Akisada M, Tani S: Filarial chyluria in Japan: Lymphography, etiology, and treatment in 30 cases. *Radiology* 90:311, 1968.

Akisada M, Tani S: Lymphangioadenopathy of filariasis. *Trans R Soc Trop Med Hyg* 64:885, 1970.

Date A, Shastry JCM, Johny KV: Ultrastructural glomerular changes in filarial chyluria. *J Trop Med Hyg* 82:150, 1979.

Koehler PR, Chiang TC, Lin CT, et al: Lymphography in chyluria. *Am J Roentgenol Rad Ther Nuc Med* 102:455, 1968.

Rajaram PC: Lymphatic dynamics in filarial chyluria and prechyluric state: Lymphographic analysis of 52 cases. *Lymphology* 3:114, 1970.

INDEX

Numbers in *italics* refer to pages on which illustrations appear.

Coagulation factors, 11
Cobra, 185
Coccidioides immitis, 163–164, *176, 177*
Coccidioidomycosis, 163–164, *176, 177*
Colitis, ulcerative, 213
Collagenase, 8, 11
Combined hemoglobinopathy, 199–200
Complement system, 3, 6–7, 11–12
Congenital syphilis, 117, *123*
Congenital toxoplasmosis, 17
Corticosteroid, 15, 212
Coxsackievirus, 86, 238
Crescentic glomerulonephritis, 87, *153*, 210
Crohn's disease, 210, 213
Crotalus, 183
Crotalus durissus terificus, 183
Cryoglobulinemia, mixed, 81, *101*
Cryptococcosis, 159–160, *172, 173*
Cryptococcus, 83
Cryptococcus neoformans, 160, *172, 173*
Cryptophis nigrescens, 183
Cunninghamella, 165
Cutaneous blastomycosis, 161
Cutaneous leishmaniasis, 26
Cyclo-oxygenase, 8, 12
Cyclophosphamide, 15, 212
Cyprinol, 229
Cyst
    alveolar, 70
    hydatid. *See* Echinococcosis
Cysticercosis, 70, *73, 74*
Cystitis, 232
    candidal, 158
Cytomegalovirus, 83, 85–86, *106*

D
Death cap mushroom, 227–228
Dehydrogenase, 8
Delta agent, 79
Demansia nuchalis, 183
Demansia nuchalis affinis, 183
Dengue hemorrhagic fever, 77–79, *96, 97*
    world distribution of, *95*
Dengue shock syndrome. *See* Dengue hemorrhagic fever
Dermatitis, 43
    cercarial, 61–62
Dermatologic cream, mercury-containing, 228–229
Diffuse endocapillary proliferative glomerulonephritis, 85, *106*, 149–150, 201
Diffuse interstitial nephritis, 130
Diffuse mesangial proliferative glomerulonephritis, 70, 82
Diffuse mesangiocapillary glomerulonephritis, 81
Diffuse proliferative glomerulonephritis, 86, 110

Diffuse pyelonephritis, 167
Diffuse sclerosing glomerulonephritis, 211
Dioctophyma renale, 54, *57–59*
Dioctophymiasis, 54, *57–59*
Dispholidus typhus, 183
Disseminated aspergillosis, 164
Disseminated mucormycosis, 165
Divicine, 228
Djenkol bean, 227
DNA, 5
Dysentery, 17, 193
    bacillary, 128

E
Echinococcosis, 69–70, *71–73*
Echinococcus granulosus, 69–70, 72
    life cycle of, 69, *71–73*
Echinococcus multilocularis, 70
Echinococcus oligarthrus, 70
Echis carinatus, 183, 185
ECHO virus, 86, 238
Elastase, 8, 11
Electrolyte depletion, 193
Elephantiasis, 41
Endocapillary glomerulonephritis. *See* Diffuse endocapillary glomerulonephritis
Endocarditis, 134
    Brucella, 130
Endoperoxide, 8
Enhydrina schistosa, 183
Entamoeba histolytica, 17–18, *40*
Enteric fever, 127
Enterobacteriaceae, 127
Enterobius vermicularis, 55
Enterovirus, 83, 86
Epidemic hemorrhagic fever. *See* Hantavirus
Epidemic nephropathy. *See* Hantavirus
Epidemic typhus, 110
Epididymitis, 41
Epimembranous glomerulonephritis, 228
Epstein-Barr virus, 84–85, 231
Escherichia coli, 127, 129, 131–133, *137*, 238
Eustrongylus gigas, 239

F
Falciparum malaria, 13–15
Falciparum malarial nephropathy, *21–22*
Fava bean, 201
Fibronectin, 2
Filarial nematode infection, 41–44, 239
Filariasis, *244–246*
    Bancroftian, 41–42, *45–50*
    Brugian, 41–42, *45–50*

Malacoplakia, 131–133, *140–143*
Malaria, 4, *20–25*, 201, 207, 213, 231, 239
   epidemiological assessment of status of, *19*
   falciparum, 13–15
   malariae, 13–15
   quartan, 3, 5, 14, *23–24*, 208
Malariae malaria, 13–15
Malarial nephropathy, 13–15
Malignancy, in tropics, 231–232
Malta fever. *See* Brucellosis
Mango fly, 42
Mansonella ozzardi, 41
Mansonella perstans, 41
Mansonella streptocerca, 41
Marking-nut tree, 227
Measles virus, 86–87
Mebendazole, 70
Mediterranean fever. *See* Brucellosis
Megalocytic interstitial nephritis, 132
Membrane attack complex, 6–7
Membranous glomerulonephritis, 42–43, 62, 79–81, *97–98*,
   123, 229
Membranous nephropathy, 117
Mercury nephropathy, 228–229
Mesangial glomerulonephritis, *225*
Mesangial IgA nephropathy, 210–212, *220–224*
Mesangial proliferative glomerulonephritis, 79, 83, 149–150,
   190
Mesangiocapillary glomerulonephritis, 2–3, 6, 42, 62, 66–
   67, 70, 79–80, 82, *148*, 210
Mesangium, 3, 10
Metabolic derangement, 191–193
Meurer's clefts, 13
Michaelis-Gutmann body, 131–133, *140–142*
Mite, 209
Mixed cryoglobulinemia, 81, *101*
Monocytes, 1, 7, 10–12
Mortierella, 165
Mosquito, 13, *20*, 41, 46, 77–79
Mucocutaneous candidiasis, 158
Mucocutaneous leishmaniasis, 26
Mucocutaneous lymph node syndrome. *See* Kawasaki
   disease
Mucor, 165
Mucormycosis, 165–166, *179–180*
   disseminated, 165
Mumps virus, 86, 238
Muroid virus nephropathy. *See* Hantavirus
Muscle injury, 191–192
Mushroom, 227–228
Mycetoma, 131, 164, 167
Mycobacterial infection, 149–151
Mycobacterium, 132

Mycobacterium avium-intracellulare, 83, *104*
Mycobacterium leprae, 149–150
Mycobacterium tuberculosis, 150–151
Mycoplasma, 83
Myeloperoxidase, 9
Myoglobinuria, 54, 127, 184–185, *194–195*
Myonecrosis, 184
Myositis, infectious, 191
Myxovirus, 238

N

NADPH oxidase, membrane-associated, 8–9, 11
Necator americanus, 55
Necrosis, caseation, 151, *156*
Necrotizing pyelonephritis, 166
Necrotizing vasculitis. *See* Polyarteritis nodosa
Nematode infection, 53–55
   filarial, 41–44
   intestinal, 54–55
Nephritic syndrome
   in filariasis, 42
   in leprosy, 149
   in mesangial IgA nephropathy, 211
   in treponematosis, 117
Nephritis
   acute interstitial, *30*, 76, 131
   acute tubulointerstitial, 84, *186*
   bacterial, 129
   chronic interstitial, 150
   chronic tubulointerstitial, 228
   diffuse interstitial, 130
   diffuse sclerosing, 211
   focal interstitial, *96*
   immune complex, 211
   interstitial, 42, 149
   megalocytic interstitial, 132
   quartan malarial, 15
   transient, 84
   tubulointerstitial, 2, *49*, 117, 133
Nephropathia epidemica. *See* Hantavirus
Nephropathy
   epidemic. *See* Hantavirus
   falciparum malarial, *21–22*
   IgA, 6, 210–212, *220–224*
   IgM, 212, *225–226*
   lupus, 209
   malarial, 13–15
   membranous, 117
   mercury, 228–229
   mesangial IgA, 210–212, *220–224*
   muroid virus. *See* Hantavirus
   reflux, 129
   toxic, 227–229

Sulfonamide, 163, 167
Sulfur granule, 166
Superoxide anion, 8–9, 11
Superoxide dismutase, 9
Suppurative pyelonephritis, 166
Swimmer's itch, 62
Syphilis, 117–118, *123–125*
  congenital, 117, *123*
Systemic blastomycosis, 161
Systemic candidiasis, 158
Systemic lupus erythematosus, 6, 210

T
Tacaribe virus, 76
Taenia echinococcus, 239
Taenia nana, 239
Taenia solium, 70, *73–74*
T cells, 10–12
Thalassemia, 200–201, *205*
Thrombin-activating protease, 8
Thromboxane, 8, 11–12
Tick, 77, 109, 116
Tiger snake, 183
Tityus, 184
Tityus serrulatus, 184
Togaviridae, 77–79
Torulopsis glabrata, 157, 159, *170*
Torulopsosis, 159, *171*
Toxic nephropathy, 227–229
Toxin, plant, 227–228
Toxoplasma gondii, 16–17
  life cycle of, 16–17, *26*
Toxoplasmosis, 16–17, *36–39*
  congenital, 17
Transient glomerulonephritis, in malaria, 14
Transmembranous glomerulonephritis, 2
Trematode infection, 61–63
Treponema pallidum, 117–118
Treponematosis, 117–118, *123–125*
Trichinella spiralis, 53–54, *56*
Trichinosis, 53–54, *56–57*
Trichuris trichiura, 55
Trihexyphenidyl, *194*
Tropical extramembranous (membranous)
    glomerulonephritis, *217*
Tropical extramembranous (membranous) nephropathy,
    208, *217*
Tropical nephropathy, 207–208, *215–216*
Tropical splenomegaly syndrome, 213
Trypanosoma cruzi, 16, *34*
Trypanosomiasis, American, 16, *34–35*
Tuberculosis, 150–151, *156*, 213, 239
Tubulointerstitial lesion, 1

Tubulointerstitial nephritis, 2, *49*, 117, 133
  acute, 84, *186*
Tula fever. *See* Hantavirus
Tumor cell necrosis factor, 11
Typhoid fever, 127–128, *135–136*, 193
Typhus
  epidemic, 110
  scrub, 110

U
Ulcerative colitis, 213
Undulant fever. *See* Brucellosis
Urinary bladder, carcinoma of, 232, *236*
Urinary tract, lymphatics of, *243*

V
Varicella, 85, *106*
Varicella zoster virus, 85
Vasculitis, 109–110, *112*
  necrotizing. *See* Polyarteritis nodosa
Vasoactive amine, 3, 11
Venomous snakebite, 183–184, *186–188*
Vibrio, 127
Vibrio cholera, 128–129
Vicis favus, 228
Viral hepatitis, 79–82, *97–103*
Viral infection, 75–87, *88–107*
Visceral leishmaniasis, 15–16, *27–33*
von Hansemann histiocyte, 132

W
Wasp sting, 184, *190*
Water
  contaminated, 17, 70, 127
  radiolysis of, 8
Weil's disease, 115
Wuchereria bancrofti, 41–42, 239
  life cycle of, 41, *46*

X
Xanthine oxidase, 8
Xanthogranulomatous pyelonephritis, 133–134, *144–147*

Y
Yaws, 117
Yeast lake, 162
Yellow fever, 77–78, *93*
  endemic zone in Africa, *91*
  endemic zone in the Americas, *92*
Yersinia, 127

Z
Ziemann's dots, 13
Zygomycosis. *See* Mucormycosis

273